Caring and Responsibility

Caring and Responsibility

The Crossroads Between Holistic Practice and Traditional Medicine

June S. Lowenberg

upp

University of Pennsylvania Press
Philadelphia

Acknowledgment is made for permission to quote from published
works. A complete listing appears at the end of this volume, which
constitutes an extension of the copyright page.

Library of Congress Cataloging-in-Publication Data

Lowenberg, June S.
   Caring and responsibility : the crossroads between holistic
practice and traditional medicine / June S. Lowenberg.
       p.   cm.
   Bibliography: p.
   Includes index.
   ISBN 0-8122-8174-8
   1. Holistic medicine—Social aspects.   I. Title.
   [DNLM: 1. Holistic Health.   2. Philosophy, Medical.   W 61 L917c]
R733.L68   1989
610—dc19
DNLM/DLC
for Library of Congress   89-5283
                                                                              CIP

Contents

Figures

Acknowledgments

Many people provided the support and resources that enabled me to complete this research project and book. First, I want to thank the staff at "Mar Vista Clinic" and at the holistic dental office for their willingness to grant me access for the research. These physicians, nurses, and other health providers generously gave of their time, their privacy, their ideas, and their hospitality during the months I spent in the setting. The open access they provided, with so little to gain, testifies to their deep commitment to improving the provision of health care. The other health professionals interviewed and the patients in the settings also generously shared their time and experience.

Scholarly work is always a collaborative undertaking, and I remain grateful for the intellectual climate and support within the Sociology Department at the University of California, San Diego. I am particularly indebted to my dissertation committee. Fred Davis generously provided the type of intellectual guidance and mentorship every doctoral student hopes for. Our discussions helped me clarify the theoretical arguments developed in this work. Kristin Luker and Richard P. Madsen also went far beyond any "professional duty" in providing both intellectual and supportive input throughout the period of the dissertation and book. I am also deeply grateful to Joseph R. Gusfield, Bennett M. Berger, Hugh Mehan, Charles Nathanson, Jacqueline Fawcett, Clifford Grobstein, and Lola Romanucci-Ross for sharing their ideas, critiques, and encouragement at various stages of the process. Many other colleagues provided support and feedback during the development of the research, among them Alexandra Dundas Todd, Marcine Cohen, Joseph Kotarba, Judith Liu, Ashley Phillips, and Kathleen Murphy Mallinger.

Financial support from several sources also facilitated the research and writing culminating in this book. The initial research was aided by both a National Research Service Award (Nurse Fellowship Program, Department of Health and Human Services) and a Dissertation Fellowship awarded through the Sociology Department at the University of California, San Diego. I was also fortunate to receive intramural research funds from the University of San Diego while extending the analysis and writing the book. My research assistant, Karen Szafran, provided impeccable research and computing assistance throughout the preparation of the book manuscript (her enthusiasm also helped replenish mine). And Patricia Smith of University of Pennsylvania Press provided supportive feedback when it was most needed. Her expertise and enthusiasm, along with that of Alison Anderson, made a difficult undertaking far more tolerable.

My parents, Ben and Sally Slavkin, gave me the love of learning that led to this undertaking, as well as their continuing encouragement throughout the process. There is no way I can adequately thank them. Most of all, I appreciate the often heroic measures provided, as well as the everyday trials and tribulations endured, by my husband, Paul, and my son, Aaron. Without their constant support and unfailing humor, this project could never have been completed.

I

Introduction

Americans are interested in holistic health. They may be flagrantly for it or against it. They may be abstractly speaking of incursions of the new health oriented, preventive, and participatory approaches to medical care into their lives. Or they may be trying acupuncture or visualization for a chronic illness, or incorporating nutritional changes and exercise into their daily routines to improve their health. This book will examine a range of issues subsumed under the term "holistic health" in an attempt to understand this phenomenon and its implications for the broad context of health care.

There are a multiplicity of ways to structure definitions of health, illness, and healing interactions. Each society organizes the experience of health and illness, as well as the provision of health care services, in ways congruent with its dominant values and institutions. According to Wallis and Morley, most societies have historically been medically pluralistic. They elaborate: "Practitioners of various curing arts employing distinct concepts and techniques have competed for a clientele which accord to none of them a status as uniquely competent or efficacious over the general domain of human illness" (Wallis and Morley, 1976:10).

In contrast, advanced industrial societies have been characterized by the dominance of scientifically-based, allopathic medicine. This emergence of a broad consensus of an organized medical profession has promoted the rise of various forms of so-called marginal medicine. Wallis and Morley describe and summarize the characteristics of these forms: "Almost inevitably marginal practitioners conduct their practice not merely outside the profession, its facilities and privileges, but also on the basis of divergent beliefs concerning the causes and appropriate practices for coping with illness" (ibid:13–14).

Both medicine and the goal of health are relatively sacrosanct in contemporary America (Freidson, 1970a:51). Freidson describes the medical profession as "an officially approved monopoly of the right to define health and illness and to treat illness" (Freidson, 1970b:5). Starr concurs with Freidson's assessment, portraying medicine during the twentieth century as embodying the professional ideal in American culture (Starr, 1970:177).

However, recent years have seen the emergence and strengthening of increasing numbers of alternatives to traditional allopathic medicine in the United States. Mechanic asserts that a new paradigm is emerging in the health services and that its encouragement is essential (Mechanic, 1975:vii). And Carlson argues a more radical scenario: "The end of medicine is near. Medical care as provided by physicians and hospitals is having less and less impact on our health" (Carlson, 1975:1).

Although holistic health is but the newest challenger among many other marginal groups such as osteopathy or chiropracty, there are several reasons it warrants further study. First, it presents a challenge from the inside. Many physicians who graduated from highly regarded, traditional medical schools are advocating the new model. Second, the holistic health model represents a new world view, rather than being more specific and bounded. For example, the advocates of osteopathy or laetrile confine their divergent beliefs to the causes and appropriate treatments for illness. Holistic health is thus potentially more broadly subversive, challenging the ideological infrastructure of traditional allopathic medicine. Third, it can be argued that marginal competitors like osteopathy and supporters of laetrile segment out their clientele, while holistic health practitioners are competing for the same broad base of clientele as allopathic medicine. Finally, one can argue that the challenge of holistic health is more likely to succeed in at least modifying the traditional medical model because its historical timing may be fortuitous.

This book will examine the holistic health model as a form of healing and health care diverging from the dominant allopathic medical model. It takes the growing pervasiveness of the new model as a given. Specific practices at the radical end of the spectrum, while they provide an empirical data source to further understanding, are not the focus; rather, the emphasis is on the pervasiveness of new model beliefs and modalities as integrated with more traditional forms of practice.

Articles and images in the mass media, as well as reports in the professional journals and continuing education programs for health professionals, continually attest to this shift towards a more holistic, preventively oriented medical model. References are increasingly made to concepts of health, wellness, preventive approaches, lifestyle change, responsibility, stress reduction, and mind-body continuity. Bio-feedback, acupuncture, exercise and nutrition regimes are finding their way into traditional medical programs and practices. Comprehensive programs and clinics for "health enhancement" are becoming commonplace at prestigious medical institutions such as Scripps Clinic and the University of California, Los Angeles Medical Center.[1] In short, we are witnessing a social transformation as it is reflected in the health care system.

In this book I attempt to answer several questions in relation to this transformation. I analyze the social consequences of this shift towards a more holistic, participatory model of medicine. The primary question is: what are the changes in the enactment of the sick role in the holistic health model, and why are they so problematic?[2] Does holistic health actually transform the sick role? If so, how is the sick role modified when the new model is carried out at the practice level? The primary focus of that examination will be on the shifts in the provider-patient interaction and the attribution of responsibility for illness. A closely related question is how a movement grounded in humanism can come to at times have such antihumanistic consequences in terms of patient blame and guilt.

Background Assumptions of the Study

A major assumption underlying this analysis is that it is *non evaluative*. The approach here will derive from an initial examination of the strengths and weaknesses of both models of illness and their relevance for what is conceived of in medical sociology as "the sick role." Thus the more preventive, participatory holistic health model will be depicted in contrast to the traditional, allopathic medical model. Rather than an evaluative stance postulating the superiority of one conceptual model over the other, I see each as having its specific set of strengths and strains. In other words, I am not interested in analyzing the two models with a view of determining which provides "better" outcomes. Instead, I examine the limits of the two models from the perspectives of both the participants and the sociologist.

This approach also assumes the moral character of both illness and medical interactions; thus this research treats issues of morality and moral reasoning in examining how the specific definitions change. The definitions of what it means to be ill are never value free. Subtle implications of stigma and processes of labelling occur in relation to the range of problems that a culture refers to as illness. A large body of literature in Medical Sociology focuses on the moral attributions attached to illness or handicap, defining illness as a deviant role (Parsons, 1951; Freidson,

1965; Davis, 1972). This approach focuses on how illness phenomena become stigmatized, and examines the interplay between individual and collective levels of moral attribution as the societal moral designations around illness change.

More specifically, many of my underlying assumptions in the areas of deviance and social control derive from a symbolic interactionist perspective, and are most clearly articulated in similar contexts in the work of Gusfield and of Conrad and Schneider (Gusfield, 1981; Conrad and Schneider, 1980). First, I take it as given that America is a highly pluralistic society with extremely diverse beliefs, values, and behavior related to health and illness (Zborowski, 1952; Mechanic, 1962; Zola, 1966; Kosa et al., 1969; Twaddle, 1972). Second, I assume that any examination of deviance and social control also studies moral reasoning. Morality and values come to be presented as taken-for-granted, factual, and derived from science through processes which are essentially political (Gusfield, 1981; Conrad and Schneider, 1980). For example, since physicians have disproportionate amounts of status in this society, I would expect their definitions, with both the underlying cognitive and moral assumptions, to heavily influence the way the problem is ultimately conceptualized at the public level. This of course assumes that their self-interests as a group must be considered to understand the larger phenomenon.

Obviously, such an approach in examining the two models assumes a relativistic, *social constructionist* view of social phenomena. Rather than focusing on objective "fact" and "science," I see those phenomena as social constructions with political, economic, and moral roots. As Luker has demonstrated in relation to the abortion debate, such conflicts do not revolve around "facts," but instead arise from differing interpretations of the same "facts," which in turn derive from radically different world views of the participants (Luker, 1984). Similarly, I view "science" as a social enterprise, where the claims of moral neutrality cover ethical and political assumptions and values that are taken-for-granted (Gusfield, 1981).[3]

Although the focus of this study will be on the interactional level, by necessity the social structural aspects of the phenomena must be considered to make sense of both function and process. Medicine is seen as dealing with imputed deviance, and the moral designations comprising such attributions vary by both culture and specific historical and spatial location. As Gusfield writes, "Sociological definitions of public problems, unlike psychological ones, raise issues of group interests and moral commitments and move into public and political arenas" (Gusfield in

Conrad and Schneider, 1980: viii). I assume that locating the phenomenon in the broadest possible context will result in the most adequate interpretation, despite the complexity.

This study thus attempts to go beyond an examination of the two medical models, to analyze the transformation of subtle moral meanings that occurs with a shift towards a more holistic, participatory model of health and illness. Thus there is emphasis on change, flux, and transition as well as interaction. Such a focus on transition highlights discrepancies, paradox, and inconsistency as participants attempt to make sense of contradictory cognitive and moral elements in their daily lives. In focusing on the process of change that occurs in the intersection of different world views, I am interested in the negotiations that take place both between people and within a single individual's cognitive framework. As a sociologist, I will focus on both the continuities and discontinuities that arise. Which phenomena change, and which remain constant? How do participants make moral sense in such contradictory situations?

I initially hypothesized that, despite the humanistic ideology, I would find in the new model a moralistic attribution of blame and stigmatization of patients. However, the actual clinical interactions and their moral consequences proved far more complex, and they often were in direct conflict with the prevailing rhetoric.

The empirical questions derive from this focus on the interaction between the two models. Does a more holistic, participatory health model actually change the way people enact the sick role? Despite evidence of changing societal definitions of responsibility and patient participation, there has not yet been any empirical documentation of actual shifts in the sick role. I am most interested in the shifts in responsibility and participation, and the implications this would have for the sick role.

If the sick role is significantly altered with a shift towards the new model, how can that change be described? Furthermore, why did these notions change? And why are these ideas and changes in behavior arising at this point in time? Even more crucial is the question of how and why a movement grounded in humanism can be interpreted as having nonhumanistic consequences.

While I am interested in all facets of the changing sick role, the central theme here is that of the attribution of responsibility. As individuals increasingly come to be seen as "responsible" for their level of health and illness, are they "blamed" and stigmatized when they become ill? How do changing notions of responsibility affect the welfare of patients and the organization of provider-patient interaction?

Methodology

The research focus evolved through successive stages. It began as an exploratory study focusing on the broad outlines of the Holistic Health movement. I then focused on the interactions in two specific holistically oriented settings. Finally I used intensive interviewing of holistic practitioners, leaders in the Holistic Health movement, and patients seeking care in such settings.

At each stage of the research process, the focus was on learning, understanding, and analyzing the symbolic meanings, beliefs, and values of participants, while simultaneously observing and analyzing those participants' interactions in concrete, clinical situations. The underlying assumption was that a phenomenon can only be understood if the normative meanings, symbols, and ideology of participants are first comprehended.

Attention to the symbolic aspects of the question included observations of language use, as well as the symbolic representations of ideas in participant dress and the appearance of the settings themselves. As Conrad and Schneider write, "The social world is thus both interpreted and constructed through the medium of language. Language and language categories provide the ordered meanings by which we experience ourselves and our lives in society" (Conrad and Schneider, 1980:21). For example, whether participants used the word "patient" or "client" was an important distinction I analyzed. Similarly, the use of purple or burnt orange sheets on the examining tables in the primary clinic symbolized core values that contrasted markedly with, for example, white disposable sheets. These symbolic meanings were analyzed to understand the concepts of participants of what constitutes a good life, health, a good doctor, and a good patient.

Basically, I learned how these practitioners and patients interpreted the world, and specifically the phenomena of health, illness, and healing. This included understanding the moral meanings attached to these interpretations. Isolating the content of the constitutive ideas, or the ideology of participants, was necessary to see how these ideas get transformed in the process of concrete interactions between practitioner and patient.

Especially in studying a movement or phenomenon in transition, individual variations noted in both healers and patients were often marked. Discerning the patterns without losing sight of the diversity represented by such conceptualization remains a problematic aspect of the sociological task. Not only are there highly divergent interpretations of "holistic health," there are always major differences between the ways new ideas are implemented by the initial prophets and leaders, those who carry the vision out, and those who integrate aspects of the vision into their prior framework. Ideal typical representations were constructed to allow the coherence needed to contrast against other models or to develop other conceptual constructs.[4]

To make sense of the analysis of these phenomena, links between the micro and macro sociological levels of analysis had to be developed. For instance, the analysis of shifts in the attribution of responsibility for illness to patients depended both on the changed meanings of responsibility held by individual providers and patients and on factors at the macro level, such as the growing economic constraints on health care. Cultural influences and social structure must be related to variables at the micro-sociological level to understand these phenomena in any meaningful way. The focus remained on the interrelationships of ideas, cultural styles, and concrete interactional behavior during a period of transition. Because of the breadth of this endeavor, some portions of the analysis will be more speculative than those derived from the more focused ethnographic data.

Rationale for the Research Approach

The specific offices I chose for the field study, as well as the practitioners I located for interviews, fit stringent requirements. These providers were all attempting to integrate what they saw as the best of holistic approaches with the best of conventional allopathic medicine, the system in which they had all received their medical training. In addition, I did extensive groundwork to ascertain the "standing" of these practitioners and their practice in the community, ultimately including in the study only those practitioners seen by insiders to the movement as highly competent practitioners. There were several reasons behind this decision.

First, I felt that the practitioners at the extreme end of the continuum would have much less effect on the direction of future health care. Over time, it appears likely that holistic approaches will be increasingly incorporated into the health delivery system; however, it is highly unlikely that a model rejecting scientifically based allopathic medicine will become predominant. The practitioners combining the models would come closest to modeling future health care practice.

Second, I wanted to avoid the far-out, "flaky" end of the holistic continuum. Within both allopathic and holistic medicine there is a wide range of competence of practitioners (this is true of any healing system). Since I was not attempting a study of poor quality medical care, I wanted to insure that I had practitioners with standards of high quality care.[5] When I found strains or limits in the model, I wanted to be sure those problems derived from the model itself, rather than from an inability to carry the model out. Although locating this group turned out to be much more cumbersome and time consuming than I had anticipated, the results would have been ambiguous without that careful selection process.[6]

Third, I was specifically interested in the social consequences, not only of the implementation of the new model, but also of the attempted integration of the two conceptual models. This provided the opportunity to analyze the problematic aspects which derived from the process of transition itself. For instance, I suspected that I would see patterns of "routinization of charisma." That is, the attempt to integrate the new model would be eroded as it became institutionalized. As it turned out, the intersection of the models led to more complex outcomes than such a unilinear model postulates. Observing the attempt to integrate two world views, or two conceptual models, provided an opportunity to study the unintended consequences that accompany change.

Another reason for undertaking this study relates to the available literature on holistic health. Although the last ten to twelve years has seen an explosion of both articles and books related to holistic health, most of the literature is undocumented by empirical data. Ideology and rhetoric are everywhere; however, there is only sparse research relating ideological convictions to concrete data. This gap is most visible at the level of practitioner-client interaction.

Additionally, most of the available material is heavily biased, whether in favor of traditional medicine or holistic health.[7] The proponents of holistic health write persuasively of the amazing consequences in terms of improved health, longevity, and decreased cost of medical utilization which will derive from a switch in more holistic, preventive directions (Ardell, 1977; Brenner, 1978; Bloomfield and Kory, 1978; Miller, 1978; Simonton et al., 1978; Gordon, 1981). Health policy experts echo these claims of potential benefits, often placing more stress on effective health utilization and cost containment (Fink, 1976; Lee, 1976; Knowles, 1977; Hayes-Bautista and Harveston, 1977). On the other side, detracters from both medicine (Relman, 1979; Oppenheim, 1980; Geyman, 1984; Angell, 1985) and the social sciences (Crawford, 1978; Guttmacher, 1979; Kopelman and Moskop, 1981; Shapiro and Shapiro 1979; Scarf, 1980; Taylor, 1982; Freund, 1982; Glymour and Stalker, 1983; Arney and Bergen 1984) warn of numerous dangers of holistic approaches.

While the basic parameters of the ideology behind holistic health, along with the modalities, have been delineated fairly comprehensively, the data on interactional behavior is extremely sparse. I needed to learn what practitioners and clients said, and what these same participants did in concrete clinical situations. By observing interactional behavior over time, I studied how they attempted to carry out their convictions in everyday life situations. How often were they able to practice what they believed, and what problematic areas arose with conflicting beliefs? In ascertaining their beliefs, values, and behavior, how did they explain the discrepancies, and what other possible explanations presented themselves?

Given the large body of literature on the allopathic medical model and the sick role, I needed to elaborate the similarities and contrasts in practitioner-client interactions in contexts incorporating holistic concepts and modalities. Like the established data, this data then needed to be related to the concrete social, cultural, political, and economic context.

Description of the Field Setting

The research approach was that of participant observation and field research (Lofland, 1971, 1976; Schatzman and Strauss, 1973; Bogdan and Taylor, 1975). Various phases of ethnographic research continued over a period of four years.

First, throughout the research project, but especially in the early stages, the broader cultural field served as the arena of field research. Cultural materials such as books and journal articles (both those meant for professional and lay consumption), material portrayed through the electronic and print media, and listings of continuing education offerings for health professionals were used for qualitative analysis, as the salient trends and meanings in the holistic health model were ascertained. During this period I also attended numerous courses, conferences, and workshops on holistic health for health professionals, immersing myself in movement activities and joining the Association for Holistic Health.

Gradually this focus narrowed to an exploratory participant observation study of a holistic dental office, a more extended study of a holistic family practice clinic, and formal interviews of providers and leaders in the local holistic health field. I conducted a three month exploratory ethnographic study in a holistic dental office.[8] This early study provided extensive empirical data relating to the major differences of a holistic approach, as contrasted to more traditional dentist patient interaction, in both the organizational and interactional areas.

Later, after much investigative work, I obtained access to do field research in a family practice clinic stressing holistic, preventive approaches. To learn what the model actually looks like in practice, I observed its enactment in a clinic that identifies itself as belonging to the movement. This portion of the study was conducted over an eight to nine month period and constituted a fairly typical participant observational experience. I observed and questioned practitioners and patients in broad, open-ended questions in the initial period. After establishing more trust and becoming more taken-for-granted in the setting, I focused both observations and my questioning in more specific directions.

In addition I conducted twenty-five intensive formal interviews outside the settings. These were carried out between September 1981 and June 1983, and consisted primarily of providers and leaders in the holistic health movement in the Southern California area (four patients were also included). These interviews lasted between 25 minutes and over four hours, averaging an hour-and-a-half. Initial interviews covered broad areas. The focus narrowed during the research period, so that more specific, focused and probing questions dominated the final set of interviews. Although I brought a prepared list of topic areas to introduce with open-ended questions for each interview, I left them intentionally open-ended and encouraged participants to elaborate on the issues they saw as important. The interviews were also structured so that questions eliciting how practitioners viewed their practices in their linguistic terms came earlier than questions focusing on differences in practice among providers I had observed.[9]

Three of the methodological issues that were most salient during the research were access, representativeness, and the insider-outsider dilemma. *Access* presented two problems. First, it was difficult to locate the practitioners meeting the criteria I had established. Second, it proved considerably more difficult to convince physicians in private practice to grant entree to all aspects of their interactions with patients, than it would have been to initiate a comparable study at a research or teaching institution. The fact that these practitioners were willing to grant a researcher such free access with so little to gain is a testimony to their commitment to both research and improving health care.

In a broad study such as this, the issue of *representativeness* of the setting I studied must be treated. It would have been tempting to conduct a comparative study (I considered it early in the course of the research), spending three months in each of three settings: one a traditional general or family practice office, a second holistic health office, and a third attempting to integrate approaches. Ultimately such a selection would still not have controls for representation (each of the three ideal typical categories could have had providers who were atypical of that category).

Additionally, in field research, a great deal of time is spent familiarizing the researcher with the setting and gaining participants' trust. A three month period of observation would be likely to provide only superficial observations because of my own lack of familiarity and the participants' guardedness against an outsider. I opted to carefully locate one medical setting as representing an "ideal typical" or "exemplar" case and then explore it further in both depth and breadth.

This setting, then, was chosen to represent the ideal-typical case of competent providers attempting to combine allopathic and holistic medicine. Thus this portion of the data does not necessarily reflect the holistic health movement as a whole, or even how the holistic health model is played out in a specific practice in, for example, Omaha or Chicago. I basically observed a setting to see what this type of care actually looked like at the level of practice. I used the secondary settings and the external interviews to insure that the primary setting was interactionally fairly typical. I then used the extensive data from the ideal-typical setting to abstract a model of the social consequences of that care.[10]

A third area, that of the *insider-outsider dilemma*, has to be briefly mentioned in terms of my stance as a researcher in the setting. Methodologically, I value the need for a self-conscious balancing of insider and outsider status for sociological analysis. Since I have already advocated a relativistic, constructionist perspective, I need to make my stance more explicit for readers to judge how strongly my biases may have influenced the analysis. Although I was aware of those biases, and explicitly tried to keep them from affecting the work, they invariably colored my perceptions. Fortunately, I came to the study with a balanced tension in my preconceptions. I had strong sympathy for attempts to change the medical model in more humanistic, as well as holistic, directions. Simultaneously, I had such a strong grounding in the allopathic, scientific medical model that I was extremely cautious in relation to new approaches. This grounding included both undergraduate and graduate preparation and a faculty position in nursing at two University of California campuses (this preparation preceded my doctoral work in sociology). This interdisciplinary background enabled me to balance and synthesize a wide variety of perspectives on these phenomena.

This research attempts to extend our awareness in the area of health care models at two levels. First, it illuminates the social consequences of the shift towards a more holistic, participatory model of health and illness at the level of everyday practitioner-client interaction. At a policy level, it analyzes the implications of such a shift for the institution of health care in our society. This is particularly salient within the present crisis context of cost containment and consumer dissatisfaction with medicine. Awareness of the potential dangers and limitations, as well as strengths, of the new model can assist both health planners and professional providers of health care. Thus it analyzes the implications of the holistic health movement for future health care delivery patterns. Although it raises almost as many questions as it answers, it significantly extends our knowledge of the direction and complexity of such changes.

Some of the theory generated by the study has dual implications for policy planning and theory in Medical Sociology. For example, the results illustrate how functional maintaining some distance is for caregivers. In other words, although these practitioners became more involved with their patients than do traditional providers, there were still limits on the involvement of caregivers with their patients' experience. Similarly, the analysis demonstrated how important the gatekeeping role of physicians may be for society as a whole.

In terms of extending sociologial theory on a broader scale, the analysis attempts to more fully illuminate processes of change and transition in our highly pluralistic society. Beyond studying how meanings are negotiated during periods of change by analyzing concrete instances where individuals attempt to make sense of paradoxes and contradictions from the intersection of two world views, it further demonstrates a process of moral syncretism based in a particular historical and societal context.

Sequence of the Book

Chapter II develops the broad outline of the new "holistic health" model, contrasting its underlying beliefs and approaches with the assumptions of the traditional allopathic medical model. The two models are sketched and elaborated as a prelude to the rest of the book. Holistic health is defined and elaborated, presenting the paramount ideology, meanings, and values shaping participants' views and practices.

Chapter III grounds the holistic health movement historically and contextually, examining the movement's roots in the 1960s and summarizing the continuity of ideas and personnel that extend to the present day movement. The context of the health care crisis and consumerism is also related to the holistic model, demonstrating the alliance of economic and humanistic pressures pushing for a shift in this direction. This chapter also considers the relationship of the new model to the allopathic, public health, nursing, and behavioral medicine models of health, illustrating how both psychology and nursing may derive more power within the health system from a shift towards a more holistic model of health and illness.

The study then considers the implications of such a shift for the enactment of the sick role, asking how the holistic model is actually carried out in concrete practice settings. Chapter IV focuses on the implications for the sick role of the shift towards the holistic health model. To provide a context in which to view specific changes at the concrete interactional level of clinical practice, a brief description of the primary ethnographic setting is followed by an overview of the conceptualization of the sick role. The enactment of the sick role in the traditional and new models are contrasted by examining the most salient areas of divergence: the meaning of illness, mind-body continuity, the more egalitarian practitioner-client relationship, and the shift of personal responsibility for illness to the patient.

Chapter V focuses in considerable detail on the changes in the practitioner-client relationship. Here the tension is explored between holistic health movement ideology and the actual behavior of the participants: the way ideology is actually manifested, or sometimes evaded, in practice situations. In the process, the limits of reducing the power differential between professionals and clients are assayed. Although the actual practitioner-client relationship in the new model is definitely more egalitarian, the change represents only a partial shift within definite limits of continued physician control of the interactions. The interactional situation also does not fit the description of a "consumerist" model, because it incorporates much broader affective components and less specificity than either the traditional medical or the consumerist model postulates.

Chapter VI extends the analysis of the sick role enactment by addressing the shift in the attribution of responsibility to the individual. The consequences of that attributional shift are analyzed at the societal, interactional, and individual levels. My findings contrast markedly with the view of responsibility presented in movement ideology: holistic doctors continue to absolve patients in a process closely paralleling the absolution function of more traditional physicians. I outline the mechanisms that allow this group of practitioners to absolve patients from guilt, while emphasizing responsibility. I then demonstrate how patients are experiencing blame and guilt outside these settings with the diffusion of holistic concepts into mainstream medicine and the society at large. Finally, two crucial questions are explored: why practitioners want this shift, and why patients are willing to accept it.

Chapter VII concludes by analyzing the themes developed in Chapters IV through VI. The implications of uniting the parts of the model are demonstrated. For example, the shifts in attribution of responsibility can only be understood when analyzed simultaneously with the shift towards a more egalitarian physician-patient relationship. The potential of a widespread moralistic lifestyle crusade is presented. I argue that the decreased gatekeeping function of the physician may set the stage for moral condemnation of the ill to limit illness in a period of diminished economic resources.

Interpretations of the potential moral lifestyle crusade also need to take into account the intersection of two different world views or belief systems. I demonstrate how the wide translation of Eastern philosophy into Calvinistic terms of utilitarian individualism promotes views of individual guilt and blame for illness. This process reflects a far broader societal transition and illuminates processes of social change. The implications of such a framework for processes of change and transition in general, as well as for a wider societal shift towards incorporating a partial Eastern world view, are also discussed and summarized.

2

The New Model

Presenting even a superficial overview of the Holistic Health phenomenon is a highly problematic undertaking. "Holistic health" has come to
be used as a vague, "umbrella" term which incorporates highly diverse
ideas, values, and treatment modalities. In addition, the proponents of
holistic health range from the most esoteric healers to quacks to prominent members of the medical, health policy, and academic establish-
ments. A sampling of definitions is presented to highlight their global
nature:

> the balanced integration of the individual in all aspects and lev-
> els of being: body, mind and spirit, including interpersonal re-
> lationships and our relationship to the whole of nature and our
> physical environment. (statement of purpose, Association for
> Holistic Health [AHH, 1979])

> The concept in its original sense relates to the integration
> and growth of the individual. There really is no holistic ther-
> apy . . . ; but rather there is an approach, a concept, and a
> process to bring about and focus the healing forces and energies
> within the individual for the integration of body, mind, and
> spirit. (Richard H. Svihus, M.D., Dr.P.H., past President of
> the Association of Holistic Health [Svihus, 1978])

> In the last several years holistic (sometimes spelled wholistic)
> medicine has come to denote both an approach to the whole
> person in his or her total environment and a variety of healing
> and health-promoting practices. This approach, which encom-
> passes and is at times indistinguishable from humanistic, be-
> havioral, and integral medicine, includes an appreciation of
> patients as mental and emotional, social and spiritual, as well

as physical beings. It respects their capacity for healing themselves and regards them as active partners in, rather than
passive recipients of, health care. (James S. Gordon, M.D.,
formerly at NIMH [Gordon, 1980:3])

Many Americans, particularly in the urban centers of the West
and East coasts, have become increasingly interested in a variety of health practices grouped under the rubric of "holistic
health" or "holistic healing," or, sometimes, "holistic medicine." Some of these practices are ancient, derived from Chinese and Indian medical and religious systems. Others, such as
biofeedback, are the products of modern psychological research. Still others are derived from folk and "primitive"
healing systems and from marginal healing systems, such as
chiropractic and homeopathy. What binds these diverse practices together is a philosophy of health—a way of viewing the
person in a particular environment as a whole person who
may be afflicted with disease. (Phyllis H. Mattson [Mattson,
1982:1])

The phenomenon of holistic health at times refers to a social movement, at other times to a set of treatment techniques, and at times to a
core set of beliefs and a way of approaching health, illness, and healing. To further complicate the problem of definition, the meanings and
approaches labelled "holistic health" often overlap, or are used inter-
changeably, with models called wholistic medicine, behavioral medicine,
humanistic medicine, comprehensive or client-centered medicine, psychosomatic medicine, integral medicine, and alternative health care
(Gordon, 1981:114; Benson, 1979:viii; Frank, 1981:1; Fink, 1976:23;
Jaffe, 1980:5). There are also large areas of overlap with professional
nursing, transcultural nursing, family medicine, preventive medicine,
and both transpersonal and health psychology.

Furthermore, with the overuse of the holistic terminology, combined
with the highly charged emotional and political connotations and distor-
tions that have come to be attached to the term, more participants are
avoiding the term, creating new problems for arriving at a consensual
definition (Carlson, 1975, 1984; Svihus, 1978:1; Weil, 1983:181; Gordon, 1984:546).

Since the holistic health movement is so amorphous, its cohesiveness derives more from its underlying meanings and definitions of health,
illness, and treatment than from its structural and organizational aspects.

Similarly, the modalities utilized are far less important than the symbolic meanings framing their use.

Seven salient parameters, or sets of core beliefs, can be abstracted from the vague and highly pluralistic diversity of definitions attached to the concept of holistic health. These characteristics, including their underlying assumptions and metaphorical content, unite the range of participants in the holistic health movement. Together they comprise the model of holistic health; additionally, they outline the ideology and constitutive ideas of adherents to the new model. In this chapter I summarize these parameters and their major underlying assumptions. These core parameters include: holism, health promotion, the meaning of illness, individual responsibility, the practitioner stance, cultural diversity in healing practices, and a constellation of values and meanings comprising an alternative world view or consciousness.

In this chapter I describe each of the seven parameters, including an overview of the specific structure and underlying assumptions of each. This model of holistic health practice was initially developed from an extensive literature review, supplemented with data gathered from holistic organizations, conferences, interviews with participants, and field observation in the holistic clinics (various portions were gathered between 1977 and 1984). I analyzed the holistic health literature, along with the data from participants, ultimately dividing the primary beliefs and values into the seven areas. Thus the parameters represent *what adherents claim and believe* in relation to the new model. In other words, I am describing, rather than assessing, participants' claims. In later chapters, I will analyze how these ideas and values come to be implemented at the concrete behavioral level of clinical practice. In this chapter, however, the aim is to portray clearly the model in terms of the participants' views. Some contradictions and paradoxes within the abstracted model will become evident; however, the focus remains primarily descriptive.

It must be remembered, however, that any such conceptual scheme is an abstraction or ideal typical representation, and that considerable ambiguity and overlap occur between specific practitioners and in the concrete situations where the meanings are applied and negotiated.

While defining and elaborating the holisitic health model, facets will often be presented in opposition to the traditional Western allopathic model of medicine.[1] This highlights the major points of divergence of the two models of health and illness.

Thus this chapter presents and analyzes the core beliefs, meanings, and values shared by the diverse group of holistic health practitioners and participants. These parameters portray the values and beliefs underlying practice that uses a holistic paradigm.[2] Later chapters will focus on how this model is carried out in actual practice. In other words, this analysis focuses on the ideological, rather than behavioral and interactional level of practice.

Holism

The first parameter characteristic of holistic health is, perhaps obviously, that of holism. By "holism" several things are meant. In general, holistic health practitioners view their client as a person in his or her totality. They assess and treat the entire person, rather than a specific set of symptoms or a disease. This derives partially from humanistic concerns and partially from a model of the interrelationship of the physical, mental, emotional, and spiritual dimensions of man. A further assumption views humans as dynamically interacting with their environment. Mythical views of the individual in harmony with nature and the environment and a romanticization of nature underlie these meanings. Several central assumptions underlie this parameter of holism, particularly concepts of uniqueness, underlying unity, process, and an ecological view. This section will focus on those component meanings, and the ways that related scientific developments, such as recent research on stress and the placebo effect, have promoted them.

Focus on a Unique Individual

One of the primary derivatives of holism is the focus on a unique individual at a specific point in time. Individual differences in genetic, physiological, and psychological makeup are stressed and positively valued. Thus two people with similar presenting symptoms might be treated very differently from each other in a holistic paradigm. As Otto and Knight write, "Wholistic healing recognizes and values the unique individuality of each person and is opposed to the dehumanization inherent in a perspective where the focus is on the treatment of an organ . . ." (Otto and Knight, 1979:10–11). Mattson's chapter on holistic health principles also contains a section detailing "The fundamental value of each individual." She sees the goal of social interactions as "accepting others as they are, as unique personalities on different life paths, rather than identifying people by their roles or deciding what they 'ought' to be" (Mattson, 1982:44).

All these descriptions of the focus on "holism" emphasize the value placed on uniqueness. Viewing each individual as unique constrasts starkly with the emphasis in the allopathic medical model on viewing aggregates. From a holistic framework, such aggregate studies are defined as dehumanizing. Practitioners also do not see people as part of statistical aggregates. For example, it would be less important to look at percentages in terms of the survival rate for breast cancer than to focus on the potential positive outcomes for a particular woman. This deviates markedly from the traditional allopathic medical model; American medicine has made most of its advances through a quantitative, statistical approach. Thus there is an implicit attack on scientism underlying this approach.

This focus on a unique individual also emphasizes flux, movement, and transition rather than viewing static conditions and phenomena. Growth and learning are highly valued as part of reaching one's unique potential. For example, a crisis is viewed in terms of its potential for growth.

Underlying Unity

Beyond the focus on the unique individual, the core dimension of holism is the *interrelation of the physical, mental, emotional, spiritual, and social dimensions* of the human state. Each person is seen as a unified system, rather than as consisting of a body, a mind, emotions, and a soul. A basic "unity" is postulated which not only characterizes each person, but describes an underlying relationship between individuals and between each individual and his or her environment.

Most authors attribute the impetus behind the recent rise in holistic approaches to Jan Christian Smuts' book *Holism and Evolution*, published in 1926 (Deliman and Smolowe, 1982; Gordon, 1980; Carlson, 1980; Blattner, 1981). Smuts developed his philosophical concept of holism in reaction to the prevailing reductionism he observed in the sciences. Another more recent source of the holistic approach of unity is the newer theoretical developments in physics. One of the most frequently quoted sources on holism is Fritjof Capra's *The Tao of Physics*, which postulates an essential unity of all things and events (Capra, 1975).

This focus on the unity aspect of holism is probably the single most pivotal concept in holistic health. Still, many leaders, practitioners, and writers in the field are increasingly reacting to and avoiding the term "holistic" because of its overuse and misuse (Carlson, 1980, 1984; Weil,

1983). For example, Carlson describes the term "holistic" as one of the most overly used and abused words in our language, and describes how often it is glibly applied and trivialized (Carlson, 1980:485–490). Similarly, most of the practitioners I interviewed spontaneously expressed negative reactions when I used the term.

The literature continually emphasizes this unity component of holism. For instance, in Connelly's book describing the traditional acupuncture system, she consistently uses the term "*bodymindspirit*," and warns against segmenting the "bodymindspirit" (Connelly, 1979:3). This attempt to alter language use to reflect connectedness closely parallels George L. Engel's formulation of the "*biopsychosocial*" model (Engel, 1977). Similarly, Deliman and Smolowe describe this central aspect of holism in their introductory essay in *Holistic Medicine: Harmony of Body Mind Spirit*: "the ideal in holistic practice is to be integrative, to form a more complete, coordinated whole of the client" (Deliman and Smolowe, 1982:5). Effie Poy Yew Chow and Ardell also describe the concepts of holism and the interrelation of all forces and entities as central (Chow, 1979:409; Ardell, 1977:55).

An assumption underlying the emphasis on unity is that *process, transition, and interrelatedness* are more important than discrete parts and causal relationships. As Dossey writes, "human beings are essentially dynamic processes and patterns that are fundamentally not analyzable into separate parts—either within or between each other. Like health and disease, they are spread through space and time, and it is their interrelatedness and oneness, not their isolation and separation, which is most important" (Dossey, 1982:113–114).

It could be argued that "holism" is simply an extension of psychosomatic theories to a somewhat broader arena. Proponents of holistic health, however, argue that "psychosomatic" has often meant "it's all in your mind," rather than a true interactional model. The biomedical model has continued to search for organic causes of disease.

Theories of *mind-body continuity* remain the simplest level at which this essential unity can be seen. The evolution of research findings in conventional medicine and psychology has resulted in a gradual switch towards beliefs incorporating mind-body continuity. Often, however, these views in the mainstream postulate a simplistic, unilinear relationship: mind and emotions affect physiological functioning. The practitioners with a strong commitment to holistic health extend this to a more complex set of constantly changing interactions between mind, body, emotions, spirituality, and relationships with others.

Beyond the problems of simplistic interpretations, the adherents of the holistic model see the area most often missing in mind-body para-digms as that of *spirituality*. It has been easier for traditional physicians to accept and incorporate cognitive or emotional dimensions into concep-tualizations of health and illness than spiritual dimensions. Spiritual well-being and its relationship to health and illness are an integral part of the holistic approach. As Stone writes:

> Wholistic healing includes the spiritual area . . . The work of Jung was pioneering in this area, and his work on the arche-types and the transpersonal self led into the work of Assagioli and the psychosynthesis movement leading eventually into the meditative disciplines and their attempt to tap into transper-sonal elements (Stone, 1980:36).

This holism or basic unity is the opposite of viewing the individual from a mechanistic paradigm. The Cartesian duality underlying the allo-pathic model not only separates body and mind, but separates the body into discrete organs. Ng et al. argue that this separation historically en-abled scientists to study the body without invading the troubling realms of mind or soul (Ng et al., 1982:45). From the holistic health perspec-tive, allopathic medicine treats the human body as a machine. The pri-mary metaphor in the biomedical model is that of body as machine. Once a problem develops, the person is taken to doctors for "repair" of the malfunctioning part or organ. In fact, the metaphor of car repair is fre-quently used in descriptions or critiques of allopathic medicine. As Svi-hus writes, patients see their bodies much like their cars, which they bring to a mechanic to be repaired (Svihus, 1978:1). Interestingly, while holistic practioners usually decry this mechanistic approach, a common metaphor some use to describe the need for prevention is that of preven-tive maintenance for an automobile.

Thus, the allopathic medical model is seen by holistic advocates as firmly rooted in Cartesian duality, which divides nature into two separate realms, mind and matter (Capra in Dossey, 1982:ix; Cassell, 1986). This is consistent with viewing organisms as machines. Jerome Frank, M.D. summarizes the biomedical view:

> Biomedical medicine is based on the world-view of scientific materialism—a view that holds that the world of matter is a complete, self-contained causal system consisting of objects lo-cated in space and time and related to each other solely by the laws of cause and effect. Space is a fixed framework and time

proceeds only in one direction, with causes always preceding their effects. . . . biomedical medicine considers psychological and spiritual experiences to be irrelevant to the causal chain (Frank, 1981:2).

In contrast, the proponents of holistic health see a much more complex interrelationship than a simple mechanical one. Dimensions of mind and spirituality are fused with material and physical aspects. This view is also diametrically opposed to medical specialization. Advocates of a holistic model view organisms as having too many complex interrelationships to divide them into component parts.

The closest Western concept to this more unitary view of man is that of *systems theory*. Models of systems, *homeostasis*, *adaptation*, and balance come closest to describing this state of unity postulated by the new model. The system as a whole is seen as going beyond any addition of the component parts.

Both beliefs about the cause and treatment of illness derive from this emphasis on holism. The "cause" of illness is rarely seen as either organic or psychological. Instead, an input to the system at any point affects all parts of the system, so that it becomes very difficult to talk about "a cause." Causation, if it is discussed, is seen in multifactorial terms. As Jaffe states, "most diseases stem from not one but a long chain of contributing factors, which intensify and multiply over a period of months or years. Our behavior, feelings, stress levels, relationships, conflicts, and beliefs contribute to our overall susceptibility to disease. In essence, everything about our lives affects our health" (Jaffe, 1980:3–4).

Similarly, treatment can be directed at many points in the system, resulting in transformations throughout the entire system. Healing in one area can lead to positive changes in others, thus the practitioner or patient can intervene at any point: nutritional, emotional, spiritual, etc. With this multifactorial approach, practitioners may treat symptoms even when they cannot locate the direct cause.[3]

An example of the complexity of interrelationships postulated in a holistic approach is that of nutrition, an area rarely discussed in allopathic medicine. A high quality nutritional intake is seen as affecting not only physical health, but cognitive and emotional health as well. On the other hand, a person's emotional state is seen as affecting the absorption of nutrients. Thus, by improving nutrition, a practitioner could strengthen a person emotionally and increase her energy level, so that she could initiate further health changes on her own (Ballentine, 1982).

Rudolph Ballentine, M.D. adds even more factors to an example of a holistic view of nutrition:

The variables that affect the nutritive value of what we eat are complex indeed. Vitamin, mineral, and protein content vary not only from food to food but also from foods grown in one area to those grown in another. The value of the protein, for example, also depends on the way in which various foods are combined, and the amount of carbohydrate we need depends on our activity and way of life. Moreover, each person's needs vary according to his individual makeup, his personality, and his way of reacting to situations around him, so some people have higher requirements for one vitamin and lower requirements for another. The amount of food assimiliated from that which is taken in depends to a great extent on the functioning of the digestive system. This varies from person to person, but it may also vary from day to day or even hour to hour, depending on our emotional or mental state. We may secrete more enzymes or less, depending on our state of mind and on our attitude toward the food, what it might mean to us, or whether it looks and tastes appealing. Climatic and seasonal variables also enter into the picture and have an effect on our requirements (Ballentine, 1982:41).

Ballantine goes on to write that the interactions between a person's food intake and the mind form complex downward or upward spirals. Thus, as the mind and emotions become disturbed, an individual becomes more irritable and eats more erratically (fails to eat on time, skips meals, or overeats). Poor dietary intake then leads to poor nutritional status and deficiencies, which in turn makes the person even more irritable (ibid:41–51).

Research on Stress, Resistance Resources

A growing body of studies in medicine, behavioral medicine, psychology, and sociology have increasingly pointed towards a mind-body link, and this research has strongly influenced the approach of holistic health. Since Hans Selye's classic work on stress and the generalized adaptation response, a large body of research linking stress and illness has developed (Selye, 1956, 1979; Benson, 1975; Holmes, 1980). One of the earliest holistic books overviewing this research in relation to a wide variety of organic illness categories was Kenneth Pelletier's *Mind as Healer, Mind as Slayer*. He explored disorders from ulcers to hypertension as maladaptations to psychosocial and environmental stressors (Pelletier, 1977). In his later book, *Holistic Medicine*, Pelletier affirms his original thesis: "A new medical model must also recognize the role of life stress. In interaction with biochemical imbalances and genetic predispositions, stress is a major determinant of the time of onset, the severity, and the course of treatment of a disorder" (Pelletier, 1979:33).

Two major series of studies initially helped legitimize research linking stress to susceptibility to illness. First were Meyer Friedman and Ray Rosenman's studies linking Type A behavior and heart disease. The second was the research conducted by Thomas Holmes, which resulted in the Holmes/Rahe scale, which rates forty-two common life changes and is used to assess individual susceptibility to disease at a given point in time. Another set of studies frequently quoted by holistic proponents are those demonstrating the increased mortality rates after death of a spouse (Engel and Schmale, 1967; Parkes, 1972). Other studies, such as those attempting to develop a cancer personality profile, led in similar directions (LeShan, 1959, 1977; LeShan and Worthington, 1956). Research such as the Harvard prospective study reported by George Vaillant, M.D. in the *New England Journal of Medicine*, demonstrated that even physically healthy persons who react poorly to stress run a significantly higher risk of developing serious health problems or dying by the time they reach their fifties (Vaillant, 1979).

More recent research programs defining the links between stress and emotion and physical illness derive from the field of psychoneuroimmunology. Articles by Ornstein and Sobel and by Weschsler review this emerging area, describing the range of studies demonstrating links between an individual's immune functioning or disease course and his emotional status and stress (Ornstein and Sobel, 1987; Weschsler, 1987; Rosch and Kearney, 1985).

These lines of research located stress within the individual as causative of illness; however, the sociological and social psychological research on the buffering effects of social support in stressful situations further moves causation to a social and interactional level. Studies on social support and illness stress the importance of relationships, family interaction, and community ties for an individual's level of health and illness (Pearlin et al., 1981; Turner, 1981).[4]

In the mid to late 1970s, research efforts began to shift towards studies of resistance resources that act to buffer or neutralize the effects of excessive stress levels. For example, Kobasa et al. developed the concept of "hardiness" to account for the fact that many people do not become ill, despite exposure to high levels of stress. Viewing resistance resources as including a range of variables such as health practices, social contact, and family illness patterns, they found that the personality traits connected with hardiness (commitment, control, and the tendency to accept challenge) function to reduce the effects of stress on susceptibility to illness (Kobasa et al., 1982). The studies investigating the importance of locus of control also stress the importance of individual traits in buffering the effects of stressors.

Once research efforts moved to resistance resources, the holistic view was further expanded. Not only does the experience of stress result in physiologically measureable changes in the body, but social relationships must be taken into account as both cause and effect. For instance, Antonovsky's work argues that early social-structural, cultural, and child rearing factors influence an individual's resistance to stress throughout life (Antonovsky, 1980). Similarly, an expanded emphasis on the secondary gains an individual derives from illness draws attention to family and social factors in maintaining illness (Brenner, 1984:184; Jaffe, 1984:216–217).

Primacy of Mind, Attitudes, Belief Systems

Although a wide range of bodily, social, spiritual, and environmental factors are considered in the holistic model, when compared to the biomedical model the primary difference is that there is far more primacy placed on aspects of mind: attitudes, belief systems, and emotions. Both C. Norman Shealy and Eric Cassell claim there is a rising consciousness among health care professionals and the public of the effect of the mind and emotions on health (Shealy, 1979:vii; Cassell, 1986:34). And Rene Dubos writes, "The body's defense against infection depends in large part on the mechanisms of humoral and cellular immunity, but these mechanisms themselves are influenced by the mental state—as demonstrated by the effect of hypnosis on the Mantoux test (for tuberculosis)" (Dubos, 1979:19).

Two areas of research that have contributed to this development are the studies, largely anecdotal and clinical, on the "will to live," and the growing research based on biofeedback and similar techniques that develop voluntary control of involuntary bodily functions. As Jerome D. Frank writes in *Persuasion and Healing*, hopelessness can retard recovery or even hasten death, while mobilization of hope plays an important part in many forms of healing (Frank, 1974). In the holistic model, the will to live, hope, and faith are seen as crucial variables affecting both recovery from illness and maintenance of health.

Biofeedback and scientific studies of patients voluntarily controlling heart rate, blood pressure, and muscle tension also facilitated the acceptance of views emphasizing the major role of the mind. Biofeedback is based on the psychophysiological principle: every change in a person's emotional or physiological state affects the other. Herbert Benson's relaxation techniques were derived from research on meditators (TM), which demonstrated volitional changes in autonomic functioning, such as blood pressure and heart rate (Benson, 1975).

Much of the holistic approach tries to educate clients about such effects and to set up expectancies, as well as teach techniques, that give the individual more voluntary control over bodily function. As the Simontons write, "We also work to help them believe that they can influence their condition and that their mind, body, and emotions can work together to create health" (Simonton et al., 1980:11).

Some holistic techniques go beyond educational approaches to attempts to change belief systems. "The Course in Miracles" is a set of books, on which many other holistically oriented books and conferences are based (Jampolsky, 1979; Mattson, 1982). It has techniques to help teach and reinforce a new belief system that views the individual as creating his perceptions. Belief systems screen perceptions, which determine emotions, which then affect physiological and emotional functioning. This approach definitely gives primacy to the individual's creation of reality through his belief system.

As this paradigm becomes more widely accepted, it raises numerous issues beyond the importance of treating the whole person and teaching techniques to decrease stress. If individuals actually create their reality through their minds, they can change their feelings and health through alterations in their belief system. This raises complex issues in relation to belief systems. Can belief systems be easily changed? To what extent does healing require belief in its efficacy? How can deeply ingrained mental attitudes be transformed? This raises ethical issues of mind control. One could even question whether commonly accepted "preventive" approaches such as routine breast examination are liable to become self-fulfilling prophecies.

Placebo Effect

The placebo effect raises further questions in relation to holism. Allopathic medicine has persistently discounted the placebo effect rather than attempting to use it. Actually, physicians use it in many taken-for-granted ways, such as symbolism and what we call "bedside manner." Belief, placebo, and healing are related to expectation, symbolism, and power in modern medicine as much as in nonindustrialized cultures (Moerman, 1980).

Jerome Frank wrote the classic work investigating the placebo phenomenon (Frank, 1963). As he asserted more recently in relation to holistic health, "a considerable proportion of the effectiveness of all remedies depends on the so-called placebo effect—the evocation of the patient's expectant faith by symbols of the physician's healing power" (Frank, 1981:12). Like Moerman, he argues that most physicians are unaware of the extent to which they inadvertently mobilize healing in their patients: "The paraphernalia of modern medicine, by symbolizing the miraculous healing powers of scientific technology, have psychological effects similar to those of religious images at a healing shrine" (Frank, 1981:13; Moerman, 1980).

Researchers from a variety of disciplines are beginning to recognize the importance of the placebo phenomena for health and recovery, and a number of studies attempting to locate the mechanisms underlying the effect, such as the release of endorphins, have begun to improve our understanding of the process (Pelletier, 1979; Benson and Epstein, 1980). The holistic approach attempts to use the placebo effect, in its broadest sense, very consciously.

For example, Carlson poses the question, "If cures can be achieved by a fusion of the patient's belief in the treatment and the manifestation of symbols of healing, we must ask if it is possible to use equally effective but less expensive symbols" (Carlson, 1975:19). Similarly, Brenner writes, "If a placebo works 35% of the time, why not use more nothing" (Brenner, 1978:65). Holistic health has used the placebo effect as a concept that demonstrates the validity of a holistic approach. As Pelletier writes, "Frequently, holistic methods are dismissed by attributing any positive outcome to the placebo effect. It is far more constructive to seriously consider methods by which the placebo effect can be systematically enhanced" (Pelletier, 1979:36).

Ecological View

The holism accepted by adherents of the holistic health movement goes beyond the view of an isolated human to a concept of humans dynamically interacting with the environment. This view, taken to its ultimate conclusion, postulates a unified universe.

Initially many outside observers of the movement, especially those espousing a radical critique of the medical system, saw holistic health as

self-oriented to the exclusion of a sense of social and environmental responsibility (Berliner and Salmon, 1979; Guttmacher, 1979; Freund,
1982). However, the central focus on holism includes the interconnectedness of individuals to each other and to all of nature and the world. As
Fritjof Capra writes:

> We live today in a globally interconnected world, in which bio-
> logical, psychological, social, and environmental phenomena
> are all interdependent. To describe this world appropriately we
> need an ecological perspective, which the Cartesian world view
> does not offer (Capra in Dossey, 1982:ix).

Similarly, Dossey writes: "We cannot separate our own existence from
that of the world outside. We are intimately associated not only with the
earth we inhabit, but with the farthest reaches of the cosmos" (ibid:116).
Kane also argues that illness is basically a social statement, which can
not be separated from the person's family, cultural, and environmental
relationships (Kane, 1983:3).

Environmental concerns are therefore both central and prevalent
within the holistic health model. Not only are many of the practitioners,
leaders, and clients often politically involved with environmental issues,
but aspects of nutrition, stress, and the concern with environmental tox-
ins are central concerns.

One example of the strength of this linkage is that Mike Samuels,
M.D., the author of one of the landmark holistic health books, *The Well
Body Book*, along with several later holistic books, more recently re-
leased a publication called *Well Body, Well Earth: The Sierra Club Environmental Health Sourcebook* (Samuels, 1973, 1974, 1982, 1983).
Published by Sierra Club Books, it has sections titled "How the Earth's
Health and Human Health Are One," "All Diseases Are Environmen-
tal Diseases," "Systems Theory and Environmental Health," "Human
Health as a Barometer of the Earth's Health," and "Lifestyle and Environmental Health." The major section, "The Sourcebook," has chapters
on radiation, chemicals, water and air pollution. Similarly, the eighth
annual Mandala Conference, sponsored with the Association of Holistic
Health in August 1982, was titled "Healing Ourselves, Healing Our
Planet."

Moving down from the global level, connectedness and interaction
between individuals is heavily stressed. Because of this, social and interactional aspects of health and illness are highly visible in the holistic

health model. Thus the family of the ill person must be pivotly considered in both assessment and intervention. As Jaffe writes, "sickness is definitely a family affair, which both affects and is affected by family bonds" (Jaffe, 1982: 117).

Similarly, concepts of community are central and prevalent, and the modified structure of the provider-client relationship is predicated on their underlying connectedness. This is reflected in the emphasis on interdisciplinary collaboration, partnership with the patient, and especially the value of a close, caring community. There is also a positive value placed on physical touch as an expression of caring in both healing and collegial relationships.

Focus on Health Promotion

A second parameter of holistic health is the importance placed on health promotion. A component assumption is the emphasis on health rather than disease and symptom amelioration. Practitioners and clients focus on the goal of positive wellness. Health itself is viewed as more than the absence of disease. A closely related assumption of health promotion is its preventive focus. A preventive, rather than crisis, orientation pervades the holistic health outlook. Practitioners emphasize nutrition, exercise, stress reduction, lifestyle patterns, values and belief systems in working towards the goal of high level wellness.

Health-promoting lifestyle patterns and habits are stressed heavily in holistic health, while those health habits have been regarded as more peripheral in the biomedical model (Ardell, 1977; Crawford, 1980; Frank, 1982: 10–11). Most allopathic physicians have only minimal knowledge of nutritional needs in illness, for example, and even less background on the nutritional requirements to attain or maintain optimal health.

A brief sampling of titles of books on holistic health demonstrates the emphasis on wellness and health promotion that dominates the literature:

The Well Body Book (Samuels and Bennett, 1973)
Wellness Workbook (Travis, 1977)
High Level Wellness (Ardell, 1977)
Health is a Question of Balance (Brenner, 1978)
Health For the Whole Person (Hastings et al., 1980)

Health as Balance/Integration/Harmony

Usually both health and illness have been defined in absolute terms. Additionally, Ng et al. point out that health has traditionally been defined by what it is not (Ng et al., 1982:44). Once the focus shifts to a goal of health and transition, the problem becomes that of defining health. Attempts are not yet completely unitary, but most of the holistic definitions share components such as balance, harmony, integration, sense of well-being, and energy to work and play. "Health" derives from the English word for "wholeness," and this derivation is reflected in most holistic definitions. Psychological, social, and spiritual well-being are emphasized equally with bodily well-being.

The holistic health literature contains frequent references to the World Health Organization definition of health as "a state of complete physical, mental, and social well-being, and not merely the absence of disease or infirmity"; however, many practitioners see that definition as too vague and simplistic and attempt to go beyond it (WHO, 1947).

Health as balance, harmony, and integration are probably the most prominent themes in holistic definitions of health. For example, one of the early holistic health books was Paul Brenner, M.D.'s *Health is a Question of Balance* (Brenner, 1978). Effie Poy Yew Chow describes the concept of balance as the fundamental precept of Chinese Medicine, which has strongly influenced the holistic health model (Chow, 1979: 404–405).

Jaffe's description of health also focuses on harmony and balance: "Good health—in its broadest sense—occurs when we live in harmony with ourselves and our environment, maintaining a balance in the face of changes, growing with challenges, and developing our innate healing powers. In essence, to be healthy is to be integrated and whole" (Jaffe, 1980:5). Like many others in holistic health, he writes of the possibility that a healthy person can become ill (ibid:15). Dossey adds the process element to such definitions: "The idea of health as harmony, of harmony as a quality of perfectly moving parts, suggests, as we have seen, a kinetic quality of health" (Dossey, 1982:184). These definitions of a fluid balance are closely related to models based on evolution or personal growth.

Bloomfield and Kory's definition of "positive wellness" reflects similar views. They go on to describe specific components of health such as vigor, alertness, joy of living, "ruddy cheeks," optimism, high energy, physical fitness, and fulfillment (Bloomfield et al., 1978:20–21). These authors also attempt to define spiritual health:

Within holistic medicine, spirit is a pragmatic concept, not religious or mystical. . . . Spirit refers to that which gives meaning and direction to your life. Important signs of spiritual health are satisfaction with work, an untroubled home life, and a sense of deep inner happiness. Although spiritual growth may contribute to a religious life, it may also be experienced and understood in terms of the actualization of an inherent human potential. In any case, through spiritual growth you experience a personal connection to a greater reality, be it Nature, God, or History (Bloomfield and Kory, 1978:50).

Health comes to be seen as a continuum with transitional states. Pelletier thus describes health as a dynamic and ongoing process (Pelletier, 1979:17). In looking at the potential for positive movement on the health continuum, the holistic assumptions lead to the view that wellness initiatives in one area of a person's life will support health enhancing behaviors in other areas (Ardell, 1977:6). The goal of this view then becomes *high-level wellness* or *super health* (Ardell, 1977; Gordon, 1980:17; Crawford, 1980:366).

This view of health places more value on the *quality of life* than on quantity, and references to this crop up throughout the literature, as well as coming out of many comments practitioners and clients make. As Dossey writes, "We no longer insist in the new view that length of life is of critical importance. Long-lived existences have no intrinsic value over short-lived ones. A short life is not tragic—although we continue to act to preserve life" (Dossey, 1982:176). This again places emphasis on the meaning of life and highly value-laden concepts.

Preventive and Promotional Focus

Holistic health advocates agree with critics of the health system like Dubos and McKeown who assert that ecological factors play a larger role than the medical care system in determining the level of health of a population (Dubos, 1959; McKeown, 1979). As McKeown concludes, a focus on nutritional, environmental, and lifestyle changes leads to more effective and less expensive outcomes than does intervention once disease is present (McKeown, 1979:vii).

Holistic health advocates consistently espouse this view that the health care system must shift its emphasis towards prevention and health promotion. There is frequent acknowledgement that the effectiveness of technological medical care is limited, and that future health care improvements will come from environmental and lifestyle changes (Knowles, 1977a; Pelletier, 1979:2). Pelletier differentiates the way in which the holistic preventive approach differs from prevention in the biomedical framework:

> Traditional preventive medicine consists of immunization, arresting the spread of disease through epidemiology and public health measures, multiphasic examinations, monitoring health care organizations, and related measures. The primary orientation is toward detection of signs, symptoms, and disabilities. As necessary as such an approach is, it still functions within a biomedical model, viewing health as the relative absence of pathology. Holistic approaches move beyond this neutral position to work toward increasing health and optimum health (Pelletier, 1979:87).

In response to this emphasis, an increasing number of wellness and preventive health centers have emerged. John W. Travis, M.D. founded what is probably the most well-known of these, the Wellness Resource Center, in Mill Valley in 1974, which influenced much of the thinking in holistic health. Clients in this program (many of the early clients were health professionals) complete numerous assessment tools, including a wellness inventory, health hazard appraisal, life change index, computerized dietary inventory, physical fitness assessment, and a purpose-in-life test (Travis, 1977, 1978; Ardell, 1977:12–15; Gordon, 1980:472). Beyond the large number of practitioners who attended workshops and were influenced by the center, Travis' *Wellness Workbook*, along with his *Wellness Workbook for Professionals*, influenced the perspectives of countless professionals in diverse disciplines, especially medicine and nursing.[5]

Several major issues derive from this emphasis on health. First, prevention and health promotion, whether advocated by practitioners of traditional allopathic medicine or holistic health, invariably focuses on basic lifestyle change. Thus it can easily evolve into a moral crusade. Early indications that this scenario may be developing will be discussed in detail in the final chapters of the book.

A second issue raised by this focus is that it elevates health to an even more central life concern. Even when healthy, a person should take the responsibility of actively working to maintain or improve that state of health and well-being. As Blattner writes, "If a person takes responsibility for creating a healthy lifestyle, everything that person does is directed toward or away from that goal" (Blattner, 1981:40). This view relegates concerns not directly related to health to a low priority. American society has often been criticized for already elevating health and disease concerns to too high a level; this emphasis within holistic health moves us even closer to a virocracy. The pursuit of health becomes an infinite quest.

A third and closely related paradox is that, once health comes to be defined so broadly, the push to manage so many areas of everyday life conflicts with the Eastern stance of passive acceptance, which is also part of the movement stance. In fact, it constitutes an interventionist bias, closely akin to that critiqued in the biomedical model by movement adherents.

Meaning of Illness

A third parameter is the meaning of illness within a holistic health model. Within the framework of the traditional medical model, illness signals a breakdown in bodily functioning and initiates a characteristic sequence of events to attempt to reverse that breakdown. In contrast, illness within a holistic health model is viewed as a message that the person needs to readjust his way of living. Unlike the negative connotations attached to illness in the medical model, the holistic health paradigm views illness as an opportunity for positive growth. As Brenner writes, "What is happening in your life to allow illness?" (Brenner, 1978:16) and "Illness has the potential to place one in a higher state of consciousness. It may provide the opportunity to exercise options and establish priorities— It's an internal psychiatrist—use it—you paid for it" (ibid:19). Similarly, Samuels and Bennett have an entire section in their *Well Body Book*, titled "Disease as a Positive Life Force" (Samuels and Bennett, 1973:15–16).

Illness as Imbalance/Dis-ease

In the allopathic medical model, illness is conceived of as a random event which comes from outside the person. Metaphors of illness as an external enemy accompany this concept. For instance, we think in terms of "catching a cold." As Jaffe writes, "Most of us regard illness as an external invader, attacking a body that was previously healthy" (Jaffe, 1980:3). Deriving from this notion is the view of curative action also coming from external sources. Thus, for example, a specific organism invades a person's body; the physician may then prescribe an antibiotic that inactivates that organism.

Again, the underlying assumptions of each model determine the meanings attached to illness. In the biomedical model not only is the cause of illness particularistic, but so is the treatment; this is basically the doctrine of specific etiology. Similarly, the symptoms are seen as bounded in both time and space. In contrast, in a holistic model both individual causes, symptoms, and treatments receive less priority than the broad contextual picture.[6]

Becoming ill has very different symbolic meanings within a holistic model. Just as health means balance and integration, illness signifies a breakdown of that balance. Micro-organisms are seen as part of our natural environment. An individual who is out of balance develops lowered resistance, so that an infection might develop. The curative emphasis is on assisting the person to regain a healthy balance, so that his or her own healing powers are activated in overcoming the infection. Even when an antibiotic is used, in a holistic model it is seen as assisting the patient to regain enough strength so that internal defenses can then take over. Thus pharmocological agents are viewed as facilitating healing, rather than "curing."

Holistic practitioners frequently talk about illness as *dis-ease*. Various degrees of discomfort are seen as lying on a continuum with severe illness. Rather than waiting until a problem is defined as severe enough to be labelled "illness," it is considered preferable to initiate self-healing measures or to seek help at the mildest indication of dis-ease.

It seems that holistic conceptions bring illness beliefs closer to many traditional folk beliefs. Similarly, the holistic conceptions emphasize the illness experience over the medical categorizations of disease (within medical sociology, "disease" refers to the physical or biological condition, while "illness" refers to the individuals's subjective experience and response to disease). This view of illness thus assumes that the patient's subjective experience of dis-ease or illness is paramount (Salmon and Berliner, 1980: 198), and it lends more credence to that experience than to "objective" medical determinations.

Treat Cause, Not Symptoms

Once a problem of dis-ease is determined, the treatment focuses on the underlying imbalance within the person or between the person and others, rather than focusing on discrete symptoms or organs. According to this model, if an individual is healed by an external medication, such as an antibiotic, unless she then makes changes that get to the cause of the imbalance, she is likely to become reinfected or develop alternate symptoms in the future.

Specific symptoms are not ignored, however, in the holistic model. Symptoms are often seen as having particular symbolic meaning for that individual, and this can guide that person to an understanding of why illness occurred (Kane, 1980; Brenner, 1978). As Ardell argues, "it is important that healers be sensitive to and interested in helping you unmask the meaning of your illness" (Ardell, 1977:56).

Two additional sources, or contributing causes of illness, must be mentioned here. First, many holistic advocates view illness as learned behavior. As a child, the individual had limited coping resources, and illness was one of the only ways to gain either attention or relief from overwhelming responsibility within the family context. Becoming sick became an unconscious, learned pattern of responding to stress.

A closely related source is the view of explicit secondary gain in illness. Many holistic practitioners discuss the benefits derived from illness in more volitional terms. Letting go of responsibility and relaxing are often stigmatized as "weakness" in our achievement-oriented society; yet, it is permissible and even valued when a person becomes ill.

Jaffe sees the primary quality of secondary gain as the person's unconscious use of his illness to exert control over others, particularly family members, without assuming responsibility for those actions. He advocates family therapy to help that person learn to achieve those goals without the cost of illness (Jaffe, 1984:217).

Illness as Opportunity

This assumption represents a major departure from the allopathic medical model. Illness in our society traditionally has had a fairly unambivalent negative connotation. Since illness in a holistic model functions as a bodily message of an underlying imbalance, it is interpreted as an opportunity for growth. As Dossey writes:

> In the new view of health we cease to see disease as entirely negative. Health, too, is not altogether positive for us. The fact is, the distinctions between health and disease at a point begin to blur. . . . In the new view we attach little value to health and disease. Rather than seeing them as either good or bad to us they seem to be simply a statement of the way things are (Dossey, 1982:145).

Similarly, Gordon writes that holistic medicine views illness as an opportunity for discovery as well as a misfortune (Gordon, 1980:21). Phyllis Mattson concurs with this view of illness as opportunity in the holistic model: "the illness itself is not necessarily considered bad fortune—it is but a step in life's journey, one's karma or destiny" (Mattson, 1982:11). If the message of illness is not heeded by the person, however, proponents see the body giving "louder" messages until the person either responds to those messages or becomes incapacitated.

Dis-ease or illness means that something needs to be changed in some part of an individual's life, so it essentially requires some form of life reevaluation. As Jaffe writes, "Once you recognize that disease is not simply a physical struggle but may also involve psychological, spiritual, and social dimensions, then it becomes clear that the appearance of any physical symptoms—especially a serious or chronic one—ought to evoke a deep personal inquiry into your life" (Jaffe, 1980:18). This includes examining the ill person's work situation and family interactions, as well as his patterns of rest, exercise, nutrition, stress reduction, and recreation. A meaningful sense of purpose is also seen as necessary to reverse disease, as well as to avoid becoming ill.

The person should ask herself why she became sick and why it happened at this particular time. For example, a person may be "pushing too hard," ignoring the need for rest and nurturance. She might come down with a cold at that point, and that would serve as a reminder that she should respect her needs. If that individual, however, continued to work even harder, ignoring the cold, she would be likely to develop increasingly severe physical problems until she was "forced" to rest. Irving Oyle writes of that type of situation, arguing that most people take over-the-counter drugs to continue "pushing" when they develop minor symptoms. He advocates paying closer attention to the bodily communications, so that such problems could be resolved in their early stages (Oyle, 1979:97).

The potential for growth derives from the ways that individual could learn more about her needs and how to take care of herself. She might plan to incorporate more rest or use stress reduction techniques during the high pressure periods. This is seen as placing her at a higher level of consciousness about herself, as well as moving her lifestyle in more health-promoting directions. Thus disease can motivate an individual towards more self-awareness and self-understanding (both are highly valued in holistic health). Pelletier cites examples such as spontaneous remission from ostensibly terminal cancer to argue that illness can serve as a precondition for a profound self-transformation (Pelletier, 1979:17).

Faith, the will to live, a rediscovery of meaning in life, and symbolic forms of rebirth and transformation again imply growth leading to a healthier outcome.

Individual Responsibility

A fourth feature prominent in the holistic health model is the belief that health care is primarily a matter of individual responsibility. This derives from a synthesis of the views of holism, health promotion, and the meaning of illness. The client is seen as bearing the primary responsibility for his or her own decisions and the resultant level of health. As Gordon writes, "Holistic medicine emphasizes the responsibility of each individual for his or her health. The practitioners of holistic medicine feel that we have the capacity to understand the psychobiological origins of our illness, to stimulate our innate healing processes, and to make changes in our lives that will promote health and prevent illness" (Gordon, 1980:18). This view is echoed by Ardell:

> You Are the Chairperson of Your Own Well-Being. You can carry the key to your own physical, emotional, and mental well-being in the way you choose to live. Doctors and others can help you, can give you advice, can save your life in certain instances, and can usually make things easier, but in the overall analysis, you have the responsibility for whatever goes well or poorly; for your own health and well-being (Ardell, 1977:49).

Mattson also portrays self-responsibility as one of the foundations of holistic health, extending it to the case of illness: "Taking responsibility for health includes taking responsibility for illness, too. If one gets sick, for example, one says to oneself, 'I created this illness for myself, and only I can create getting better' " (Mattson, 1982:37). Mattson goes on to remind us that self-care probably accounts for the major part of medical care in all societies (ibid:41).[7]

The individual is responsible for maintaining health promoting health habits when well, and for seeking the knowledge necessary to implement them. Once he becomes ill, he is responsible for not only seeking help and cooperating with the healer and healing program (these responsibilities also accompany the biomedical model), but he should also actively participate in decisions on the healing regime, and, most importantly, make himself receptive to healing. In addition, the patient is seen as the one with the most knowledge about the self and the life situation; therefore, the sick person is the one who can best determine the personal meaning of the illness at this point in time. In other words, the client has major responsibility for both assessment and intervention in illness.

This area of responsibility increasingly brings together holistic practitioners with physicians in family medicine and health policy experts (Knowles, 1977; Fink, 1976; Ardell, 1976). As Jeter writes in his article on holistic health and family practice: "Getting patients and families to take charge of themselves, and therefore their illness, and recognizing the individual's or family's role in triggering or exacerbating the condition is in consonance with family medicine's ideology and practice" (Jeter, 1982:79).

Two major assumptions underlie this parameter of individual responsibility. The first appears to be a move towards *privatization* with a decreased reliance on hospitals and bureaucratized, technological organization. This is closely related to the more general movement of deprofessionalization and deexpertization (Lopata, 1979:128).

A second assumption underlying individual responsibility is that of *illness as stigma*. The assumptions of illness as stigma and attribution of blame are highly problematic in both the medical and holistic health models. The complexities of this area will be analyzed in detail in Chapter VI; however, it is important to note here that the view of self-responsibility often becomes translated into terms of blame and guilt. Once illness is no longer assumed to derive from natural, external causes, as it is in the allopathic medical model, the sick person is often seen as intentionally causing his illness.

Talcott Parsons already recognized the patient's participation in becoming ill, although he saw it in terms of unconscious processes. Because of this view of unconscious participation, he saw the responsibility as balanced with the caring and compassion of health professionals, as long as the patient kept her side of the bargain in terms of her responsibilities to seek care and cooperate with the physician's regime. Thus illness was structured so that it would remain limited and under the control of the medical gatekeepers, who served an important societal function in maintaining those limits (Parsons and Fox, 1958).

The holistic stance on responsibility varies widely. While some proponents like Polidora (1977) talk of our creating our total reality in our minds (thus we bear total responsibility for our state of health), many others recognize dangerous ambiguities in the concept and attempt to avoid placing blame on the ill person. For instance, Irving Oyle moderates his discussion of how people create their own illness:

> But suppose you're not one, but two . . . One side of you wants to be sick, while the other wants to get well. One part of you creates and actively maintains the illness. The complementary opposite side sincerly and honestly wants to be rid of it. It is the responsibility and the task of the physician to help shift the balance from one side to the other (Oyle, 1979:96).

Another view that maintains the view of responsibility, yet avoids blame, is that of Dennis Jaffe:

> By accepting responsibility for your well-being, you need not assume blame for your illnesses. If you are sick, you need not feel guilty. Guilt will not change the past or the present, or enhance your chances for a healthy future. Your energies should instead be focused upon acquiring an understanding of the factors that may have helped cause or aggravate your illness, and changing them. Rather than feeling helpless, hopeless, or guilty when you become ill, you must begin to explore what you can do to make yourself healthier (Jaffe, 1980:90).

Those studying holistic health show the same divergence in their interpretations of responsibility as practitioners do in their writing. For example, Kopelman and Moskop, Shapiro and Shapiro, and Crawford write of the dangers of self-responsibility, while Fink, Knowles, and Mendelsohn welcome it (Kopelman and Moskop, 1981; Shapiro and Shapiro, 1979; Crawford, 1980; Fink, 1976; Knowles, 1977; Mendelsohn, 1979). Neither group presents solid empirical evidence to support their contentions in terms of the interactional outcomes.

Another interesting paradox is raised by the emphasis on self-responsibility. The holistic health approach encourages bodily awareness, sensuality, and nurturing oneself; yet, self-responsibility often means strict self-denial in those same areas. Many forms of self-nurturance that are common within this society, for example eating rich or sweet foods, become defined as self-destructive indulgence. This ignores the emphasis on "holism," since eating those foods may also nurture the person emotionally in ways that promote health. Thus physical and emotional effects of food intake need to be weighed. This same self-denial in relation to lifestyle also conflicts at times with the value placed on quality over quantity of life. Again, these paradoxes and the ways they are translated into practice will be analyzed in considerable depth in later chapters.

Practitioners as Educators, Consultants, Facilitators

Fifth, practitioners function as health educators, consultants, and wellness/healing facilitators. This characteristic of holistic health derives from the recognition of the client's responsibility; furthermore, it advocates a democratic, egalitarian relationship between the practitioner and client. The pervasive emphasis on egalitarian relationships within the holistic health movement highlights core values of the participants. Both egalitarianism and cooperation are stressed prominently within movement ideology. Cooperative, collaborative relationships extend to both practitioner-client encounters and the interactions between practitioners. Several dimensions of this role will be highlighted.

In the holistic model the provider shares her expertise and knowledge about health and illness. She explains the problem and outlines the various options; then the client makes the actual decision alone or in collaboration with the practitioner. Because most Americans in this society know so little about health principles such as adequate nutritional intake and stress reduction measures, much time is spent discussing such areas and teaching about them and their relationship to health. Mattson writes, "The healee is assumed to be the healer, in fact, while the practitioner is considered a guide, counselor, or facilitator. The healee has responsibility for the healing, and must be an active partner in the process" (Mattson, 1982:45). And Gordon describes this type of role in the holistic model:

> Holistic health centers emphasize education and self-care rather than treatment and dependence. Practitioners tend to believe that each person is his or her best source of care, that their job is to share rather than withhold and mystify their knowledge, to become "resources" rather than authorities (Gordon, 1980b:471).

This movement to viewing the practitioner relating in a teaching, facilitating role also parallels the emerging emphasis in family practice (Jeter, 1982:79).

Practitioner Mobilizes Innate Healing Capacity

Rather than a view of an authoritarian physician making assessments and intervening on behalf of a patient, the practitioner is seen as a healer who mobilizes innate healing capacities residing in the client. The client's healing is facilitated by the practitioner, whether through providing information or applying healing interventions.

Jerome Frank sees the holistic and biomedical approaches as having the potential to benefit each other. He writes that holistic health should remind the biomedical physician that the ultimate source of healing is the recuperative power of the patient. The chief function of whatever medical procedures are used is to facilitate or maximize this power (Frank, 1981:19–20).

Warmth, "Caring" Highly Valued

The practitioner is seen as part of the client's environment, and his or her job is to create a setting conducive to healing for the patient. This environment again helps mobilize the patient's inner healing capacity. Gordon summarizes the general environment holistic health settings strive for:

> Holistic health centers maximize the therapeutic potential of the setting in which health care takes place. The centers are generally both physically and interpersonally inviting and tend to inspire trust rather than fear or awe. . . . The design leans heavily toward open spaces and attractively decorated, plant-filled rooms. Those who come for help are generally called clients rather than patients and are often encouraged to call staff members by their first names and to see the center as a place for education, volunteer work, and socializing as well as care in health and illness (Gordon, 1980b:474).

Thus, visible warmth and caring, as well as empathy, are considered essential for a practitioner. Many practitioners talk of transpersonal or unconditional love as initiating or facilitating healing within the patient. Another way model adherents conceptualize such affective aspects of the relationship relates to their views of healing as dealing with energy transference between the healer and healee.

Touch and physical contact between practitioner and patient is also seen as an essential component of mobilizing healing (Krieger, 1975;

Gordon, 1980:19). Dolores Krieger has done research on the phenomenon of healing through therapeutic touch, as well as teaching large numbers of nurses and other clinicians, over the past thirteen years (Krieger,
1975, 1984). The exploratory study of holistic physicians by Goldstein
et al. found that, when asked what differentiated them from other physicians, they reported "touching clients more" as a consistent difference
(Goldstein et al., 1987:104).

This implies emotional involvement of practitioners, which is far
more highly valued than is emotional neutrality or "professional distance" (Blattner, 1981:21). Kane, for instance, advocates a stance of
physician compassion, empathy, and involvement with patients: "The
trick is not to sidestep involvement, but to maximize it and stay centered
at the same time" (Kane, 1983:3). This emotional involvement also
extends to interactions between staff members. Warm, caring, demon-
strative interactions between practitioners are also highly valued and frequently visible, so that often holistically oriented centers have a definite
feel of "family" or "community."

Egalitarian Relationship

The relationship between practitioner and client is also described by
participants as being far more egalitarian than in that involved in the
biomedical model. The doctor-patient relationship has traditionally en-
compassed a definite status differential, and an attempt is made to minimize this inequality in holistic settings.

One example of the shift towards a more egalitarian relationship
between the provider and client is the language used by those writing
about the holistic health model. Rather than using the term "patient,"
most authors and practitioners refer to a "person" or "client," or even a
"consumer." Similarly, informality often extends to practitioners, as well
as patients, so that the former are frequently addressed by first name,
rather than by their professional title. Ardell's book, *High Level Wellness*, has a section headed "It's Better to Be a Client than a Patient"
where he articulates the rationale for this stance:

> The term patient connotes a subservient quality in the nature of
> your relationship with a physician; as a client, on the other
> hand, you are the responsible party in transactions with the
> provider. (That's because in the wellness framework, the pro-
> vider is a facilitator of learning, an ally, and a guide in the

healing process—not an authority figure.) The distinction is more than a rhetorical gesture: the ethic of active self-responsibility for your well-being is the foundation of a wellness philosophy, and the idea that you are the sovereign of your own well-being is simply easier to recognize when you are respectfully treated as a client than it is when you are condescendingly managed as a patient. The patient takes the doctor's orders; the client considers his or her advice (Ardell, 1977:53–54).

Again, this egalitarian stance extends to collegial relationships, whether within or between disciplines. The holistic model is more receptive to, and more positively values, interdisciplinary collaboration than does allopathic medicine. The literature portrays an attempt to minimize a hierarchical structure in holistic practice. Physicians and nurses in a holistic setting often work closely with nutritionists, body awareness and fitness experts, psychologists, acupuncturists, and at times ministers. Similarly, more egalitarian relationships between men and women are valued.

Mutuality in Interaction

Another shift in the practitioner role goes beyond egalitarianism in the relationship between provider and client, to *mutuality*. A provider is not seen as objectively intervening and affecting change in a passive, nonresponsive client. Rather, the healing encounter involves two active systems interacting and ultimately changed. Both the practitioner and the client are seen as growing through the encounter. As Dossey describes this view:

> Patients are no longer seen as objects "to whom" or "for whom" something is done. In the new view patient and therapist form a unit through the processes that connect all beings. Patient-oriented therapy is a boomerang, affecting the therapist at the same time. From the modern therapist's perspective, thus, patient therapy is self-therapy. To heal another is to heal oneself (Dossey, 1982:145).

Similarly, Brenner discusses healing as a cocreative process in which the person being healed simultaneously heals and teaches the healer (Brenner, 1984:181). This notion is very close to Jung's "Wounded Healer."

Practitioner as Role Model

Lastly, in the holistic model practitioners are frequently described as role models. Providers try to carry out the health measures they advocate to patients in their own lives. Transcendental awareness and spirituality is highly valued in the practitioner as well. For instance, Robert Gerard believes that healing techniques are not as important as the quality of the healer's own being (Gerard, 1978). And Ardell argues, "It seems to me that physicians who themselves pay little regard to the importance of nutrition, exercise, stress management, and self-responsibility are highly unlikely to promote lifestyle reform to you and me" (Ardell, 1977:50). Mattson concurs: "Healers are supposed to be role models also, and patients are encouraged to look carefully at their healers to see if they are living what they preach" (Mattson, 1982:47).

References to this dimension appear repeatedly in holistic practitioners' statements as well. For example, Walt Stoll, Medical Director of the Holistic Health Centre in Lexington, Kentucky, describes encouraging all the practitioners in his clinic to "practice what they preach and serve as examples of wellness to the clients who come to the Centre" (Read, 1983:384). Janet Moll writes that nursing may have difficulty in its attempts to promote high-level wellness because of the absence of high-level wellness in nurses themselves (Moll, 1982:61). Similarly, Jeff Kane describes most of his fellow doctors as "lackluster advertisements for our craft," citing the high mortality rates and risks of alcoholism, substance abuse, and suicide among physicians (Kane, 1983:1). And Goldstein et al.'s research comparing members of the American Holistic Health Association with a group of Family Practitioners found that the holistic physicians were significantly more likely to be personally involved in a rigorous health promotion program (Goldstein et al., 1987:113).

Cultural Diversity in Healing Practices

A sixth parameter of the holistic health phenomenon is the celebration of cultural diversity in healing practices. Frequently components of Eastern philosophical and healing systems coexist or are integrated with Western healing modalities. Native American and a variety of folk medicine healing systems are also frequently encountered. The resultant array of healing forms are united primarily by their respect for the body's innate healing capacity and their emphasis on natural and less intrusive healing approaches. As Gordon writes:

> A holistic perspective respects the ways culture shapes patho-physiology and distinguishes between the anatomical lesions that constitue a "disease" state or diagnostic category and the individual's experience of "illness." This kind of perspective leads to a respect for culturally sanctioned views of illness and its treatment and to the incorporation of indigenous healers where their services are appropriate (Gordon, 1981:116).

Healing modalities commonly encountered in holistic practice include: guided imagery and visualization, meditation, biofeedback, nutritional therapy, massage, yoga, acupuncture, reflexology, homeopathy, Shiatsu, and autogenics. An attempt at a complete listing would overwhelm the remainder of this book.

The holistic health model is described as being more receptive to alternative systems, seeing value in the many modes of healing used in various cultures. This assumes a cooperative approach, so that a family practice physician might work alongside a traditional acupuncturist in healing a patient. In another instance the family practice physician might utilize acupuncture along with more traditional medical approaches.

The primary underlying assumption is the value placed on *multicultural pluralism*. In particular, Eastern philosophical and health systems are highly valued. Many of the central modalities utilized in holistic health are derived from Oriental approaches, while others, such as yoga, were more common in India.

For example, both traditional acupuncture as a holistic treatment approach, and pulse diagnosis as a holistic diagnostic tool, derive directly from Chinese medicine. Similarly, the range of meditational approaches derived strongly from both Buddhist and yogic approaches in the East. Benson's studies at Harvard Medical School leading to his concept of the relaxation response began with his research demonstrating physiological changes in long-term practitioners of Transcendental Meditation, a technique derived from India and "packaged" in Western form (Benson, 1975; Benson et al., 1981).

Many holistic health practitioners also see yoga and ayurvedic medicine as adjuncts to healing. For instance, Jeff Kane, a former Medical Director of the Berkeley Free Clinic, wrote an article in *Yoga Journal* called "Yoga and Medicine: A Healing Partnership?" (Kane, 1980).

Similarly, Grisell writes, "As practiced from day to day, this (kundalini) yoga is physical-psychological preventive medicine, but there exists an array of techniques to readjust imbalances and to help the mind-body heal itself" (Grisell, 1980:441).

Native American cultural healing systems are also used frequently, as are other folk medicine systems. These approaches and modalities, like the Eastern approaches, are seen as more in touch with nature and natural measures than allopathic medicine. For instance, Sun Bear, a Bear Society Chippowah medicine chief, spoke at an Association of Holistic Health/Mandala Conference on the native American healing approach. He spoke of being more interested in "holistic life" than holistic health, describing how medicine to native people means "everything." He interpreted modern society's problems as stemming from our disconnectedness from nature and creation (Sun Bear, 1982). Various Western faith healing approaches are sometimes included as well. Chow depicts the core value of harmony pervading this range of alternative cultural systems:

> The monitoring of body/mind energies toward a state of being attuned with the harmony of universal forces is practiced, not only by the Chinese people, but in other cultural and theoretical systems as well. Curanderismo, Indian shaminism and herbology, Philippine healing and Black folk medicine are only a very few of the cultural healing systems that are based on principles of balance and harmony of vital life forces as related to a higher universal power (Chow, 1979:409).

Not only do all these Eastern and folk approaches respect the person's own healing capacity, but they are also attractive to holistic health practitioners because they rely more on self-care for preventive health than does allopathic medicine. These approaches also share a focus on more natural, less intrusive approaches to healing. Drugs and surgery, as well as "intrusive" diagnostic techniques such as x-rays, are used much more sparingly, in favor of more natural procedures.

Again, the wide diversity of modalities contrasts sharply with a more standardized approach in the allopathic model. Most holistic practitioners feel there are many alternative approaches that assist healing and movement towards more optimum health. They at times cite research like the study by Kleinman and Gale, demonstrating that patients may derive benefits from folk healing comparable to physician treatment, according to both self report and research staff evaluation (Kleinman and Gale,

1982). They also feel that strengthening the patient in any area has a synergistic effect, so that there are many valid ways to approach the same problem. Which approach is ultimately used in a situation again depends on the particular patient/client and the particular healer.

Pervasive Influence of Chinese Medicine

The single most pervasive influence on the holistic health model is that of traditional Chinese medicine. Tsun-Nin Lee, M.D. spoke at an Association of Holistic Health conference, discussing Chinese Medicine as a "paragon of holistic health" (Lee, 1978). Similarly, David E. Bresler, Ph.D. wrote in an article on "Chinese Medicine and Holistic Health":

> One of the earliest systems of holistic medicine was practiced by the ancient Chinese more than 5,000 years ago. Traditional Chinese medicine did not distinguish between mind and body but viewed physical and mental symptoms as manifestations of a unitary underlying energy imbalance that affected the entire organism. Thousands of years ago, Chinese physicians recognized the critical importance of environmental influences, diet and exercise, and preventive medicine. An ancient aphorism states "the superior physician cures before the illness is manifested. The inferior physician can only treat the illness he was unable to prevent" (Bresler, 1980:407).

Effie Poy Yew Chow, R.N., Ph.D. also depicts the Chinese system as the primary source of holistic health, and the East-West Academy of Healing Arts she founded in San Francisco has been highly influential in the holistic health movement. In an article on the contributions of Chinese medicine to holistic healing, she details the influence of Eastern ideas, demonstrating how concepts of holism, balance, moderation and harmony are derived from the fundamental precepts of Chinese medicine (Chow, 1979:403–406). She describes the parallels between Chinese medicine and holistic health as even more obvious when looking at the treatment approaches used: "Methods of treatment rely on the monitoring of body/mind energy patterns and the modification of life habits and behaviors to maintain (or regain) the ultimate harmonious balance essential to well-being" (ibid.:412).

Beyond the direct influence of Chinese medicine on the holistic paradigm, its influence is observable in more diffuse views and values discussed by holistic practitioners. These shifts will be discussed in the next section on the alternative world view. Yet another sign of this influence is the frequency of quotes from Eastern, and particularly ancient Chinese, texts that appear in holistic works. For instance, Herbert Benson, a cardiologist at Harvard Medical School, begins the first chapter of his book *The Mind/Body Effect* with a quote from *The Yellow Emperor's Classic of Internal Medicine* (Benson, 1979:1–2). Dianne M. Connelly opens her book on traditional acupuncture with another quoted conversation between Ch'i Po, an acupuncture master, and the Yellow Emperor from the same classic (Connelly, 1979:frontispiece). Besides numerous quotes from ancient Chinese philosophers such as Lao Tzu and Chuang Tsu, holistic literature frequently contains sayings from other Eastern traditions, such as the Sufi (Idries Shah's works are most often used) and Yogi traditions. For example, Larry Dossey, M.D. begins one of his articles with a Sufi fable of Nasrudin (Dossey, 1982:1).

Alternative World View/Consciousness

A seventh parameter of the holistic health model postulates a fundamentally different world view of participants. The nature of reality and the meanings attached to life, health, and healing are seen as differing dramatically from the traditional Western world view. This component of the holistic health movement is by far the most vague and difficult to identify or describe; yet, it is the most important to the determination of the movement's core meanings and values. An interconnected web of shared definitions of experience unite the practitioners who are involved in implementing a more holistic model of health.

While "consciousness" is a word frequently evoked by holistic adherents, defining its precise meaning is problematic. Robert Ornstein's work, *The Psychology of Consciousness*, presents only a rudimentary conceptualization of the results of recent research in the two modes of consciousness available to man. The second mode derives primarily from "right hemisphere" brain function; it operates primarily in a spatial, simultaneous mode which is predominantly non-linear, non-sequential and intuitive (Ornstein, 1975). A shift towards this mode most closely approximates the meanings discussed by participants. Pelletier also attempts to describe this consciousness shift:

> Today there is a profound alteration taking place involving the nature of human consciousness. . . . (and the) transformation of our most fundamental belief systems. . . . Questions are

being raised concerning the essential nature of reality, from quantum physics to the emerging science of consciousness (Pelletier, 1977:301).

Joseph Gusfield's conceptualization of the "consciousness of kind" clarifies the type of process postulated here. After describing "community" as a social construction, he writes:

> Within the emergence of a consciousness of kind is the rise of a collective experience; a sense of participating in the same history. . . . Community might almost be defined as people who see themselves as having a common history and destiny different from other. . . . (An) aggregate of people (with) a common history ensures the sharing of symbols, legends, names and events that are unlikely to others. . . . It is even much more than that, however. It also involves shared attitudes toward events, both past and present (Gusfield, 1975:35).

Several meanings and symbols permeate the particular world view or consciousness shared by those involved in the holistic health movement. Many of them emerge from, and overlap with, the first six parameters; however, they extend far beyond the circumscribed areas of health and illness. Many of their features, additionally, approximate "right hemisphere" brain function. A brief listing, which will be further elaborated in Chapter III, includes: an anti-technological and at times anti-scientific stance; a distrust of basic institutions such as medicine, government, and corporate business; an anti-bureaucratic bias; a resurgence of humanistic concerns; an egalitarian stance; an emphasis on cooperation and community; a tolerance and encouragement of diversity of lifestyles; a desire to live closer to nature and in harmony with the environment; a valuing of sensory experience and intuition above conceptual knowledge; an emphasis on present time orientation over future orientation; a devaluing of detachment and objectivity in favor of involvement; an existential stance stressing individual choice and responsibility; and a transcendental, spiritual world view which is anti-materialistic. Other closely related core values found in holistic participants include sensuality, authenticity, and expressiveness.

There is also a set of meanings that suggest a more Eastern stance in relation to the self. The Eastern self is more passive, less controlling and interventionist, and more connected with its environment (both other people and the physical environment) (Marsella, De Vos, and Hsu, 1985). Thus Jim Polidora advocates learning how to "surrender" and "let go." A person should work towards learning to be more passive and receptive, rather than always active and intervening (Polidora, 1978).

The emphasis on a present time orientation is also partially derived from Eastern views. Dossey describes the shift in time perception, portraying the holistic way of perceiving time in a static, nonflowing, nonlinear way (Dossey, 1982:176). He contrasts this perception to the usual perception of time in our society: "a sense of urgency is associated with the perception of time as a linear process of past, present, and future. Our modern sense of this urgency is expressed by our feeling that there is not enough time" (ibid.:179). Mattson concurs with his view: "Holistic health advocates attempt to be "here and now" oriented. They wish to live in the present, aware and participating to the fullest every moment, whether it is pleasant or not" (Mattson, 1982:51).

Another set of meanings and values relates to the devaluing of detachment and objectivity, in favor of more subjective, intuitive, and involved ways of relating to others and gaining knowledge. Oyle describes the prevalent holistic views on objectivity: "Elimination of the barrier (the differentiation between the observing scientist and the observed data) makes untenable and obsolete one of our most common and most entrenched illusions—the concept called objective reality" (Oyle, 1979:70).

Similarly, altered states of consciousness are frequently discussed in holistic literature, and they are valued as one means to attain spiritual and emotional growth. A variety of meditational and experiential techniques are utilized in an attempt to move the individual to such altered states through "natural" means, rather than resorting to the use of psychedelic drugs.

Many holistic health leaders and practitioners refer to Thomas Kuhn's *The Structure of Scientific Revolutions* in describing the "paradigm shift" to a new medical holistic model. Additionally, there are frequent references to authors describing the research findings from the "new (quantum) physics," especially Fritjof Capra's *The Tao of Physics* and Gary Zukov's *The Dancing Wu Li Masters* (Kuhn, 1970; Capra, 1975; Zukov, 1979; Cassell, 1986). Also frequently quoted in holistic literature and conferences are leaders from the self-actualization and human potential movements. Abraham Maslow's theories on self-actualization are frequently encountered, along with numerous references to Sidney Jourard and Fritz Perls.

Phyllis Mattson concurs with my conclusion that these more global meanings encompass a larger arena than holistic health. She argues that the ultimate goal of holistic health is a transformation of world view: "Although most advocates of holistic health state that its goal is to make people healthy, there are many who suggest that this goal is but one step in a societal transformation toward a new world view, new social institutions, and a change in national lifestyle" (Mattson, 1982:129–130).

Summary

These seven parameters of the holistic health model are visible in the massive proliferation of books, courses, and healing programs increasingly available over the last twelve years. In fact, an observer of the movement is struck with the uniformity of the meanings that are expressed almost repetitively throughout the literature. For example, a multitude of books attempt to translate research supporting this approach into practical knowledge and techniques for self application. One of the first, *The Well Body Book* by Mike Samuels, M.D. and Hal Bennett embodies the previously discussed characteristics of holism, health promotion, illness as message, individual responsibility for health, use of practitioners as consultants, cultural diversity in healing practices, and the different world view or consciousness. It has lengthy sections presenting techniques of preventive medicine and stress reduction. The authors discuss disease as a "positive life force." Techniques for physical examination are presented, followed by a lengthy "how to" section for self-diagnosis and treatment. Finally, the book describes ways to use one's doctor, as well as drugs, as further "resources" (Samuels and Bennett, 1973). More closely integrated with the traditional medical model are books such as Herbert Benson's *The Relaxation Response*, Kenneth Pelletier's *Mind as Healer, Mind as Slayer* and *Holistic Medicine: From Stress to Optimum Health*, Arthur C. Hastings et al.'s compilation *Health for the Whole Person*, J. Warren Salmon's *Alternative Medicines*, and James S. Gordon et al.'s *Mind, Body and Health: Toward an Integral Medicine* (Benson, 1975; Pelletier, 1977; ibid., 1979; Hastings et al., 1980; Salmon, 1984; Gordon et al., 1984).[8]

Courses for both public consumption and health professionals have also increased exponentially. For example, included here is a brief sampling of course titles offered to nurses as a basis for credit toward professional relicensure in California between 1978 and 1980:

Stress and Illness
Stress Reduction
Healing the Healer
On Healing the Whole Person
Holistic Health for Nurses

The Psychology of Consciousness
Positive Wellness: Health, Love and Effective
   Communication
Stress and Tension: Cancer/Death and Dying
Therapeutic Touch as a Preventive Modality
The Patient's Responsibility for Health
The Healing Brain

Each year between 1975 and 1985 the Mandala Society and the Association for Holistic Health have joined, several times with either the University of California, San Diego, School of Medicine Continuing Education division or the California State University, San Diego, Continuing Education, to present a major symposium on holistic health. The 1977 conference, titled "Experiencing the Medical Model of the Future—An In-depth Survey of Holistic Health" represented a range of highly divergent positions. Out of the 28 speakers, ten held M.D.s and seven Ph.D.s. Speakers such as Jonas Salk, M.D. shared the podium with spiritual healers and the Pir of the Sufi Order. Interestingly, although no nurses spoke during the formal program, the vast majority of conference attendees were nurses (physicians comprised the smallest group represented at the early conferences, although they were prominently represented as speakers).

These examples should assist in placing the salient characteristics of the holistic health model in a more concrete framework. Uniting the seven parameters that have been elaborated in this chapter provides a description of the new model. In addition, these parameters represent the constitutive ideas, symbolic meanings, and values of adherents to the model.

Thus the new holistic model has been described by focusing on the core parameters which comprise the holistic health model: holism; the focus on health promotion; the meanings attached to illness; individual responsibility for health, illness, and healing; the practitioner's role as health educator, consultant, and wellness facilitator; cultural diversity in healing practices; and an alternative world view or consciousness.

Before focusing down to the specific consequences of implementing this model, the holistic movement will be examined in relation to its social and historical context. Chapter III will locate holistic health in relation to major cultural and historical trends, as well as more clearly highlighting its areas of overlap with and divergence from the more traditional allopathic medical model.

3

The Larger Context

This chapter locates the holistic health model within its broader social context, relating it both to the major critiques of the present health care system and to the broader social movement from which it derives its constituency. The development and growing appeal of the new model can only be understood within this sociological framework. Initially the chapter focuses on the component features of this health care crisis which compellingly suggest the need for major restructuring of the system. Next, it examines the historical roots of the holistic health movement, considering both the societal changes which occurred during the sixties and the larger Romantic, humanistic tradition. Third, it briefly documents the relationship of the holistic health model to the allopathic, public health, nursing, and psychological models of health and disease.

The Health Care Crisis and Consumerism

Health policy experts comprising the entire political spectrum have joined forces in their critique of the inadequacies of the present system. Paul Starr describes this health care crisis as existing since 1965, adding that both conservative and radical critics have come to see medicine as contributing less to health than either environment or lifestyle (Starr, 1970:175–179). And James S. Gordon, M.D. writes that the paradigm of holistic medicine has evolved "in tandem" with the critique of modern biomedicine (Gordon, 1981:116). Widespread perceptions of prohibitive costs, diminished effectiveness, and dehumanization, as well as the growth of the consumer movement, appear to be contributing to this crisis view. Each of these subsidiary components of the health care crisis will be briefly described in this section.

Accelerating Costs and Limited Resources

Accelerating costs and a diminished cost/benefit ratio comprise one of the major criticisms of the present health care delivery system. During the 1960s health policy was oriented towards extending the provision of medical care. Starr describes the dramatic shift in emphasis by the mid-1970s from the improvement of medical care towards efforts to save money (Starr, 1970:190). By that period in the mid-1970s, a broad consensus among health policy experts called for massive interventions to cut expenditures (Ardell, 1976; Carlson, 1975; Crawford, 1981; Fink, 1976; Knowles, 1977; Lee, 1976). Predicted increases in mandatory resource allocation and rationing decisions are extensive (Evans, 1983a, 1983b). Carlson presents the typical argument: "the 'limits' of medical care are being reached in the United States. . . . The sustained growth and development of a 'services' approach to health throughout the world will bankrupt treasuries everywhere" (Carlson, 1975:61).

John H. Knowles, past-president of the AMA, echoes these concerns in a frequently quoted 1977 editorial in *Science*: "The individual must realize that perpetuating the present system of high cost, after-the-fact medicine will only result in higher costs and greater frustration. . . . Meanwhile, the people have been led to believe that national health insurance, more doctors, and greater use of highcost, hospital-based technologies will improve health. Unfortunately none of them will" (Knowles, 1977a:1103).

Many other physicians publicly acknowledge the pressure that is being applied to shift towards a more holistic and preventive model on the basis of cost containment (Lee, 1976; Masi, 1978; Todd, 1977). For instance, Masi writes, "Understandably, the government and other institutions are advocating Health Maintainance Organizations (HMO's) and other cost incentive plans for health maintenance, early diagnosis and ambulatory care as alternatives to previous emphasis on more expensive hospitalization" (Masi, 1978:565–566).

The *structure of health insurance*, as it relates to economic factors, is also under attack. Increasingly, health planners such as Philip Lee and Donald Fink emphasize the ways in which what we call "health insurance" is actually a set of benefits concerned strictly with illness episodes (Fink, 1976:27; Lee, 1976:1). The insurance structure contains incentives built around illness for both providers and clients. As Ng, Davis, and Mandersheid write:

the health care system provides economic incentives for sickness rather than health, in that people receive financial rewards from most health care plans only when they are ill. Physicians are paid only for treating illnesses, and there is no incentive to focus on methods for promoting health. . . . Such practices not only fail to reward those who are healthy or who make an effort to stay healthy, but also implicitly penalize them (Ng et al., 1978:448).

Jeff Kane, M.D. echoes these concerns from the perspective of a holistic physician, noting that the medical insurance system essentially provides a de facto penalty for those actively working to maintain their health (Kane, 1979:146).

These issues around accelerating costs and limited resources are usually seen as the most overriding force promoting change in the health care system. Most health policy experts point to these limits as increasingly forcing a national policy shift towards health prevention (Boulding, 1966:219; Lee, 1976:5; Ng et al., 1978). For instance, Philip Lee, after describing the major obstacles of shifting from the present health care strategy to health promoting strategies in health planning, concludes, "Despite the obstacles, the growing constraints on the resources that can be devoted to health care will act as a counterforce and move us toward a strategy based on health maintenance and health promotion" (Lee, 1976:5). Similarly, George Yahn, M.D.,Ph.D. describes the growing impact of holistic medicine and holistic health concepts in an editorial in the *Journal of the American Medical Association*, adding that governmental agencies are impressed with the low-cost results of such medical groups (Yahn, 1979:2202).

Perceptions of Diminished Effectiveness

Perceptions of diminished effectiveness of medical care is a second major component of the present health care crisis. Beginning in the early 1960s, a variety of commentators began to claim that allopathic forms of treatment had been far less effective in combatting morbidity and mortality than was formerly believed (Ehrenreich, 1978:10; Gordon, 1980a:6). Until that time, there had been a fairly unambiguous consensus among health policy experts, health professionals, and the public that advances in allopathic medicine were responsible for the gradual improvement in the general level of health within the population. Kenneth

Boulding, an economist in the center of the political continuum, summarizes the prevalent view of this problem of the effectiveness of medical activity and research:

> Probably only in the last hundred years has the medical profession done more good than harm in promoting health. Now, although the direction of the effect is not in doubt, a certain amount of doubt remains about its magnitude. Certainly the most spectacular productivity of human activity in the production of health is only indirectly related to the medical profession as such (Boulding, 1966:218–219).

Just as economic restraints buttressed support for preventive approaches, the entire range of health policy planners focus on the need to shift towards more preventive directions in relation to the diminished effectiveness of medical care (Fink, 1976; Lee, 1976; Ng et al., 1981). For example, Philip Lee emphasizes that lifestyle and environmental factors remain the most important factors in contributing to further decline in mortality rates (Lee, 1976:3). Similarly, Aaron Wildavsky argues:

> According to the Great Equation, Medical Care equals Health. But the Great Equation is wrong. More available medical care does not equal better health. The best estimates are that the medical system (doctors, drugs, hospitals) affects about ten per cent of the usual indices for measuring health: whether you live at all (infant mortality), how well you live (days lost due to sickness), how long you live (adult mortality). The remaining 90 per cent are determined by factors over which doctors have little or no control, from individual lifestyle (smoking, exercise, worry), to social conditions (income, eating habits, physiological inheritance), to the physical environment (air and water quality). Most of the bad things that happen to people are at present beyond the reach of medicine (Wildavsky, 1977:105).

Prominent physicians add their critiques of the effectiveness of the present system to the health policy experts (Duval, 1977; Fink, 1976; Knowles, 1977; Masi, 1978). For instance, Louis Gluck, M.D., a Professor of Pediatrics at the University of California, San Diego School of Medicine, issued a statement of support for holistic health in *Holistic Health Focus*. Listing the reasons behind his contention that we need an alternative to modern medical practice, he asserts, "There is no question that our modern practice of medicine fails to give more than temporary relief of symptoms in perhaps 80 to 85 percent of diseases" (Gluck, 1978:2).[1]

The radical critics, such as Ivan Illich, Rick Carlson, and John and Barbara Ehrenreich, raise even stronger protests against the results of medical care (Carlson, 1975; Ehrenreich, 1978; Illich, 1976). Illich takes these arguments to the most extreme position in his book *Medical Nemesis*. In dramatizing the iatrogenic effects of medical care, he writes:

> The medical establishment has become a major threat to health. The disabling impact of professional control over medicine has reached the proportions of an epidemic (Illich, 1976:xii). Unfortunately, futile but otherwise harmless medical care is the least important of the damages a proliferating medical enterprise inflicts on contemporary society. The pain, dysfunction, disability, and anguish resulting from technical medical intervention now rival the morbidity due to traffic and industrial accidents and even war-related activities and make the impact of medicine one of the most rapidly spreading epidemics of our time (ibid:17).

Ehrenreich differentiates between the more traditional radical critique of medical care and the more recent "cultural critique." He describes the traditional radical critique, which is strongly based in Marxian theory, as seeing the private ownership and control of medical and paramedical institutions as the root of the problem. The goal was seen as changing the inequitable distribution of health services deriving from a capitalist system. The cultural critique, instead of attacking the inequitable distribution of a desired service, devalues the services itself. The implications of the new approach challenge any efforts to expand access to something considered worthless (Ehrenreich, 1978:1 6).[2]

These arguments derive most recently from the environmental or ecological perspective proposed by Rene Dubos in *Mirage of Health* in 1959.[3] Medical technology had been credited with major gains in reducing both mortality and morbidity from infectious disease. Dubos first developed the argument that the dramatic drop in incidence of contagious diseases was a direct result, not of improved medical intervention, but of changes in sanitary and hygienic conditions (he details the cases of tuberculosis and polio among his examples)(Dubos, 1959:144–182). Thomas McKeown also concludes that the major influences on level of health in a population are nutrition, environment, and lifestyle behavior, all outside the medical system (McKeown, 1976; 1978).[4]

The recognition of the influence of environmental and lifestyle factors on health status was still further supported by the LaLonde document, "A New Perspective on the Health of Canadians." Although the Canadian national medicare program made health services available to all Canadians, follow-up research demonstrated that it had very little impact on Canadian morbidity and mortality rates. Analysis showed that environmental and lifestyle factors made the greatest contribution to morbidity and mortality reduction (Gordon, 1981; Ng et al., 1981:47).

Paul Starr grounds the critique of the effectiveness of medical care in a broader historical perspective. Like Ehrenreich, he writes that the main issue for liberals during this century was that of equal access to medical services. The effectiveness of medicine was not questioned until the past few years:

> However, in the past few years, almost all the questions about medicine that had been closed since the nineteenth century have been reopened. . . . there is, once more, widespread questioning of the ultimate value and effectiveness of medicine. . . . In the nineteenth century, some leading scientists held that virtually all existing drugs and treatments were of no use, and that the sick had no other hope than the healing power of nature. This doctrine was known as therapeutic nihilism. Today disbelief has returned in a new form: now the net effectiveness of the medical system as a whole, rather than particular treatments, is called into question. The most serious critics of the system now doubt that it does much good for our health (Starr, 1981:435).

This raises an important epistemological question. Many experts and lay people are defining the problem as "decreased effectiveness" of medical care. The research does not actually support that contention.[5] Instead, there have been *major changes in the beliefs and perceptions of the effectiveness of allopathic medicine*, and this shift of perceptions has led to other major changes now affecting the health care system. Empirical data only indicate that medical care accounts for less improvement in the health level of a population than was formerly believed. The beliefs have changed; however, the level of medical effectiveness has remained relatively stable. Still, the consequences of these changed perceptions remain almost as tangible as if the level of effectiveness had in fact decreased.

Two arguments postulate an actual decrease in the level of effectiveness of medical intervention. First, medical care within a biomedical framework appears to be less effective with chronic and disabling than acute conditions. With the proportional increase in chronic conditions within the population, the net effect may be lessened effectiveness.[6] Second, the more radical critics argue that the iatrogenic side effects of an increasingly technological and specialized medicine have come to outweigh the original benefits.

Although it is difficult to ascertain how much of this shift is due to alterations of perceptions and beliefs, and how much is due to an actual decrease in the net level of effectiveness of medical intervention, the ultimate result remains clear. This increasingly widespread belief that the effectiveness of technological medical care is limited, and that future health improvements will come from environmental and lifestyle changes, has now spread beyond these policy experts and health providers to major segments of the public.

For instance, David Hayes-Bautista writes that at both ends of the socioeconomic scale, many people are now rejecting the medical model (he distinguishes this type of marginality from physical marginality, where barriers such as income keep patients from regular use of the medical system). Hayes-Bautista sees this phenomenon as especially prevalent among college age and highly educated people who become marginal to the mainstream health care delivery system by choice. This group believes that many aspects of personal health cannot be achieved through medical care (Hayes-Bautista, 1977: 36–39).

In response to the accumulating evidence of spiraling costs and the perceptions of diminished effectiveness of medical care, health policy experts appear almost united in advocating a preventive and health promotional focus (disagreements do exist in the ways they view the state, medicine, or the individual as implementing those preventive measures). There appears to be widespread agreement that new technological advancements will only exacerbate the problems. Instead, lifestyle changes have come to be seen as the most productive approach to change the national level of health (Kasl, 1986; Taylor, 1982). The 1980 document, *Promoting Health, Preventing Disease: Objectives For The Nation*, prepared by the Department of Health and Human Services, speaks symbolically to this national commitment (Kasl, 1986: 359).

Dehumanization and Fragmentation of Care

Beyond prohibitive cost and diminished effectiveness, a third major component of the current health care crisis can be termed "dehumanization." The single, most overriding conflict inherent in proposed directions of change within the health care system is the polarization between humanistic and technological advances. This tension pervades all attempts to improve care. Pelletier discusses the "resurgence of humanistic concerns in the midst of the proliferation of industrial and biomedical technology. Advances in the material sciences and technology have failed to bring the panacea they promised. At hand now is the task of integrating technological sophistication with humanistic values and an improved quality of life" (Pelletier, 1977:302). A diversity of interests echo this concern with medical care as reductionist, specialized, fragmented, and professionalized.

One component of this dehumanization appears to be the increasingly *bureaucratized nature of the delivery of health services*. Freidson views professional authority as presenting more similarities to bureaucratic authority than is generally recognized. He argues that the outcome of medicine's use of such authority is similar to the problems of bureaucracy (Freidson, 1970:209). Furthermore, medical care occurring in hospital, clinic, and alternate institutional settings is provided within a bureaucratic structure. The increasing bureaucratization of the larger society is paralleled in the medical system. Weber's theory of a cyclical balance between institutionalization and charisma can be seen as applicable here. The resurgence of humanistic concerns and the holistic health movement can be viewed against the backdrop of bureaucratized expediency and depersonalization.

Thus, Gartner and Riessman argue that the self-help approach is gaining influence because of what they describe as a strong anti-bureaucratic, anti-Leviathan, populist trend in our society. They see the small self-help group orientation as operating as a countervailing force, which reduces alienation (Gartner and Riessman, 1979:7).

Specialization and fragmentation of care is a second area closely related to these concerns. Carlson discusses this problem:

> Historically physicians functioned not only as healers, but also as counselors, confidants, and friends, roles that display the anthropological side of medicine. But with the advent of new and more sophisticated medical hardware, and the specialization that characterizes today's medicine, the technical aspects of the physician's practice are emphasized. . . . specialization and assembly-line processing of patients has become inevitable. The patient can no longer be treated as a whole person because few physicians are equipped to do so (Carlson, 1975:35).

And Masi writes, "The unprecedented expansion of medical knowledge, especially in the past quarter century, has led to specialization, which combined with social changes, have attenuated the cherished and therapeutic patient-family-physician relationship" (Masi, 1978:564).[7] Taylor concludes that the most consistent theme in consumer dissatisfaction with medicine is dissatisfaction with the current physician-patient relationship (Taylor, 1984:204).

A third area contributing to dehumanization is *perceptions of medicalization* of increasing areas of modern life. The arguments of Illich, Zola, John and Barbara Ehrenreich, and Carlson merge with those of the radical psychiatrists such as Laing and Szasz, as they view medicine as slowly appropriating areas of individual responsibility (Carlson, 1975; Conrad and Schneider, 1980; Ehrenreich, 1978; Illich, 1976; Zola, 1978). Ehrenreich and Ehrenreich describe the process by which the medical system replaces lay sources of help with professional dependency (Ehrenreich and Ehrenreich, 1978:54). Increasingly birth, death, aging, parenting, and sex are defined and managed by medicine. As Zola writes:

> medicine is becoming a major institution of social control, nudging aside, if not incorporating, the more traditional institutions of religion and law. . . . Moreover, this is not occurring through the political power physicians hold or can influence, but is largely an insidious and often undramatic phenomenon accomplished by "medicalizing" much of daily living, by making medicine and the labels "healthy" and "ill" relevant to an ever increasing part of human existence (Zola, 1978:80).

As in the discussion on efficacy of allopathic medical treatment, this section deals with widespread *perceptions* within the society. An argument can easily be made for the humanizing consequences of medicalization; however, the constituency of the holistic model strongly equate medicalization with dehumanization.

This component of dehumanization, including the diverse effects of bureaucratization, specialization, and medicalization, remains a major focus of diverse critics of the health care system. It may constitute the major impetus for change of proponents of the holistic health movement. The growing concern around this issue, beyond the holistic advocates, is reflected in works such as the interdisciplinary attempt to define the parameters of the problem contained in the volume *Humanizing Health Care*, edited by Howard and Strauss (Howard and Strauss, 1975). Howard's attempt to operationalize the ingredients of humanized health care highlights many of the dominant concerns of the holistic health movement as well. For example, she lists inherent worth, irreplaceability (uniqueness of the individual), holistic selves, symmetry in professional-patient interactions, freedom of action, status equality, and empathy (Howard, 1975:72–87).

Public Dissatisfaction with Medicine

A fourth major component of the health care crisis relates to public dissatisfaction with medicine. This growing distrust of the profession of medicine and personal dissatisfaction with physicians extends to all the areas previously discussed: the rising costs, the perceptions of decreased effectiveness, and dehumanization and fragmentation of care. Ng et al. point out the irony of this phenomena:

> The biomedical model of disease and its treatment has been successful beyond all expectations, but at a cost. It is an irony of history that at the very time that we are witnessing major strides in molecular biology and genetic research, we are simultaneously experiencing a crisis of confidence in the ability of medical science to improve the health status of our post-industrialized society (Ng et al., 1982:45).

Yet there are numerous indications that this public dissatisfaction exists, and that it often results in an adversarial relationship between physician and patient. Perhaps the most visible symptom is the massive increase in malpractice litigation during the last decade. Another tangible sign is the movement towards requiring various forms of institutional or governmental review over medical work (Freidson, 1986:67).

Betz and O'Connell trace the dissatisfaction, along with the decline in public respect, as increasing since 1950 (Betz and O'Connell, 1983: 85). Mechanic asserts that two-thirds of Americans are losing their faith in physicians in general, although he argues that most people have more faith and trust in their personal physicians. He concludes that this erosion of physicians' public image is likely to accelerate in the future (Mechanic, 1985:181–182).[8]

This growing public attitude can be partially related to the tremendous increase in expectations for medicine (Ehrenreich and Ehrenreich, 1978:53; Thomas, 1979:103). The public has come to feel that medicine should be able to "cure" any problem. When these expectations are not met, people respond with what Starr describes as "free floating public hostility towards medicine" (Starr, 1970:178). Starr relates this loss of confidence in medicine, along with a "new agnosticism" towards physicians, as part of a cyclical pattern of influence exerted by allopathic medicine (ibid:175).

Growth of Consumerism

A closely related factor contributing to the health care crisis is the growth of consumerism, along with the emergence of the self-care movement. Reeder links the public dissatisfaction with medicine with the growth of consumerism as a broad social movement. He elaborates:

> During the decade of the sixties a new concept came into prominence in the delivery of health services in this country. This was the concept of the person as a consumer rather than a patient. . . . Indeed, it is now generally recognized that we are in the early stages of the "age of the consumer" (Reeder, 1978:113).

Schwartz and Kart relate this growing consumerism to a demand for accountability and a growing public suspicion that, "neither the expertise nor the goodwill of the professional are to be taken on trust, at face value" (Schwartz and Kart, 1978:108). Closely related is Helena Lopata's description of the revolt of the client against expertization, as a more general societal phenomenon as well as a shift within the medical arena (Lopata, 1979).

Haug et al. have documented the rise in the consumerist perspective as it relates specifically to health care. Their research demonstrated that, at least in attitudinal terms, a substantial portion of both the public and physicians currently take a consumerist perspective (both groups gave self-reports of behavior not always matching those demands, however). The findings also pointed to a group of younger, more knowledgeable lay people who were convinced of their right to control health care decisions (Haug et al., 1981:213–222). Additional empirical support for this view of a growing consumerist perspective emerges from Freidson's data on physicians' negative reaction to the new "demanding patient" who claims services on the basis of contractual rights (Freidson, 1973). Freidson believes that the growing group of college-educated middle income professionals pose the major problems to physicians. Not only are they knowledgeable on medical matters, but this group understands their contractual rights and pursues them through appropriate bureaucratic channels (Freidson, 1982:74–75).[9]

Both the public dissatisfaction with medicine and this new consumerism are also supported by Kotarba's study of patients undergoing treatment by acupuncturists. He found the patients perceived themselves as having a physical problem which medicine could not alleviate "to their satisfaction" (Kotarba, 1975:154). He summarizes his findings:

> Patients with chronic pain problems seek acupuncture to relieve them either from pain or from dependency on analgesic drugs. They do not undergo acupuncture because they are ignorant of contemporary "scientific" medicine or because they have not been properly socialized in the culturally accepted meanings of suffering and health care. All have previously sought help from accepted or normal medicine; they were not satisfied with the result (ibid:173).

The participants in the holistic health movement definitely reflect this dissatisfaction with the allopathic medical model and with physicians as a group. For example, Goldstein et al. found that their sample of physicians with membership in the American Holistic Medical Association, while extremely diverse on many dimensions, consistently expressed dissatisfaction or disillusionment with allopathic medicine (Goldstein et al., 1985). While the specific nature of this dissatisfaction varied, they write, "Many emphasized that doctor-patient relationships in mainstream medicine were too narrow and artificial to be either effective or personally satisfying" (ibid:325).

Most patients I observed in the primary ethnographic setting spontaneously spoke in characteristic, almost ritualized ways about traditional medicine. All had previously gone through the traditional medical system, and they were now highly critical of both the medical profession and its assumptions. Two of the most frequent comments were that "physicians only treat symptoms, not causes" and that physicians "think they're God."

Similarly, a great deal of anti-medical sentiment was expressed at the various holistic health conferences. At three Mandala/Association for Holistic Health conferences I attended, there was frequent and consistent cheering after comments presenters made, charging that "medicine only treats symptoms" or that we needed a new medical model. For instance, at the eighth annual Mandala Conference, Lawrence Weed, M.D. spoke on the status of the computer for optimizing health. He told a joke about

South Dakota having the highest life expectancy and the lowest per capita physicians. Almost everyone cheered, laughed, and clapped. Similar strong anti-medical expressions continued throughout the conference, despite the fact that most of the speakers were physicians who often advocated an alliance between traditional and holistic approaches. Samuel S. Epstein, M.D. spoke on an ecological perspective in medicine. When he mentioned that the health care system had very strong linkages to the pharmaceutical industry, the audience spontaneously broke out into loud applause. Another outburst of applause interrupted him when he continued by saying, "We're talking not about the medical profession, but the medical *industry*." [10]

The *shift towards self-care and advocacy* is closely related to the growth of holistic approaches, and there is much overlap between both the practitioners and adherents/clients of the two movements. Masi indicates that patients are becoming more interested in self-care, and cites over 500 different health and self-care books published between 1973 and 1975 alone (Masi, 1978:565). [11] Similarly, by 1979, Andrews and Levin estimated that over 500,000 mutual aid groups existed in relation to health and medicine (Andrews and Levin, 1979:45). Ferguson reminds us that most health care is, and has always been, self-care. Along with other commentators, he sees a great deal of overlap between self-care and holistic health, and argues that both represent a move away from excessive dependence on experts in health care (Ferguson, 1980:87–89; Gartner and Riessman, 1979; Guttmacher, 1979; Mattson, 1982).

Alliance Between Economic and Humanistic Interests

Basically, holistic health interests are promoted by an alliance of those representing economic and humanistic concerns. The pressures from the dual sources sometimes unite to advocate holistic approaches; however, since there are many points of divergence between the two kinds of pressures, it remains to be seen whether that alliance can be maintained. Advocates argue that a shift in the direction of self-care will result in both increased quality of care and economic savings. Again, can this coalition last, or will the economic and humanistic bases diverge or come into direct conflict?

In response to a combination of all these critiques, the health care system as a whole has been shifting towards a renewed emphasis on prevention and chronic disease. Thus the combination of all these contextual changes in the health care system, and in the larger societal arena, supports the emergence of a new model of health and disease. These factors of prohibitive costs, diminished effectiveness, dehumanization, fragmentation of care, and the public dissatisfaction with medicine have combined to set the stage for receptivity to a more holistic, participatory model of health care.

Historical Roots in the Sixties

While the holistic health movement developed in reaction to the crisis in the health care delivery system, it did not evolve in isolation. The movement can be viewed as an extension of the larger social movement originating in the sixties. This section will examine how it relates to other such cultural phenomena.

Ehrenreich suggests that the receptivity to more holistic and multiple-causal models of disease, as proposed by Dubos, Selye, and others, derives from the movements of the sixties: the black movement, the environmental movement, and the counterculture (Ehrenreich, 1978:13). And Bloom and Wilson locate related changes, "in a period when, in the United States, all the most basic values of the society were being challenged. Racial discrimination, poverty, and war catalyzed a collective consciousness that shook the foundations of all the nation's basic institutions, and health services were not spared" (Bloom and Wilson, 1979:288). Ferguson similarly describes the self-care movement as an extension of a broad contemporary change of consciousness; he also links its roots to the sixties counterculture, the ecology movement, and the consumer movement (Ferguson, 1980:87–88).

James Gordon, Rick Carlson, Phyllis Mattson, and David Hayes-Bautista also link the holistic health model directly to the sixties movements (Carlson, 1980:487–488; Gordon, 1980b:467–470; Hayes-Bautista, 1977:38; Mattson, 1982:56–70). As Gordon writes:

> The founders of the first alternative (health) services (in the late 1960s) resembled the earlier settlement-house workers in their idealism and humanitarianism. They differed in their commitment to the kind of participatory democracy that animated the civil rights, antiwar, youth, and women's movements of the 1960s. . . . These activist workers . . . questioned the appropriateness of professional services that labeled or stigmatized those who came for help, and in their own work they blurred or obliterated boundaries between staff and clients. . . . Determined to remain responsive to their clients' needs, these early

workers continually advocated the social changes that would make individual change more possible (Gordon, 1980b:468).

Mattson's book has a lengthy section which relates the holistic health movement to the sixties (Mattson, 1982:56). And Paul Starr extends the derivation to the mounting criticism of psychiatry which began in the late 1960s, citing the works of Thomas Szasz, R. D. Laing, and Erving Goffman, as well as the play *Equus* and Kesey's book *One Flew Over the Cuckoo's Nest* (Starr, 1981:436).

Despite divergent interpretations of the causes and specific aims of this broader movement, several recurrent themes dominate the literature. All of these carry over into the core assumptions of the holistic health movement, so that counter-culture ideology, meanings, and values exert a pervasive influence throughout it. Two major themes cut across core meanings. The first is a restorationist motif, a rejection of the highly bureaucratized, mass technocracy. The second is that of romanticism, idealism, and anti-materialism. Each of the component meanings/symbols described earlier can be traced to the sixties movements.

Coalition of Sixties Movements

This larger social movement, sometimes referred to as "secular humanism," represents a coalition of highly diverse groups. Ehrenreich views the "cultural critique" of modern medicine (his description of this phenomenon broadly overlaps with the parameters of the holistic health movement) as a synthesis of the separate lines of criticism of medical care developed by feminists, militant black community groups, radical psychotherapists, and health policy analysts (Ehrenreich, 1978:4). I found many people formerly involved in these movements participating in the holistic health movement; however, there were few from militant black groups.

The *feminist movement*, which began late in the sixties, had a powerful impact on the development of the larger movement. The women's movement both publicized the ways in which the physician-patient relationship reinforced male domination and began to question the actual technical competency and efficacy of doctors. Feminism also contributed to public awareness of iatrogenesis. Initially the feminist movement exposed the dangers of the oral contraceptives in the late sixties. Simultaneously women began to learn about their bodies as an attempt to gain control of medical technology (Ehrenreich, 1978:9–14). One of the primary aims of the feminist health movement was the demystification of medical knowledge. Another central aim was to transform the ideas behind routine obstetrical and gynecological care from a medical model based on acute illness to a natural, developmental view (Ruzek, 1981: 563). Gordon describes the women's health movement as providing both a catalyst and a model for the broader base of health care consumers to emulate (Gordon, 1980:13).

The *human potential movement* also held a central place in this informal coalition. Considerable overlap exists between both the philosophies and techniques ultilized by the self-actualization and holistic health movements. The stance of holistic health practitioners often is closely allied to a permissive psychotherapeutic approach, such as that advocated by Carl Rogers. Abraham Maslow's ideas, beginning in the 1950s, popularized the idea of self-actualization. Deliman and Smolowe see this approach as promoting the concept of personal responsibility (Deliman and Smolowe, 1982:7). Many activists of the anti-Vietnam war movement participated in this movement during the seventies (Jerry Rubin was one of the most visible).

The most visible psychological emphases in the holistic health movement are Gestalt, humanistic psychology, and transpersonal psychology. Gestalt psychology developed in reaction to atomistic approaches in psychological theory. Clark describes the field of Transpersonal psychology, which incorporates spiritual dimensions and is strongly based in an Eastern perspective: "Transpersonal psychology aims at synthesizing Eastern wisdom and Western science, and is exploring new ways of transforming consciousness of both self and society" (Clark, 1978:276).

Gordon specifically traces the emphasis on sensuousness and sexuality within holistic health to its links with the human potential movement:

> Modern holistic practitioners have been heavily influenced by Reich's work and its adumbration of the "human potential movement" of the 1960s and 1970s and have incorporated its insights and techniques into their clinical practice. . . . All tend to be more concerned with the quality of their patients' sexuality and their capacity for sensuousness (Gordon, 1980:21).

Two specific movements centrally concerned with demedicalization activities also participate in this coalition. Both death and birth are more commonly occurring at home, avoiding institutionalized medical control. The *death with dignity* movement's development closely parallels that of holistic health. Often practitioners move between the two spheres of work. Also practitioners seem to share the intense, almost religious dedication underlying involvement in these two movements. Similarly, *natural birthing* and approaches such as the Leboyer method are becoming more common, along with such practices as prolonged nursing of infants, home delivery, and extensive family involvement in the birthing process. The ideology of both these movements resonates strongly with that of holistic health.

Historical Antecedents

This brief sketch of several of the groups comprising the coalition of the larger social movement should give the reader a sense of the overlap of meanings and cultural commonalities. In addition, the sixties movements must be located within a boader historical context that includes the bohemian movement, nineteenth-century utopian outlooks, and the Romantic tradition. Bennett Berger, for instance, views the hippies as only the most recent expression of the older tradition of bohemianism, starting in the mid-nineteenth century. He traces key elements of bohemian doctrine to the hippie movement of the 1960s: the idea of salvation by the child, the idea of self expression, the idea of paganism, and the idea of living for the moment (Berger, 1967: 19).

Martin Schiff, on the other hand, locates the derivation of the sixties movement in the nineteenth-century utopian outlooks, especially the New England transcendentalist movement which emerged in the 1840s. In his article, "Neo-Transcendentalism in the New Left Counter-Culture: A Vision of the Future Looking Back," he writes of the shared repugnance for the scientific technology of industrial society and the disdain for materialism (Schiff, 1973: 139–140). Ralph Waldo Emerson's essay, "The Transcendentalist," describes the fundamental concept of idealism underlying his movement, emphasizing both its anti-materialist nature and its founding on consciousness (Emerson, 1949: 18). A closely related and even more direct precursor was the popular health movement of the nineteenth century (Berliner and Salmon, 1979: 32; Weil, 1983: 181).

Gusfield and Starr ground the movements of the sixties in the broadest historical perspective, that of Romanticism (Gusfield, 1975; Starr, 1979). Gusfield traces the concept of community that underlies Romanticism to the critical opposition to nineteenth-century industrialization in Europe, the United States, and Japan (Gusfield, 1975: 100). He continues by describing the diverse forms of this Romantic sensibility. Throughout his description, ideals found both in sixties movements and within the holistic health movement are apparent: "What gives unity to such seemingly diverse activities is the extolling of sentiment and feeling as superior to but corrupted by reason, science and technical organization. In this use of 'community' there is a tendency to find in the simple, traditional folk-like society the elements of moral virtues which contrast with modern life. . . . the Romantic movement has many of the aspects of an aristocratic critique of modern life" (ibid.:100). Starr echoes these links of the counter-culture to romanticism, stressing the two primary ideals of equality and community (Starr, 1979:251–252).

Closely related to the Romantic critique of industrial and post-industrial society is the influence of the philosophical schools of phenomenology and existentialism, as they have increasingly influenced Western culture beginning in the 1930s. Deliman and Smolowe describe Martin Heidegger's influence in promoting the idea of "being-in-the-world," and its accompanying shift towards a holistic view and a rejection of the prevailing Western dualism. They also discuss Jean Paul Sartre's influence on the holistic model's emphasis on personal responsibility (Deliman and Smolowe, 1982:7).

The concept of *secular humanism* represents this more general movement between the levels of abstraction of the specific movements and the broad historical tradition of Romanticism. Herman Kahn initially coined that term to encompass the cultural changes occurring at a level above the more specific countercultural movement, yet below the level of generality of the broad historical movement of Romanticism. He views secular humanism as a longer cultural tradition that waxes and wanes (Kahn, 1967).

Strands of Continuity

This portion of the chapter will focus on demonstrating strands of continuity linking the core meanings of the sixties movements with the holistic health movement of the seventies and eighties. In other words, changes in the health care system and the holistic health movement can be viewed as crystallizations of core aspects of the movements of the sixties.[12]

While the global statements of linkages between the sixties and holistic health movements comprise a tempting argument, more careful documentation is required to substantiate such claims. This section will briefly illustrate more specific strands of continuity linking the sixties movements, such as the counter-culture, hippie, feminist, civil rights, and antiwar movements, directly to holistic health. Three specific areas will be examined for strands of continuity between the holistic health movement and the movements of the sixties: continuity of political action forms, continuity of personnel, and continuity of meanings.

Continuity of Political Action Forms

Initially it appears that very little continuity exists in the forms of political action utilized by the movements of the sixties and the holistic health movement. The major emphasis in studies of the sixties movements was on protest and confrontation in an active political sense. Violence as a tactic in several of the movements was relatively commonplace.

In contrast, the holistic health movement at first appears more passive than the student or civil rights movements. The choice of tactics rejects those aimed at confrontation with political institutions for those oriented more toward the individual and aimed at cultural change. The focus of change is the individual participant; underlying this approach is the assumption that people create change through their own actions. In this sense, the holistic health movement illustrates what Gusfield terms the "privatization of social movements." He writes of the "growing concern of populations with the transformation of the self in human encounters, in religious experience and in the styles of work and leisure. Although the public arena serves to dramatize and communicate such movements, they represent a turning away from the importance of the public as the focal point of change" (Gusfield, 1978:29–30).

In this context, the choice of action form is closer to that used by the hippie movement and many of the 1960s communards. The hippies did not advocate violence; yet, they used many collective tactics which emphasized community (examples include "be-ins" and "love-ins"). Although the rhetoric of holistic health around individual responsibility makes the movement initially appear extremely individualistic, values of communal sharing and social responsibility are simultaneously in the forefront. Many of the conferences function in ways reminiscent of occasions such as Woodstock. This more passive, less confrontational approach is more inner directed and again involves elements of "transcendentalism." Paradoxically, this approach is opposed to aspects inherent in the holistic health movement which stress existentialist control over one's life.

Case and Taylor discuss this political action form within the counterculture. They argue against the prevailing view that the seventies was an era of apathy and collective narcissism, demonstrating how that decade involved attempts to create change through "counterinstitutions." They see those alternative organizations as differentiating the new left from earlier radicals in America. Both shared goals, such as reducing social inequities; however, what differentiated the new left was their belief that "the personal is political." Thus counter-culture efforts were often directed at changing everyday life and work in the New Left (Case and Taylor, 1979:4–5). Taylor sees egalitarianism and participatory democracy, along with community, as the central ideals guiding such attempts (Taylor, 1979).[13]

Starr describes the goals of these "counterinstitutions":

> It was a romantic ideal of the organization as a community, in which social relations were to be direct and personal, open and spontaneous, in contrast to the rigid, remote, and artificial relations of bureaucratic organization. The organizational community, moreover, was to be participatory and egalitarian. It would make decisions collectively and democratically and would eliminate or at least reduce hierarchy by keeping to a minimum distinctions of status and power between leaders and members, or professionals and nonprofessionals (Starr, 1979:245).

The settings I studied closely fit with Starr's description of exemplary counterinstitutions (Starr, 1979:246–247). Thus, these practitioners were trying to self-consciously change the system through change at the personal and cultural level. These people, active in the holistic health movement, believe themselves to be in that tradition, and they are attempting political change through their work in holistic health.

Ehrenreich sees these differences in tactics as being directly related to the differences between the political versus cultural nature of the changes sought. In differentiating the cultural critique from the older political economic critique, he argues:

> neither the demands growing out of the political economic critique nor the demands growing out of the cultural critique can be realized save through a mass movement. In the case of the political economic demands, this is perhaps self-evident: the vested power of the doctors, drug companies, insurance companies, etc. can only be overcome through a massive popular upsurge. [On the other hand]. .some of the demands growing out of the cultural critique—e.g., for a health system based on more self-help, for less dependency on professional care . . . etc.—do not appear to require such confrontations with eco-

nomic and political power. But they do require major changes in how people perceive themselves, their bodies, their relationships to others . . . (Ehrenreich, 1978:25).

Tipton found a similar approach to social change in his research on Zen students. He writes, "It is predicated on the monistic assumption that the society is one interdependent whole and that social change, so far as it is possible, begins with self-transformation and spreads outward harmoniously" (Tipton, 1982:166). He quoted one Zen student as explaining, "Instead of fighting to change society, like the radicals, we're trying to create society" (ibid:174). Tipton ultimately concludes that the Zen students he studied had a definite political vision of radically transforming society (ibid:243–244). Bellah also argues that sympathizers of the Oriental religions tend to be as critical of American society as politically oriented radicals (Bellah, 1976:343).

One can almost describe two levels of involvement in the holistic health movement. Those who actively participate in the movement have strong communal commitments at many levels, and these comprise a strong political identification. Those who do not actively identify with holistic health, yet whose beliefs and everyday behaviors have been modified in that direction by the diffusion of the movement into the mainstream, have a much more highly individualistic focus which could also be defined as less political. This book will argue more fully in the final chapter that, as the holistic ideology diffuses throughout the society, it is converted through its impact with more traditional beliefs underlying the Western world view and the Protestant ethic. A more radical individualism derives from the intersection between the two world views.

Continuity of Personnel
There appears to be at least a fair amount of movement of health practitioners between the holistic health movement, the free clinic movement, the human potential movement, the death/hospice movement, and both the birthing and abortion (pro-choice) movements. All represent demedicalization activities and share many core meanings.

For example, David Harris, the founder of the Association of Holistic Health and the Mandala Society in San Diego describes himself as having been active in the human potential movement and humanistic psychology. Earlier he co-founded the National Center for the Exploration of Human Potential.

The late sixties also saw the radicalization of a group of young doctors and nurses. Ehrenreich and Hayes-Bautista et al. describe the emergence of the free clinics during this period (Ehrenreich, 1978:61; Hayes-Bautista and Harveston, 1977). These community clinics not only attempted to serve groups with limited access to medical care, but they presented a radical challenge to the existing system by providing care based on a model of participatory democracy (Taylor, 1979:41; Taylor, 1984).

Williams also described the growing number of physicians in the Bay Area who, "have become disenchanted with the study of pathology and treatment of disease and are turning their quest to the wholistic school of 'health maintenance'" (Williams, 1976:30). And Gordon writes:

> Physicians, nurses, social workers, psychologists, and lay people who appreciated the interpersonal style and democratic policies of the free clinics but questioned the effectiveness of the conventional medicine practiced there began to study other approaches to health care and other traditions of healing. By the early 1970s they were stepping gingerly beyond the free-clinic model and away from their traditional training to create the services that would soon become holistic health centers (Gordon, 1980b:469–470).

Paul Brenner, M.D. represents such a career trajectory. He recounts his odyssey of leaving private practice, after working to establish a community clinic, to concentrate on health maintenance: "The inciting motivation was the Women's Movement of the late sixties which targeted gynecologists for not being responsive to the needs of women, and more importantly for not providing their patients with medical and health information" (Brenner, 1984:178).

Most of the participants in the holistic health movement appear to have been either active in or radicalized during the sixties movements. A larger scale study of both leaders and practitioners identified with the holistic health movement is needed to more precisely determine the degree of continuity of personnel with the movements of the sixties. Although that was not the primary focus of this study, the data strongly pointed in that direction. Many providers and leaders were either sensitized or radicalized by the student counter-culture and antiwar movements in particular. Most of the most visible leaders and practitioners fall within a fairly small age range, clustered between 34 and 45 years.

Two of the physicians I formally interviewed had formerly been directors of free (community) clinics; another had been instrumental in establishing one. Two others in that age group of 38–41 had also been actively involved in the student and peace movements and spoke of transferring that vision into their view of holistic health. Two of the younger physicians (33–36 years) described somewhat later involvement in the counter-culture movements during their undergraduate work, and were heavily involved with macrobiotic diets and Eastern meditational approaches during medical school. One nurse had spent time in the Peace Corps.

The first Hospice in Northern San Diego County was started and directed by a registered nurse, who was also a Founding Member of the Association for Holistic Health (Bulen, 1979:2). Another nurse who was one of the initial founders of the San Diego Hospice, and served on its board of directors, was also very active in AHH. Similarly, two physicians who were both outspoken and prominent among the obstetricians lobbying for more natural birthing and family involvement in the birthing process, left successful private practices for active participation in the holistic health movement.

Continuity of Meanings/Symbols/Consciousness

The area of symbolic meanings and world view is the primary point of continuity between holistic health and the sixties movements. Again, it becomes difficult, not only to separate out the effects of specific movements of the sixties, but to distinguish movement-related change in a direct sense from Blumer's concept of cultural drift (Blumer, 1939: 255–278). Even when the convergence of symbols or metaphors is obvious, the interrelationships between the various movements are too complex for specificity. Despite these problems, this area appears to show the most evidence of the close linkages between the holistic health movement and the larger social movement originating in the sixties.

Both Berger and Davis anticipated the cultural influence of events they observed during the sixties. Bennett Berger supported this view in his 1967 article on hippie morality. He was already observing early signs that the bohemian morality was gradually becoming legitimated (Berger, 1967). In a companion article, Fred Davis predicted the integration of cultural aspects of the hippie movement on the greater society. As Davis argued, "Indeed, it is probably through some such muted, gradual, and indirect process of social conversion that the hippie subculture will make a lasting impact on American society, if it is to have any at all" (Davis, 1967:18).

Beyond the degree that counter-culture values have begun to permeate the larger society in the seventies and eighties, their influence on the holistic health model is central and pervasive. As mentioned earlier, the two major themes which cut across core meanings are a restorationist motif and a motif of romanticism, idealism, and antimaterialism. Theodore Roszak develops these themes in his book *The Making of a Counter-Culture*. Portraying the counter-culture as rejection of the post-industrial technocracy, he writes:

> It strikes me as obvious and beyond dispute that the interests of our college-age and adolescent young in the psychology of alienation, oriental mysticism, psychedelic drugs, and communitarian experiments comprise a cultural constellation that radically diverges from values and assumptions that have been in the mainstream of our society at least since the Scientific Revolution of the seventeenth century (Roszak, 1969:xii).

While describing the core parameters of the holistic health movement, I mentioned the different form of consciousness as the most important, although the most elusive to define. This parameter derives directly from the changed consciousness/world view underlying the counter-culture movements of the sixties. Roszak analyzes the hold of technocracy over us as "the myth of objective consciousness," stressing the critical reaction against the prevailing emphasis on objectivity, non-involvement, and expertise (ibid:208–209).

Many of these alterations in consciousness initially involved either hallucinogenic drug use or adherence to forms of eastern mysticism and religion for participants in the sixties movements. Roszak sees Alan Watts as the most influential person in translating the insights of Zen into the language of Western psychology. He elaborates, "Even if Zen has been vulgarized in the translation, it embraces a radical critique of the conventional scientific conception of man and nature" (ibid:136).

Bellah summarizes these changes that emerged during the sixties as due to a significant proportion of the educated young repudiating the tradition of utilitarian individualism (Bellah, 1976:337–338). He goes on to describe the spiritual orientation of the counterculture:

> Thus the religion of the counterculture was by and large not biblical. It drew from many sources including the American Indian. But its deepest influences came from Asia. . . . In many ways Asian spirituality provided a more thorough contrast to the rejected utilitarian individualism than did biblical

religion. To external achievement it posed inner experience; to the exploitation of nature, harmony with nature; to impersonal organization, an intense relation to a guru. Mahayana Buddhism, particularly in the form of Zen, provided that most pervasive religious influence on the counterculture; but elements from Taoism, Hinduism, and Sufism were also influential. What drug experiences, interpreted in Oriental religious terms, as Timothy Leary and Richard Alpert did quite early, and meditation experiences, often taken up when drug use was found to have too many negative consequences, showed was the illusoriness of worldly striving (Bellah, 1976:341).

In describing the emergence of the counterculture, Tipton also supports its portrayal as utopian and anti-materialistic: "It assumes that what I have called a 'true inner self' beyond modern social institutions will create and express itself through the communalistic institution of an alternative social order to come" (Tipton, 1982:23). He goes on to discuss the accepting, receptive attitude of the counterculture towards reality, and contrasts it to the Western stance of activism and achievement-orientation (ibid:23). Tipton continues with an attempt to summarize the overriding world view of counterculture participants: "These alternative attitudes may be resolved into four related pairs. (1) ecstatic experience versus technical reason; (2) holism versus analytic discrimination; (4) acceptance versus problem-solving activism; (5) intuitive certainty versus pluralistic relativism" (Tipton, 1982:21). All these attitudes are consistently and centrally reflected in the meanings and values of holistic health adherents.

The last chapter has already elaborated the basic meanings and values uniting holistic health movement participants. The descriptions of the components of adherents' world view closely parallel almost all these descriptions of the emerging world view of sixties' youth. An attempt will now be made to abstract more specific strands of meaning and locate their derivation more directly within the sixties movements. Each of the component meanings/symbols described earlier can be traced back to the sixties movements. For instance, the anti-technological, anti-scientific stance, at times anti-intellectual as well, derives from the hippie, counterculture, anti-nuclear, feminist, and environmental movements of the 1960s. The value placed on egalitarianism was a core value underlying the civil rights, hippie, counter-culture, feminist, and consumer movements. The tolerance and incorporation of a diversity of lifestyles is seen in the hippies and in the civil rights movement; it can also be related to the increased interest in native American and Eastern cultures which accompanied psychedelic drug use.[14]

Any such conceptual attempt is recognized as being highly artificial; nevertheless, it can assist in establishing the continuity of the constitutive ideas. These strands are summarized in Figure 1, with each core meaning followed by a listing of the primary movements from which it derived. (see Figure 1) Obviously, most of the core meanings emerged from the constellation of movements of the sixties; however, a few seem more specific in their derivation.

Relationship to Other Health/Illness Models

Many of the central themes of holistic health are not new within health and illness models other than the allopathic. When holistic authors write that the emphasis in health care must shift towards prevention and health promotion, or that patients must become more involved in their care, they are not raising unexamined issues. Public health, pediatrics, and nursing have been incorporating these dimensions for some time. This section will briefly examine the relationship of the holistic health model to such models of health and disease, especially those of allopathic medicine, public health, and nursing. Essentially it presents the "family tree" of the holistic model.

Allopathic Medical Model

The major areas of convergence and conflict between the holistic health and allopathic medical models have already been discussed. The holistic physician is much closer to the nostalgic image of the long term family doctor, usually a local general practitioner, who came to know a family over time. Thus the holistic physician more closely approximates a general practitioner than a technologically oriented specialist.

At the present time, the holistic physician is closest to family practice physicians and pediatricians. In both pediatrics and family medicine one sees an increased emphasis on prevention and health maintenance that closely parallels the public health model. New concepts of family practice stress similar concepts and ways of relating with patients. Jeters' article on "Family Medicine and Holistic Health" documents the wide areas of overlap in the two approaches (Jeter, 1982:73–80). For instance, Jeter describes the congruent roles:

Core meanings/symbols of the sixties movements

(1) *anti-technological/anti-scientific (at times anti-intellectual) stance*
hippie/counter-culture/anti-nuclear/feminist (side effects of pill, IUD)/environmental movement

(2) *distrust of basic institutions (medicine, government, politics, big business)*
hippie/counter-culture/antiwar/anti-nuclear/feminist/environmental/consumerism/assassination of Kennedy and King/civil rights

(3) *anti-bureaucratization*
hippie/counter-culture/antiwar

(4) *resurgence of humanistic concerns*
civil rights/antiwar/anti-nuclear/hippie/feminist/student/medical policy/human potential

(5) *egalitarianism*
civil rights/hippie/counter-culture/feminist/consumer

(6) *emphasis on cooperation, harmony, and community*
civil rights/hippie/feminist/antiwar/anti-nuclear/human potential movement

(7) *tolerance of diversity of lifestyles*
hippie/civil rights/psychedelic drugs/increased interest in native American, Eastern cultures

(8) *naturalism (desire to live closer to nature and in harmony with the environment)*
hippie (back to land and communes)/environmental

(9) *sensory experience, intuition valued above conceptual knowledge*
hippie/psychedelic drugs/human potential movement

(10) *emphasis on present time orientation*
hippie / counter-culture / psychedelic drugs / human potential movement

(11) *devaluing of detachment, objectivity, non-involvement*
student/feminist/antiwar/anti-nuclear/hippie

(12) *holism: body-mind-spirit continuity*
hippie/psychedelic drugs/Eastern religions, transcendental meditation/Kennedy, physical fitness programs in early 1960s

(13) *individual taking more control, responsibility/revolt against experts*
civil rights/sexual revolution/student/feminist/consumerism/antiwar/anti-nuclear/higher tolerance for protest and civil disobedience within the society

---

Figure 1

Getting patients and families to take charge of themselves, and
therefore their illness, and recognizing the individual's or family's role in triggering or exacerbating the condition is in consonance with family medicine's ideology and practice. . . .
Taking charge of oneself and one's problems and using the
family physician as *facilitator*, *mediator*, and *expert* in breadth
is requisite for the mental and physical health of the practitioner, patients, and families" (Jeter, 1982:79).

It is interesting, however, that an observer notes a fair amount of
mutual antagonism, especially directed from some family practitioners
towards holistically oriented physicians. Vanderpool, while arguing that
the biopsychosocial approach, along with high level health advocacy, is
part of existing family medicine programs, proceeds to critique many
aspects of holistic health, including what he sees as the diversity and
imprecision (Vanderpool, 1984:774–779). Geyman's editorial in the
same issue of *The Journal of Family Practice* emphasizes that holistic
health is neither new nor coherent (Geyman, 1984:727–728).

Similarly, pediatricians have long incorporated preventive health approaches, which focused on normal developmental processes, assessing
and treating the patient within the context of the family, and dealing with
cognitive, social, and emotional issues as well as those more physiologically based. Preventive health screening and immunizations have been
accepted parts of pediatrics for several decades. Similarly, areas such as
nutritional intake are far more likely to be addressed in pediatric contexts
than in other specialty areas.

As both policy experts and consumers demand a shift towards more
holistic and preventive directions, allopathic medicine is beginning to
incorporate holistic health approaches, and many physicians are attempting to legitimate this shift in their model. The American Holistic Medical
Association was founded in 1979, and by 1982 claimed about 500 members (Gordon, 1982:546).[15] Gordon asserts that "several dozen" medical
schools offer elective courses in holistic health (ibid.). The holistic health
movement has also established inroads in Britain (Smith, 1983; Reilly,
1983).

Holistic health concepts appear to be making significant inroads
within more traditional allopathic medical practices across a range of
specialty areas. Advocates such as Gordon, see such a synthesis of approaches as crucial to the future of the health care delivery system (Gordon, 1982). Preventive approaches and a recognition of the role stress
plays in initiating or maintaining illness are pervading even very tradi-

tional practices. Additionally, many physicians already incorporate healing modalities in their practice on an intuitive level.

Thus some leading figures in both academic medicine and the
American Medical Association have supported holistic health concepts,
as documented throughout early parts of this chapter. In the early conferences of the Association for Holistic Health/Mandala Society, David Al-
len, M.D., then Associate Dean for Continuing Education in the Health
Sciences at the University of California, San Diego School of Medicine
was involved and often moderated at the conferences. The involvement
of others such as Jonas Salk, M.D. highlighted this type of support. At
least two past presidents of the American Medical Association have been
outspoken on the need to move in more health promotional and holistic
directions (Todd, 1977; Knowles, 1977).

Increasing recognition and valuing of holistic trends is also apparent
in the traditional medical journals. For instance, Lippin wrote a letter to
the editor advocating acceptance of these trends in a 1978 issue of the
Journal of Occupational Medicine:

> We hear a great deal these days about preventive and holistic
> health models as a humanistic and economically sound direc-
> tion toward which medicine is moving. It is quite evident that
> a bio-psycho-social model of health care is likely to flour-
> ish. We in the occupational health profession should recog-
> nize and accept this exciting trend. (Richard Lippin, M.D.,
> Eastern Area Medical Director, Atlantic Richfield Co. [Lippin,
> 1978:75]).

Examples such as Yahn's article in the *Journal of the American Medical
Association* and Masi's editorial in the *Journal of Chronic Diseases* also
document this trend (Yahn, 1979; Masi, 1978). As Masi concludes in
his editorial, "An holistic concept of disease allows a broader perspective than previous models and may better accommodate or help clarify
complex interactions, as well as reveal promising directions for future
studies" (Masi, 1978:568).[16]

Other responses, however, are more cautious and ambivalent. Relman's editorial in the *New England Journal of Medicine* reflects the concerns of what Freidson would describe as professional dominance (Relman,
1979). Relman reported on the first annual session of the American Holistic Medical Association. He applauds the description of the organization as interested in, "promoting an integrated, comprehensive overview
of patients as physical, mental, emotional, and spiritual beings," describ-

ing that philosophy as a return to the traditional medical emphasis on treating the whole patient. After advocating incorporation of this focus, as well as the themes of self-care and health maintenance, he attacks a publication explaining various alternative approaches to health care (for example, Shiatsu and iridology): "This is the irrational side of the holistic movement, with its mystical cults and all the paraphernalia of sectarianism. . . . But one searches in vain for any recognition of the danger to the public posed by (such) practitioners . . ." (Relman, 1979:313).[17]

A number of less ambivalent and more scathing attacks have been levied on holistic health by the allopathic medical establishment. For example, Callan's editorial in *JAMA* utilizes pejorative language in describing holistic health. Citing the attraction of "legitimate physicians" to holistic health as "remarkable," he writes: "But more recently, holism has flourished on the West Coast, fanned by the flames of the "Me," self-centered, generation and is spreading inland. Like an uncontrolled nuclear reaction, a myriad of hypothetical institutes for this, academies for that, organizations for integration of East and West, and advocates for touching, thinking, and trotting has erupted" (Callan, 1979:1156).

Perhaps the most scathing attack comes from Glymour and Stalker's editorial in the *New England Journal of Medicine*. Titled "Engineers, Cranks, Physicians, Magicians," it presents a strong critique of holistic approaches (Glymour and Stalker, 1983). For example, they write:

> A magical view of the mind and body is antithetical to the scientific viewpoint, however much holistic therapists may parade what they take to be the trappings of science. . . . Holistic medicine is a pablum of common sense and nonsense offered by cranks and quacks and failed pedants who share an attachment to magic and an animosity toward reason. Too many people seem willing to swallow the rhetoric—even too many medical doctors—and the results will not be benign (ibid: 962–963).

Stalker and Glymour, both philosophers, later collaborated on an interdisciplinary collection of critical essays, *Examining Holistic Medicine* (Stalker and Glymour, 1985). The text portends to objectively analyze holistic medicine. It is fascinating to note that, while they continually criticize and attempt to expose the rhetoric of the movement, their writing is riddled with rhetorical terms that appear out of place in an academic compilation.[18] For example, in their introduction they ask, "With so much real work to be done in the world, why bother to examine holistic medicine" (ibid.:9)? Later they state, "The essays in this book make it apparent that the science of holistic medicine is bogus; that the philosophical views championed by the movement are incoherent, uninformed, and unintelligent; and that most holistic therapies are crank in the usual sense of that word: they lack any sound scientific basis" (ibid.:10). Given their conclusion, they are obviously concerned about the numerous endorsements of various academics and health professionals.

Public Health Model

The holistic health model has a much greater degree of congruence with the public health model than with that of allopathic medicine. Three major areas of convergence include their focus on preventive endeavors, their awareness of both host resistance and environmental factors in the causation of illness, and their emphasis on health education efforts. Awareness of the importance of environmental factors, both hygienic and occupational, as well as those correlated with poverty, has been central to the public health view.

Carlson details the division between medicine and public health in the early twentieth century and describes the current lack of overlap between the two approaches (Carlson, 1975:33). And Paul Starr argues:

> Students of public health have long observed, without anyone's paying much attention, that the effect of environment and behavior on the health of populations is much greater than that of medical care. Suddenly this point is being treated, in influential circles, as if it were a major discovery (Starr, 1981:436).

The same phenomenon exists in relation to behavioral medicine. Behavioral medicine claims to raise these "new" issues, as of the mid to late 1970s, yet, medical sociology, medical anthropology, and nursing have been addressing many of those same problems for the past twenty-five years.

Nursing Model

Similarly, the holistic health model has several major points of convergence with the nursing model. This is especially true of nursing's more progressive, professionally oriented variants. Central shared concerns include their emphasis on care functions, the value placed on health education, the treatment of the client as a bio-psycho-social being, and the decreased status differential as opposed to the physician-patient relationship.

Although a comprehensive explication of "care" cannot be presented within this paper, concepts of emotional support and sensitive understanding, empathy, and assistance and education in the areas of nutrition, rest, exercise, and stress reduction have applicability to both models (Mead, 1956; Skipper, 1965; Schulman, 1958; Johnson and Martin, 1958). As Carlson writes, "But healing also occurs without sophisticated technology. A major ingredient has been 'caring' " (Carlson, 1975:20).

For example, Dolores Krieger sees the laying on of hands as an intuitive but pivotal part of nursing intervention (Krieger, 1975; 1980; 1984). Describing America as a largely no-touch culture, she sees nursing as the notable exception to the behavioral codes: "Touch, one might say, is almost a badge of the nursing profession, its imprimatur, so to speak. We are allowed to touch, we allow intimacies that no other group in our culture is permitted under formal circumstances" (Krieger, 1980:297). She continues:

> Nurses use healing by the laying on of hands quite naturally, I think, in responding with an empathetic touch to the person who is frightened or in pain, or a comforting touch for a primipara during her first birth experience, or in a quieting touch for a psychotic in frenzy. The use of touch as a therapeutic tool should be acknowledged (Krieger, 1980:299).

Professional nursing curricula have stressed concepts of "comprehensive care"; inclusion of the family and community; the cultural context of health and illness; models of stress, adaptation, and coping; and family-centered maternity and pediatric care since the early sixties.[19] For instance, from the late 1950s Helen Nahm, then Dean of the University of California, San Francisco School of Nursing, began recruiting social scientists to teach and incorporate into the curricula social science concepts relating to health, disease, the processes of care and cure, and health providers.

Nurses also have attained less of a status differential than physicians from their patients; thus, it has been easier for them to move into the new more egalitarian, collaborative practitioner-client role. In the last fifteen years many nursing curricula have increasingly emphasized the role of the nurse as patient advocate.

This convergence of the two conceptual models leads to the enthusiastic reception of nurses to holistic approaches. Holistic health basically validates what many nurses have been trying to implement in their practice. Mattson's research supports this assessment that nurses have been the most receptive group:

> Of all the cosmopolitan medical professionals, nurses are the most enthusiastic about the concepts of holistic health. They are a majority at many large symposia, and afterward they include holistic concepts and practices in their daily work. . . . Nurses in the forefront of the movement include Effie Chow (R.N., Ph.D.), who has sponsored many symposia and classes in acupressure, and Dolores Krieger (R.N., Ph.D.), who has researched Therapeutic Touch. Traditional nursing roles, with emphasis on teaching, counseling, and caring, are akin to the ideal patient-practitioner role in the holistic model. Hence it is comparatively easy for nurses to make the transition from their more orthodox training to holistic health (Mattson, 1982:114).

One example of the appeal holistic health concepts have for nursing is exemplified by Barbara Blattner's book *Holistic Nursing* (Blattner, 1981). She utilizes holistic health principles to develop a conceptual model for nursing education and practice (the model is based on one developed by the San Francisco State University Department of Nursing faculty). Core premises covered in the text include the emphasis on high-level wellness, the view of the client as the chief agent of health maintenance and illness prevention, and the value of self-care and self-responsibility. The role of the nurse is described "as that of a caring colleague with major teaching and health counseling functions" (ibid.:ix). Blattner goes on to describe caring in terms that epitimize the holistic philosophy:

> Caring is the interactive process by which the nurse and client help each other grow, actualize, and transform towards a higher level of well-being. Caring is achieved by a conscious and

intuitive opening of self to another, by purposefully trusting and sharing energy, experiences, ideas, techniques, and knowledge. Caring incorporates several major approaches and theories—the feminine principle in health and illness, humanistic philosophy and psychology, and the holistic helping and healing relationship (Blattner, 1981:70).

Numerous books and articles further document the widespread interest of nursing in holistic health approaches (Flynn, 1980; Achterberg and Lawlis, 1982; Bahr, 1982; Moll, 1982; Hine, 1982; Lockheed, 1984; Martin, 1986). One example is Patricia Flynn's *Holistic Health: The Art and Science of Care* (Flynn, 1980). Elizabeth Martin's article in the *Journal of Professional Nursing*, "Holistic Nursing Practice: An Idea Whose Time Has Come," documents the holistic influences which have historically shaped the profession (Martin, 1986). She describes in detail nursing's historical roots, beginning with Nightingale's holistic approach to patient care in *Notes on Nursing*.

One interesting issue generated here is the conflict within nursing between the striving to professionalize and the stress on deprofessionalization inherent in the holistic health model. Education for nurses has increasingly taken place within university settings, and a steadily increasing number of nurses have attained graduate preparation at the masters and doctoral levels. Nursing could gain enhanced professional status and autonomy in the provision of health care through a societal shift towards this more holistic model; yet, the ideology of holistic health brings up the humanitarian-intellectual conflict which is already problematic in contemporary nursing.

Dentistry

Dentistry must also be briefly mentioned here. Dentists have been concerned with prevention and promotional aspects of health for at least twenty years, and a number of dentists have been outspoken on the benefits of holistic health. For instance, Wollman writes that signs of internal disease are often reflected or previewed in the mucous membranes of the mouth, the tongue, or the condition of the teeth (Wollman, 1980:333). He describes how lifestyle, stress, and psychological factors relate to dental health. He concludes that dentistry has emphasized and promoted preventive health practices more than most other medical specialties (ibid:334–339).

Psychology

Psychology and Psychiatry have traditionally followed the same "illness model" as allopathic medicine. These fields have also separated mind and body as much as the medical model. As discussed earlier, even the term "psychosomatic" located the origin of illness in the mind without a model incorporating true continuity or interaction.

More recently, some psychologists are moving into the area known as "health psychology." Additionally, there is a growing shift within psychiatry and psychology from an illness model to one also intervening in health, without disease categories. The newer model stresses coping mechanisms and adaptation. Rachman and Philips describe the new field of health psychology:

> Within the medical profession there is a growing appreciation of the importance of psychological factors in what is sometimes called the "process of becoming ill." It is also agreed that psychological factors contribute to the process of recovery. Unfortunately, psychologists have been slow to recognize and respond to the need for a psychological approach to problems of illness and health, outside psychiatry. One purpose of this book is to present a case for widening the scope of clinical psychology to include medical problems as well as those of a psychiatric character. We feel that the expansion is feasible as well as desirable, and illustrate our general theme with examples from the psychology of pain, sleep disturbances, placebos, and pill taking, among others (Rachman and Philips, 1980:11).

A holistic conception of illness and treatment can thus either expand the physician's role or increase interdisciplinary collaboration. Jaffe describes how his role as a health care consultant evolved so that he now functions as the physician's partner, concentrating on family dynamics. He writes, "Just as the physician's role was to alleviate symptoms by intervening at the individual's biological and physiological level, my role was to help the family change the parts of their lives that contributed to stress, hindered rehabilitation, or led to conflicts that were likely to become expressed as physical illness" (Jaffe, 1984:212).

Behavioral Medicine

The emergence of an interdisciplinary "specialty" of behavioral medicine, like health psychology, embraces many of the holistic tenets.

Stress and stress management are central concepts in behavioral medicine (Davidson and Davidson, 1980:xiii; Holden, 1980). Many researchers in this area are working to elucidate the specific mechanisms of body-mind continuity, including the field of psychoneuroimmunology. Others focus their research on aspects of the interrelationship of the social context and health/illness phenomena, or the area of health promotion through lifestyle change.

Holden summarized the emerging field of behavioral medicine for an article in *Science* (Holden, 1980). She describes the field as treating mind and body as two ends of a continuum. As she writes:

> The core of basic research in this field is an attempt to locate the specific neurochemical mechanisms by which subjective states—specifically those associated with emotional stress—lead to disease. Ultimately, it is an approach to disease and health that spans everything from research through etiology, diagnosis, treatment, rehabilitation, and prevention (Holden, 1980:479).

Holden describes behavioral medicine as formally first recognized at a 1977 conference held at Yale University. At that conference, she portrays participants as discussing being on the verge of a "new paradigm" in medicine (ibid:479).

Park and Sheena Davidson also stress the importance of the applications of behavioral principles to problems of physical health and illness (Davidson and Davidson, 1980:xi). A sampling of articles in their compilation, *Behavioral Medicine: Changing Health Lifestyles*, illustrates the diversity of areas included. The research presented covers cognitive factors in lifestyle change, teaching coping skills, the relationship of urinary pH to the psychology of nicotine addiction, factors affecting both smoking and weight loss, attempts to promote lifestyle changes for "the whole person," preventive strategies for both child behavior disorders and alcohol abuse, physical activity in a healthy lifestyle, and the use of media in lifestyle programs (Davidson and Davidson, 1980).

An interdisciplinary panel on Behavioral Medicine, organized and chaired by Ronald W. Manderscheid, a Research Sociologist with the National Institute of Mental Health, at the 1980 meetings of the American Association for the Advancement of Science reflected a similar level of diversity in both content and disciplinary backgrounds of the participating researchers. His own paper, "Implications of Biopsychosocial Relationships," reflected many of the concerns commonly considered under holistic health. After defining biopsychosocial relationships as the "complex influences exerted by society, lifestyle, physical environment, and cognitive-affective states upon physical and mental well being," he described one of the most crucial issues deriving from this area as the question of the degree to which persons are responsible for their own health (Manderscheid, 1980:2–3).

There are many indications of the growing acceptance of the behavioral medicine approach. A number of medical schools have added departments or divisions of behavioral medicine. The *Journal of Behavioral Medicine* began publication in 1978. Similarly, a branch for behavioral medicine within the National Institutes of Health was established in the late 1970s (Davidson and Davidson, 1980; Holden, 1980; Carlson, 1980).

An interesting paradox arises in relation to behavioral medicine, and it reflects problematic issues also inherent in holistic health. Behavioral medicine, as it becomes increasingly visible and institutionalized, comes to be seen as a specialty. Thus, despite its membership from diverse disciplines and the emphasis on interdisciplinary collaboration, its image as a "specialty" conflicts with its holistic orientation.

Resultant Shifts in Power/Influence

As the new model gains wider acceptance, it allocates more power to psychologists, other social scientists, nurses, and family practitioners. If a more holistic, biopsychosocial model is accepted, then the social science research on the personal and social determinants of health and illness will become more highly valued within the health care system. Both nursing and clinical psychology appear to be attempting to enhance their role as providers within the health care delivery system through the incorporation and emphasis of holistic health services.

Legitimation and Credentialing

A further issue derives from the relationship of the holistic model to these alternate models of health and illness. How do holistic health practitioners attempt to establish legitimacy to each other, the medical establishment, and clients? Holistic practitioners will need to confront the issues underlying both legitimation and credentialing. An observer senses a fair amount of concern in relation to the issue of legitimation, at least in the more organized and visible segments of the movement. One sign of this was the choice for three consecutive years of a physician with a joint M.D./Ph.D. or M.D./M.P.H. degree as president of the Association for holistic health. The conferences sponsored by the Association also seem self-consciously to feature speakers with degrees, titles, or other indications of attained professional status (e.g.: Jonas Salk). Those holistically oriented practitioners at the more professional end of the continuum experience concern that the more "far out" practitioners will discredit the entire movement.

A fundamental conflict arises in relation to this issue. On one hand, movement ideology is anti-professionalization in its orientation. As members of the holistic health movement strive for legitimation, it inherently emphasizes professionalization. Thus, for example, Paul Brenner emphasizes his past roles and credentials (successful obstetrician/gynecologist in private practice and former clinical faculty member at the University of California, San Diego School of Medicine) to legitimate his position as an expert; yet, simultaneously he may be advocating the need to abandon the concommitant professional-client status differential and describing the need for more equal distribution of knowledge and responsibility between physician and layperson.

Credentialing derives from this conflict. Along with the move to deprofessionalize medical services, many unqualified practitioners flock to the holistic health movement. With the growth of new "specialties" like hair analysis, how do potential clients determine either the qualifications of practitioners or the efficacy of various treatment approaches? Even Rick Carlson, a lawyer who has presented one of the strongest arguments in support of the holistic health movement in his book *The End of Medicine*, writes, "The effectiveness of nonallopathic healing undoubtedly varies as much as the effectiveness of modern medical practice, and certainly relies on skill. The need for competence does not vanish outside of modern medicine" (Carlson, 1975:75).

One senses tremendous ambivalence in holistic physicians in this area. They want the respect and support of conventional medicine, and that requires professionalism; however, any move towards professionalism conflicts with basic core values of the movement. This is also problematic within nursing. Nursing has worked hard to professionalize their image; yet, the tension between professionalization and committed caring persists.

Summary

This chapter has presented the holistic health model within its broader sociological context. This overview of its relationship to major trends within the health care system, as well as its historical continuity with both the movements of the sixties and secular humanism, should give the reader a clearer picture of its location within the broader societal landscape.

The section linking the holistic model to the sixties movements and the larger romantic tradition demonstrates how much of the ideology transcends specific movement concerns. The impetus for a more holistic model of health and illness derives from a larger cultural movement, that of secular humanism.

One additional question needs to be addressed in summarizing the relationship of the holistic model to the alternate models of health and illness. Since the themes comprising the holistic health model already existed for a considerable period of time in these alternate models of health, the sudden receptivity to the holistic model at this time must be explained. In other words, why is so much more attention being paid to these issues under the new label of holistic health? There are three reasons underlying this new receptivity to the model.

First, it arrived on the coattails of the sixties. A large, youthful contingency had incorporated the world view that supported this model. This group provided a pool of both practitioners and clients who became adherents of the holistic health model. In addition, the diffusion of portions of the world view into the mainstream facilitated more widespread receptivity.

Second, once a group of physicians started advocating these themes, the public listened. When less powerful groups such as nursing and public health had represented the same themes, they did not have the equivalent impact on public perceptions.

Besides the impetus provided by the sixties movements and the added impact of physician support for these notions, a *figure-ground argument* is paramount. Once the entire medical model came under attack, the already existing concerns became more visible and received widespread attention and support. In other words, the crisis in the health care system melded with these themes, so that the figure-ground configuration was altered. The notions themselves were not new; however, the profound changes in the context acted as a stark ground contrast, creating totally new perceptions.[20] In other words, the themes underlying the holistic model were already there, and they had been addressed by both nurses and public health advocates; however, they remained invisible without the backdrop of the health care crisis.

This chapter has thus located the holistic health model within its broader social and historical context. With a comprehensive picture of the holistic model in relation to other major health and societal phenomena, we can now move to the concrete behavioral and interactional level, examining the actual social consequences of the shift towards a more holistic, participatory model of health care.

4

The Sick Role in the Context of the Clinic

The societal shift towards a more holistic, participatory model of health and illness has major implications for the delivery of health care and, more particularly, for the sick role. The specific meanings attached to health, illness, and cure affect both the individual's experience of illness and the social interactions surrounding health and illness. Alterations in the meaning of illness have numerous consequences for the interactions between patients and practitioners. The largest body of research in the Sociology of Health and Illness has focused on these social dimensions.

During the last decade, a literature has developed which purports to analyze the implications of the switch in these directions. An increasing number of sociologists have discussed what they see as probable or actual changes deriving from the new meanings around health and illness; however, most of these speculations remain unverified by empirical data, particularly data at the interactional level.

Similarly, most of the policy makers, social scientists, and physician advocates of a shift towards a more holistic model see as a desirable goal the merging of traditional allopathic and holistic approaches (Fink, 1976; Lee, 1976; Todd, 1977; Masi, 1978; Giller, 1978; Pelletier, 1979; Gordon, 1981; Jeter, 1981). Another group of social scientists anticipate dangerous outcomes from the same shifts (Crawford, 1981; Kopelman and Moskop, 1981; Starr, 1981; Kotarba, 1983; Conrad, 1984). Data are needed to substantiate what actually happens when the two models intersect.

The next three chapters portray the actual social consequences of the shift towards a more holistic, preventive, participatory model of health and illness. Earlier chapters focused on the attitudes, meanings, and values held by participants in the new model; these beliefs comprise the ideological stance of both practitioners and clients. In contrast, the next three chapters consider how the modified meanings are carried out at the interactional level: what actually happens in concrete practice settings.

Several questions can only be answered by a careful examination and analysis of the extensive empirical data provided by the field setting. Are the interactional shifts in the same direction as the values and ideological stance of practitioners lead us to believe? In other words, are the behavioral changes congruent with the ideological shifts? If those modifications are in fact documented at the behavioral level, what are the limits of those alterations? For example, if individuals take complete responsibility for their health and illness, and also for cure, there would be no need for practitioners. And how do practitioners and patients handle the limits, ambiguities, and contradictions of the ideology? This is the only way to locate both the strengths and strains deriving from the shifts currently taking place in the medical model. For example, what happens when lifestyle modification comes to be seen as the primary intervention to prevent severe disease? What happens when individual responsibility and humanistic values are combined with traditional modes of care? And, during the shift in these new directions, what paradoxes and problematic issues arise?

This chapter initially sketches the ethnographic setting, describing the physical environment, participants, and general interactional environment. Next an overview of the concept of the sick role is presented, followed by its modifications in the holistic setting. Chapters V and VI analyze the data in considerably more detail in an attempt to understand the two most crucial alterations in the sick role: the changed practitioner-client relationship and the shift in responsibility for illness and cure to the individual.

The Ethnographic Setting

The primary ethnographic site was chosen because it was a setting in which practitioners attempted to combine the best of allopathic and holistic approaches in providing health care. Thus, I examined the model at one primary clinic that sees itself as belonging to the movement, and was seen by several holistic health leaders as epitomizing this approach to health care. In addition to this preventive family practice clinic, a holistically oriented dental clinic was observed for a shorter period, and two additional holistic sites were observed very briefly. These secondary settings, along with the intensive interviews, provided further data, as well as a check to assure that the findings in the primary setting were representative.

The research focus was narrowed to documentation and analysis of modifications related to the sick role. (Readers who want more detailed ethnographic material on holistic health settings may refer to Phyllis H. Mattson's *Holistic Health in Perspective*, 1982.)[1] The primary office setting I studied closely replicated the majority of Mattson's findings, as well as the description of holistic health centers by James S. Gordon, M.D. (Gordon, 1980b).

The Physical Environment

The clinic setting is a large private practice office providing a variety of medical services. The "Mar Vista Clinic" is located in a major California city.[2] It is situated in a large, modern cluster of professional offices. Nearby offices in the complex include several other medical and legal practices, as well as offices providing a wide variety of services such as optometry, videotaping, and beautician services.

Three primary practitioners have names listed on the front door. Two of these are family practice physicians; the third is a psychologist. The psychologist's name is listed second on the door. This was one of my first observations on entering the setting, and it remains symbolic of many differences in staff interaction throughout the office. It is highly unusual for a non-physician provider to have his name appear above that of a physician in a shared private practice office.

On entering the clinic, if you did not know the underlying holistic philosophy, you might easily believe you were in any successful medical office on the west coast. Indeed, the outwardly similar neighboring office is maintained by a group of four specialty physicians held in high regard by the local University Medical School. Despite this apparent similarity, however, this office is subversively different.

Clinic staff refer to the practice to outsiders as a family practice or preventive medical clinic. They do not use the word "holistic," because they react to negative connotations others attach to the word.[3] Yet staff members identify themselves with the holistic movement, and they are identified as holistic practitioners by both leaders and providers who are self-identified movement participants. The primary physician who started this clinic, for example, is a founding member of both the Association of Holistic Health and the American Holistic Medical Association.

A brochure the clinic staff developed to describe their services to potential clients lists the clinic name, and then has the caption "partners in health" over a close-up picture of a physician checking a patient's pulses during acupuncture.[4] The brochure also lists the primary types of services provided: Family Practice, Preventive Medicine, Traditional Acupuncture, and Psychological Services. Inside the brochure, the approach and the individual practitioners are described. They present their services in terms of an emphasis on prevention and achieving optimal health levels, as well as treating both chronic and acute illness.

Warmth and Informality

Initially, the clinic interior looks like a typical family practice or internal medicine office serving a primarily middle to upper middle class clientele; however, subtle differences in both the physical and interactional environment signal the shift towards a more holistic approach. The over-all appearance and feeling within the setting appears to have been designed to communicate "warmth" and a relaxed, sociable atmosphere. Office decor was carefully chosen to create a feeling of cheeriness; simultaneously, this served to minimize the visibility of the technical equipment.

The physical environment within the clinic creates the stage for warm, affable interactions. Sociability and relaxed informality are encouraged by the colored wallpaper, the many plants, and the prints and posters on the walls. In the examining rooms, washable sheets and pillowcases in lavender, yellow, or burnt orange cover the examining tables. The gowns are also cloth, rather than disposable. Several patients spontaneously brought these features up during informal interviewing as typifying the differences they experienced in this office compared to past medical encounters.

For instance, Jeanne, an articulate business executive in her late forties, described the differences in this office to me:

> Other doctors are like the paper gowns they give you...you know, disposable. It makes me feel like I'm part of an assembly line. Here they use cloth gowns. (another patient undergoing allergy testing in the same room was nodding her head in agreement) Even things here like having this wall paper (warm tones with stripes)...even the examining rooms. They're not as sterile. There are prints and colors and plants.

While Rose, one of the nurses, positioned another patient in stirrups for a gynecological exam, the patient commented on the cloth gown and drape: "It's funny how much difference it makes!"

The symbolism to patients is a representation of humane caring versus mass-production line processing and emotional sterility, as represented by the disposable paper gown and drape in most medical offices.[5] A brief listing of some of the primary symbols includes:

> white uniforms vs. more casual dress of providers
> white walls vs. print wallpaper or cedar paneling
> white sheets vs. brightly colored
> disposable paper gowns, sheets vs. cloth
> high visibility technical equipment vs. low profile
> terms of address: last names vs. first names
> level of discourse: formal vs. informal

Those symbols represent powerful metaphorical triggers, which several clients in the setting articulated spontaneously.

Efficiency

Despite the explicit attempts to create an affectively oriented environment, the office is organized for maximum efficiency, much as one would expect in a more traditional allopathic medical practice. I had initially postulated that another major underlying value inherent in the holistic health movement, that of anti-bureaucratization, might lead to shunning any attempts at efficiency, thus decreasing the economic potential of a holistic practice. However, both this office and the secondary dental office streamlined office structure, attempting to find a balance between efficient organization and expressive, caring interactions.

The office has been so carefully organized that, despite a large number of staff, few interactions between people are visible. Most interactions take place between two individuals in the privacy of one of the rooms. Thus efficiency and organization remain highly valued, despite its devaluation in movement ideology. The nature of a large interdisciplinary team of practitioners necessitates careful coordination. They have tried to structure the situation so that organization is the vehicle to enhance and emphasize personal, non-bureaucratized interactions.

The Providers

An interdisciplinary team staffs the clinic. The primary physician, Dr. A or Dave, is board family practice certified. He attended a highly regarded Eastern medical school before completing a residency in family practice. In addition, he has a Master's degree in acupuncture. The second physician, Dr. B or John, also practices family medicine. Although he belongs to the national family practice professional association, John did not complete a residency in family practice. He attended a prestigious medical school within a prominent state university system.

Two registered nurses are an integral part of the staff. Both Rose (Nurse A) and Gail (Nurse B) hold baccalaureate degrees as well as their R.N. licensure. Rose has extensive experience in public health nursing, while much of Gail's experience has been in psychiatric nursing. Rose almost embodies the image of a highly competent and compassionate visiting or public health nurse.[6]

Two clinical psychologists also practice in the setting. Mike's (Psychologist A's) practice is fairly typical of an upper middle class practice, although he defines his approach as humanistic, existential, and transpersonal. He also has a definite health-oriented focus, and is knowledgeable about stress reduction. Shirley (Psychologist B) concentrates almost exclusively on stress reduction, meditative and visualization techniques, and other more exploratory approaches that attempt spiritual and emotionally-based healing.

Two body workers, Ann and Joe, work closely with the physicians and nurses in providing various massage and body work techniques to assist in the healing process. During much of the time I observed there was also a part-time nutritionist who did one-to-one nutritional assessment and counseling with patients.

The primary receptionist and office manager, Suzie, holds a very central place in both the team organization and the informal staff interactions. Two other receptionists, one part-time, assist with the front office work (one of these with major accounting responsibilities).

Spirituality

One important component of a description of the staff in this setting is initially not clearly visible. It took me several months to realize that all staff members considered themselves and each other to have some type of very deep spiritual commitment. If asked what religion they are, most would say none, although two identify themselves as Christian. They consider themselves spiritually involved, however, most often with Eastern religions and derivative approaches.[7]

Mattson describes one common form of spiritual involvement within holistic health as exemplified by a set of three books called "A Course in Miracles" (Mattson, 1982:18–19). Four of the staff in this office met weekly over a period of several months to discuss readings from this program. During this time Rose (Nurse A) also attended a workshop on the "Course in Miracles" at the Association for Holistic Health 1982 Conference. Thus the spiritual involvements of clinic members are sometimes shared, although most often undertaken individually.

The one staff member whose religious commitment some others were unsure of was Mike, one of the psychologists. As Gail describes it, she senses that he has a strong spiritual committment; however, he relates to the group as a whole at a more professional level. Rose, Gail, Shirley, and Ann (all were involved in the "Course in Miracles") describe themselves as definitely on spiritual paths, although only Rose is actively involved in formal religion (a Christian sect with deep convictions of charity and service). Dr. A describes himself as non-religious; in the past, however, he has been extensively involved with both the Edgar Cayce readings and Arica (both are considered New Age spiritual approaches). Dr. B is active in Eckankar (a New Age spiritual approach based on teachings from India and emphasizing soul travel). Suzie, Shirley, and Joe have similar commitments that are at times shared with other staff.

Common meanings derive from these particular spiritual approaches, and they often reflect an underlying Eastern world view. For example, at one point Shirley (Psychologist B) reflected, "Don't let your ego get in the way of what you say." Helpers-healers are supposed to be continually working on their own emotional and spiritual growth, with the goal of becoming "more evolved." In insider terms, the more evolved you become, the less your ego interferes with seeing the other person's needs.

Recruitment

One further way of describing staff in these settings is to look at what qualities are sought in recruiting staff. Staff in these settings see the recruitment process as crucial to the success of their goals. Although there are obvious areas of overlap with the qualities preferred in most allopathic private practices, there are some major differences. While many holistic physicians talked of having to use "intuition" when hiring, most had also thought about the important traits they were looking for.

During an Association of Holistic Health Conference workshop in August 1981, the psychologist founder of a large holistic health clinic discussed its staff. The "core" of the staff included a psychologist, three physicians, two chiropracters, and nutritionists. With "supporting staff" such as the registered nurses, acupuncturists, massage therapists, and physician assistants, the total staff four years after the formation of that clinic numbered 35. (It was interesting that providers in this clinic defined nutritionists as primary, while nurses were seen as ancillary; the nurses in Mar Vista Clinic held a far more central role as providers). The coordinator emphasized that they never advertised for practitioners, because they "need the practitioners to be 'in tune'." He stressed the careful personnel selection process.

In that clinic it was important that potential staff members *look healthy*. The agreements they had to make to join the staff included areas such as communicating emotions and "finding nourishment" internally, so they would "bring inspiration and joy" to their work. He saw the most important aspect as the individual's *spiritual attunement*. Everyone working at that clinic has committed him or herself to some kind of independent spiritual practice for self-renewal. The founder described this situation in terms of acceptance of a "higher consciousness," so that staff members had "less ego" and were less materialistic. He also spoke of the need for staff members to have "humility." Thus, staff are hired, at least partly intuitively, based on affective and spiritual qualities (Doty, 1981).

A physician in that same clinic also spoke publicly of the cohesiveness and close communication within the staff group. He described spiritual connection and humility, as well as being open and comfortable with not knowing all the answers, as prerequisites for working in that holistic clinic. He also described everyone at the clinic as "growing and being healed." This constellation of values closely approximates those found at both the Mar Vista Clinic and the other clinics I observed.

Clients/Patients

There is more variation among the clients, as there are different pathways by which patients arrive at this office. Clients range from those who are highly committed to holistic health as a way of life to those who stumbled into the clinic through lay referral channels. The vast majority heard about these physicians through friends, although a small percentage were referred by other holistically-oriented physicians and nurses.

The demographic picture painted by Mattson is again similar to the characteristics of clients in the Mar Vista practice (Mattson, 1982: 116–122).[8] The vast majority of patients/clients who came during my time at the clinic could be described as middle to upper middle class. Approximately 60 percent of patients seen on a given day were female (according to Dr. A, about 70 percent were female in the earlier stages of his practice). Most clients had fairly high educational levels, and were extremely sophisticated consumers in medical matters. Clients in Dr. A's practice had an average age in the mid-forties: a smattering of people in their twenties, a much larger group in their thirties and forties, and some in their fifties. Dr. A. says that although he sees a number of elderly patients, there are fewer since he moved the location of the office. Dr. B's practice had a larger group of fairly young, often more visibly "hip" patients, along with more over fifty. His practice also included a higher proportion of indigent and working class patients.

The vast majority of clients initially come to the practice for a specific problem, rather than for prevention. That presenting problem often also raises secondary prevention issues. For example, a patient may say that she or he is aware of being under a lot of stress, and wants help before the problem develops into a more major illness. Of those coming for treatment of a specific problem, approximately three-quarters have chronic, rather than acute, illness.[9] When I asked Dr. A which kinds of patients he enjoys working with most, he answered:

> I like it all, because there are times when I like to work real lightly with somebody just going over lifestyle changes and helping them with that, and they're already real motivated. Those are usually real interesting people anyway, and it's nice to be with them. And at the same time I wouldn't want to spend all my time doing it, because I have so much training helping the chronically ill person that nobody might be able to help. And of course I get burned out on doing too much of that, so I would say it's all that. It's nice to see acute problems too which will take care of themselves in a week or two. So, there isn't preference there. It depends on my mood at the time.

Obviously the clients represent a self-selected group, who can be seen as seeking a distinctive kind of service and satisfaction. Thus they are different from "straight" patients whose needs have different sources and expressions. In this section, I will briefly describe why this group came and what they want.

Dissatisfaction with Traditional Medicine: Cure and Care
Several themes emerged consistently during both patient interviews and observations. Most patients who come here have many negative feelings about traditional allopathic medicine. As soon as patients learned I was doing research on holistic health, many of them would launch into accounts of problems they had experienced with physicians. One of the most commonly repeated themes was that "physicians don't treat causes, only symptoms." Patients also frequently expressed their desire to avoid

or minimize both drugs and surgical intervention. Some patients appeared to be on a moral crusade, and attempted to convert me to all the advantages of a more holistic approach.

Most patients talked of seeking out physicians like Dave and John because of disillusionment with the traditional medical system. There are *two basic variants* of this dissatisfaction. Some clients did not receive, or rejected, *cure* within the traditional system. This situation is consistent with Kotarba's work (1975) on chronic pain patients who were sophisticated about the medical system and had gone through many of the usual routes before trying acupuncture as an alternative. Some patients chose this practice for the access to acupuncture treatment, others for the allergy testing and nutritional approaches. Another large group of patients have become disillusioned with the entire medical model, and sought out the more preventive, health conscious, and less drug- and surgery-oriented approach.

The other variant also involves past disillusionment with the medical system. Here, however, the dissatisfaction reflected a perception that the person did not receive *care* within the traditional system.[10] One patient, for example, expressed her reaction to being treated as a "non-person" without a sensitive, caring, loving, spiritual dimension.

After spending more time in the setting, I realized that many patients who elaborated reasons of lack of "cure," may actually choose this model because of perceived lack of "care." As one patient described it:

> I think what's different here is the understanding and empathy. They treat the whole person, you know...the whole thing. Dr. B's the first doctor I've really communicated with, that I'm comfortable with. The other people here are the same calibre.

Another patient spoke of having a hysterectomy in her late twenties. During the next decade she saw a variety of traditional physicians for various complaints:

> Every doctor I saw would look at the chart, with my history of a hysterectomy, and then they'd ask me what birth control I was using. I was really offended, really mad! Didn't they even read the chart?!

Other patients described how the doctors and nurses in this clinic "really talk to you." Besides the humanistic qualities patients portrayed in describing these practitioners, many of their comments directly related to the decreased status differential between practitioners and patients.

The anti-technical attitudes exhibited by many patients can also be interpreted as a reaction to a perceived lack of empathetic care in allopathic medicine. These reactions came up in the comments about paper versus cloth gowns; disposable paper gowns function as a symbol of assembly line medicine. They evoke negative images of emotional "sterility" that come to be symbolically seen as the antithesis of compassion.

The case of a third group of patients who came because no "objective" symptoms or causes were found in their illness (these were the ones who were told by other physicians, "It's all in your mind") comprise an interesting intersection of the two motivational patterns for switching to the new model. If no "cause" had been found and they were not admitted into the patient role by allopathic physicians, they came to have the original "problem" treated. They also came, reacting to the way they see themselves as depersonalized and uncared for when rejected as bona fide patients.

Most of the patients can easily describe the ideological differences in terms of "treating causes rather than just symptoms" or the use of "more natural means of treatment" and "prevention." Only slightly fewer describe as articulately the caring, affective differences in interacting with the holistic health practitioners.

Stigmatization

One other theme came up with a number of patients. The middle to upper middle class professional patients were extremely articulate in delineating the reasons they believed in this approach. This choice was a natural outcome of their health orientation, and they seemed to have a peer group who shared and validated their world view.

In contrast, several patients who were either working class or middle class, but not in professional positions, came after other physicians had either been unsuccessful in treating their conditions or had denied them entrance into the sick role. This group, while believing as strongly in the efficacy of the approach in this office, at times spoke of family, friends, or co-workers seeing a holistic approach as highly stigmatized, and many of them told others they were seeing a traditional physician. Conflict with husbands was problematic for at least three of those patients, who described their husbands as seeing some of the approaches in the office as "not scientific," and denied their wives emotional, and in one case financial, support.

Several patients described not telling at least some significant others about their choice of treatment here, illustrating the stigma still attached to it as a deviant setting. The acupuncture and emphasis on allergy and clinical ecology were most often mentioned as stigmatized (because these practitioners held traditional M.D. and R.N. degrees, it was probably less stigmatized than in some other holistic settings).

For instance, Chris described needing to be "careful who knows I'm going here." Only one person in the psychiatric setting where she works as a therapist knew. When I asked her why, she replied, "Well, most people hear acupuncture, and they right away think of voodoo, a witch-doctor." I asked a business executive whose father is a physician about his reaction to her choice of this office. She replied, "I haven't told him. He still thinks I'm seeing the other doctor. Dad doesn't even believe in vitamins." Similarly, Tina said she "doesn't advertise it," when talking of telling friends she's seeing a holistic practitioner, because "people react."

Treatment Modalities in the Setting

The specific modalities and approaches used in the setting were not the focus of the study and were not evaluated in any way. Yet, without a description of those modalities, it is difficult for the reader to have a gestalt of the context in which interactions took place. Thus a very brief overview of therapeutic activities in the setting is necessary.

Services listed in the clinic brochure included: family practice medicine, traditional acupuncture, nutritional counseling, clinical ecology, psychotherapy, biofeedback and stress reduction, structural therapy, fitness evaluation, and colon therapy. They also list a weight loss program, smoke de-addiction, pain management, and a complete wellness program. In the description of "Family Practice Medicine," it states: "careful medical examination and complete laboratory assessment in consultation with a physician. Preventive medical practices are stressed for all age groups. Homeopathic remedies are used for acute illnesses with prescription drugs given only when clearly needed."

Diagnostic and treatment activities that were observed clearly combined approaches one would expect in a more traditional family practice environment with those subsumed under holistic health.[11] Many treatments did not depart from allopathic medical procedures. For example, pap smears were administered preventively for women, and antibiotics were prescribed for acute infections. Other activities departed from traditional medicine primarily by degree. An example is the area of health promotion and patient teaching. Many progressive family practice offices have incorporated those approaches, particularly during the past ten to fifteen years. Still, there was more of an emphasis placed on those areas by all practitioners in this setting (that emphasis was carried out behaviorally as well as at the ideological level). A third area of activity would be highly irregular in an allopathic medical practice: procedures such as hair analysis or the most extreme case, colonic irrigation, fall under this category.

Health Promotion/Prevention/Teaching

Preventive care and health education are highly valued here. All the meanings around health promotion, as described earlier, are continually evident when clients are assessed and treated. Health education activities, both in relation to lifestyle and to the rationale underlying the treatment plans utilized in the office, are frequent and consistent.[12] This ties in not only with the emphasis on health promotion and prevention, but also with the value placed on self-responsibility. The patient can only take responsibility for his/her own health if he/she has the knowledge to participate in decisions. Rather than simply prescribing, or telling patients what they "should do" in this setting, conscious effort is aimed at instructing the patient in the reasons behind health practices.[13]

Basic *lifestyle change* is advocated frequently, in terms of general health promotion, as well as for specific disease problems. This also makes the emphasis on self-care and responsibility more visible. Clinic staff state that it is harder to motivate someone to make drastic changes in their lifestyle when well than when ill. Dr. A explained that when a patient has major symptoms interfering with his or her life, for example frequent migraine headaches or constant problems with diarrhea, eliminating the offending substance makes them feel so much better that they are able to maintain the dietary restrictions. Motivating a patient who does not experience symptoms to alter dietary input is considerably more difficult.

Three major points of focus relate to health and lifestyle change. Assessment and intervention in the office focuses on *nutrition*, *exercise*, and *stress reduction* in relation to a wide variety of presenting complaints. This implies an emphasis on moving each person to a higher point of wellness and balance, regardless of their initial location on a health-illness continuum. All three areas are focused on in considerably more depth and with more individual variation than in most allopathic medical offices.[14] For example, although for many clients the staff work towards modifying their diet to include more complex carbohydrates and fruits and vegetables, with an accompanying decrease in processed foods, red meat, sugar, and fats, the diet modifications focus in different directions with patients suffering from specific food allergies.

One other component of the staff approach deserves mention. Staff value highly and use intuition and intuitive approaches, along with scientific, during both the assessment and treatment process. This is probably true of all clinicians, who combine intuitive sources of information with more objective information received; however, that component is often denied, or at least ignored, in allopathic medicine, nursing, and at times psychology. Here the intuitive component is more highly valued and made more visible, although always combined with objective and scientific measurements.

Specific Treatment Modalities

In this office both physicians use traditional acupuncture. Two definite qualifiers need underlining in relation to this. First, traditional acupuncture differs from the acupuncture practiced by most physicians in the United States. The latter uses acupuncture techniques to treat specific symptoms, such as localized pain. In addition, most of those physicians usually take an intensive short course to learn the acupuncture techniques. The primary physician in this setting, Dave or Dr. A, while occasionally using acupuncture in this way, with a focus on specific symptoms, more often uses traditional acupuncture with its emphasis on restoring energy balance for the entire person. Dr. A also has much more extensive preparation in traditional acupuncture.

Allergy testing is also frequently utilized in their assessments. Clinical ecology and the avoidance of specific allergens are seen as applicable to a far wider range of clinical disorders than in most family practice offices.

The physicians in the office utilize familiar laboratory tests in diagnosing problems; however, they also incorporate some less traditional procedures. For instance, hair analysis, testing for food allergies, and an elaborate dietary intake history might accompany tests such as blood work and urinalysis. There is less use of testing procedures defined as intrusive, especially diagnostic x-rays unless they are clearly indicated.

Similarly, there is a desire to minimize drugs, hospitalization, and surgical intervention, although all three are used in acute situations. Both physicians have staff privileges at a local hospital and admit patients occasionally; they also refer to various medical specialists for further assessment and treatment.

At times the drugs one would expect in an allopathic office are prescribed; in other instances, natural remedies are used or at least tried initially. This varies not only by the level of acuity assessed by the physician, but also by his assessment of this particular patient's needs and belief system. Antibiotics are still prescribed, but much less routinely than in more traditional family practices. The ways in which such decisions are negotiated will be described in the sections on sick role modifications.

The major variable affecting such approaches was the level of acuity versus chronicity attributed to a problem. These physicians and nurses agree that the allopathic model is most appropriate and effective in acute disease episodes, as opposed to chronic disease conditions. For example, in an instance where a twelve-year-old boy came in with acute ear pain, Dr. A prescribed an antibiotic for ten days, handling the otitis media very traditionally. Similarly, Dr. B spoke of antibiotics as the treatment approach for a bladder infection. Interestingly, at times both these physicians saw the need for pharmacological agents such as antibiotics or cortisone cream, and had to justify to patients why those were the approaches of choice, rather than less traditional remedies.

At one staff conference, the entire staff had gathered during lunch to discuss several patients. While discussing a patient who had not responded to the treatment approach first utilized, Dr. A said he was thinking of prescribing Prednisone. The other physician and one of the nurses laughed and seemed to think he was joking (strong medications like steroids are a "last resort" in this type of practice). Dr. A came back with: "No, I'm not joking. I'm serious on the Prednisone. Just a couple milligrams a day. In this situation I think it's indicated."

Another adjunct to treatment, whether implemented by the physicians and nurses or by the psychologists, is various relaxation, meditative, guided imagery, and visualization approaches. Dr. A had several healing tapes professionally prepared, where classical music accompanied a soothing voice in helping a patient to relax and visualize desired healing outcomes. Individualized tapes were also prepared. One example I observed where Rose used the approach involved guiding a client who was trying to give up smoking into a deeply relaxed state, and then having her visualize herself refusing cigarettes and feeling comfortable and relaxed without them. Rose then tape recorded the session with this woman, so she could listen to the tape on a regular schedule at home. In another situation, Shirley, the psychologist, worked with a patient in his thirties with multiple sclerosis, having him use an individually designed fifteen-minute audio tape twice a day. Two of the images he concentrated on during his relaxed state were repairmen fixing his myelin sheaths and having perfect control of his bladder.

The Assessment-Treatment Process

Dr. A typically saw thirteen to sixteen patients a day during the field study period. The times allocated to specific patients varied somewhat predictably, depending on their place in a time sequence. Dr. A schedules an initial one-hour visit where he takes an extensive history and does a physical exam. Patients then obtain any required lab work, which might include blood chemistries, glucose or fructose tolerance testing, and often allergy testing.[15]

Patients also complete a form describing their own assessment of their health, their health and treatment priorities, their nutritional state, normal exercise status, and stress levels. Much of this self-assessment deals with lifestyle. This assessment form was refined from what was originally a twenty page questionaire. Dr. A found over a five-year period that the information he really wanted from patients included their goals in relation to health and the specific presenting problem, their strengths and weaknesses, whether they are able to relax and by what methods, whether they exercise, their diet, their complaints, and their medical history.

Dr. A then meets with the patient for a half-hour session, where he describes and explains all the results of the assessment, and they develop a comprehensive treatment plan together. Not only are the results presented in much greater detail than in most practices, but the meaning and rationale are explained. The terminology used by Dr. A varies considerably, depending on the patient's level of knowledge. During the actual treatment, the client might undergo a series of acupuncture treatments, set up an exercise regime, and plan specific dietary modifications. At various stages where the physician and nurse interact with the client, education and support take place. This means that several members of the team are involved in the teaching, supportive, and motivating functions, as well as the treatment plan.

While both nurses are actively involved in implementing almost all phases of both the assessment and treatment process, I tried to get a sense of the proportion of patients referred to other clinic staff. Dr. A refers about five percent of his patients to each of the two psychologists for either individual or family therapy. An additional twenty-five to thirty percent are referred for some form of relaxation training (this might be implemented by one of the psychologists or nurses). All patients are referred to the nutritional and exercise class. About a fourth of Dr. A's patients receive a series of acupuncture treatments; additionally, about a fourth undergo some form of massage or body work.

General Interactional Environment

The interactional environment of Mar Vista Clinic could best be described in terms of warm, sociable interactions. The strived-for provider stance combines the qualities of empathetic caring with professionalism. Interactions among staff, and between staff and clients, are more expressive, more social, more egalitarian, and often more humorous than in equivalent medical offices. There are frequent demonstrations of affection and caring, both verbal and physical.

Staff-Client Interactions

Staff-client interactions can be characterized by this atmosphere of *affability, caring, and rapport*. Staff interact with patients in warm, often physically expressive ways. Various forms of casual, sociable, comfortable talk is often heard between staff members and clients. In addition, there is a great deal of humorous exchange, with quiet joking and laughter audible throughout the office. Humorous exchanges are most frequently heard between patients and Dr. A, both nurses, and Suzie. Staff members seem to know many patients fairly well, and many of the exchanges are on personal and social, rather than professional subjects. It was often hard to describe how much interaction was professional and how much sociable in a given staff-client encounter. Professional and social exchanges are thus less separate here. Despite the informality, however, professionalism remains a strong value.

The clinic brochure immediately sets the tone for the staff-client relationship. As described earlier, the picture of a physician feeling a patient's pulses during acupuncture symbolizes compassion, nurturing and connection through touch. Thus, a *healing partnership* and *expressive nurturance* are crucial elements of the relationship.

More time and caring are continually evident in the relationships of staff to patient. Staff value affective "involvement" with each person they interact with. Patients often discussed how the "caring" made a difference to them. As one patient described it:

> And everyone here is warm and caring. A couple of times I've been here and felt really lousy. Gail [Nurse B] was really nice to me. I mean, more than she had to. [I asked if she could be more specific.] She made me feel I wasn't in the way, and it was okay to feel lousy. And everyone knows your name. Not just the doctors and nurses, but Suzie too. They're really human.

The relationship moves to incorporate more of Schulman's *expressive functions*, as opposed to instrumental (Schulman, 1958; Skipper, 1965). More caring laden interactions and nurturing takes place than in most allopathic offices. For instance, during one observation in the reception area, a patient who had undergone a colonic irrigation came out after getting dressed.

> Helen appeared to be in her sixties or seventies, and both Suzie [receptionist] and Gail [Nurse B] were very friendly and warm as they interacted with her. Helen and Gail gave each other a big hug, with much smiling, and Gail told her she'd see her the next Tuesday. Helen replied, "You're such a sweetheart. I love you, you know."

The degree of that type of exchange—both physically and verbally expressive and sociable—is extremely visible here, as opposed to most medical settings. There was touching or hugging with both younger patients and with elderly patients.[16]

While caring, nurturing interactions have not been unusual in nurse-patient interactions, it was more striking to note Dr. A's level of gentle nurturing. Both Dr. A and Dr. G, the holistic dentist, related to patients in ways both the researcher and patients characterized as extremely gentle, compassionate, and sensitive.

There is also less disrobing than in most offices, especially during the assessment period. This makes for somewhat less of a status differential between providers and client. A parallel difference is the more open access to information patients have in this setting. This will be more fully detailed and documented in the next chapter.

Intra-Staff Interactions

Interactions among staff members are also typified by a more egalitarian stance. They also demonstrate affective, supportive, expressive elements to a degree rarely seen in a medical office setting. Although close friendships might develop in the latter, visible expressions would not be so prominent. Additionally, the supportive relationships that do develop in more traditional settings are more hierarchical and gender isolated. Again, this must be stressed as a shift relative to the traditional norm. The women in this clinic share support more expressively and frequently than they do with the men (they also spend more time together outside the setting).[17]

I saw Dr. A as somewhat less physically expressive than the nurses, psychologists, and other staff. It was difficult to know whether that was part of his personal style or whether he still defines the physician as maintaining more of a distance to remain professional. He hugged Mike warmly at his birthday party, and he interacts very empathetically with patients. His use of acupuncture facilitates his more expressive physical interactions with patients, as well.

At Mike's surprise birthday party, for example, there was much hugging and some kissing (the men hugged without kissing). On Gail's birthday, Mike wrote a very sensitive, supportive, personal poem for her. And on a day when Suzie felt ill, I watched both Gail and Rose, the nurses, come up to her at intervals and put their arms around her, while asking how she was doing. Later they suggested that Suzie work in back where it was quieter, and let the other two staff in the reception area answer the phones.[18]

Because of the large number of team members directly involved with both assessment and treatment in this clinic, more disruptive problems can occur without increased communication and coordination. The physician cannot monopolize crucial information, as in many private practices. Besides the informal, frequent communication between staff members that took place, there were occasional staff meetings held to discuss specific patients and problems. Despite a goal of regularly scheduling such conferences, they were held sporadically, as it was often difficult to coordinate everyone's schedule. When they were held, they were informal and involved much backstage and playful, almost intimate behavior while discussing the specific patients and problems. Dave, as Dr. A is routinely called by staff, remains the coordinator of these sessions, although various staff choose patients or issues they want to discuss. Members seem to feel comfortable coming in at any point with questions, ideas, and other input.

Social gatherings of staff outside the setting were frequent and cohesive. Examples of this extension of their shared work lives during the period of the field study included a beach party, an Italian dinner at Suzie's house, and a Halloween party.[19]

Ambivalence Around Professionalization

As mentioned earlier, there are still the markings of bureaucratic efficiency in the office, although attempts are made to minimize its visibility. There are still secretaries, insurance forms, and paperwork related to billing and ordering supplies.

A fundamental conflict arises in relation to this issue. On one hand, movement ideology, with its emphasis on the value of each unique person, is strongly anti-professional and hostile to bureaucratization. Yet a shift on the behavioral level remains a partial shift that reflects much ambivalence. Staff give up many of the symbols of professionalism, but maintain others.

For instance, both patients and staff at Mar Vista Clinic go by their first names. During my time there Dr. A was routinely called Dave by other staff members, as well as by many patients (in initial visits, especially with older patients, he goes by Dr. A). At the same time, he continues to wear a white lab coat, oxford shirt, and tie. The nurses in the office wear white lab coats; however, their long slacks and shoes such as Birkenstocks are visible. In contrast, in the holistic dental office all staff members except Dr. G went by their first name. This fact particularly stood out to the researcher because, although one would most certainly expect it in a more traditional setting, in most other areas he had abandoned the symbols of his status and authority. For example, he typically wore corduroy pants and a knit shirt rather than a white jacket. Thus, although different symbols were used, the combination in each office reflected this ambivalent stance towards professionalism and formality.

The Sick Role Concept

This section summarizes the major features which distinguish the health and illness interactions that take place here from those in more traditional allopathic medical settings. One of the most useful frameworks for conceptualizing those modifications is the sick role concept.

Talcott Parsons developed the concept of the sick role, and his conceptualization has remained the normative paradigm for the last thirty years. Parsons initially labelled and abstracted the patterns of expectations and behavior attached to the sick role that accompanies illness (Parsons, 1951:428–479; Parsons and Fox, 1958). Despite the multitude of studies critiquing aspects of the sick role, it has served as a major theoretical focus in the field of medical sociology. As Fredric and Sally Wolinsky argue, "it offers the most systematic and consistent framework for analyzing the socially necessary behavior of sick individuals in American and other Western societies" (Wolinsky and Wolinsky, 1981:229).

Because of the huge volume of literature reacting to or extending Parsons' work, I can present here only an overview of Parsons' conceptual model of the sick role. It sketches the character of the traditional sick role before describing the shifts taking place with the emergence of the new model of health and illness.[20]

Parsons' concept of the sick role derives from a structural-functionalist approach; additionally, it views structure in terms of systems theory and models based on notions of equilibrium. Thus the physician-patient

Sick Role
Rights
   Nonresponsibility for causing illness
   Exemption from role responsibilities
Obligations
   Desire to get well
   Seek competent treatment and cooperate in regime

Figure 2

relationship is seen as a subsystem of the larger social system. As members of the larger society, health professionals and patients bring shared values to their encounters in the medical arena.

Patient Rights and Obligations

The patient has two contractual rights and two duties in relation to the sick role. First, the patient is not held accountable and responsible for causing the illness. The physician essentially absolves the patient from responsibility. This removes both the acquisition and cure of illness from the volitional realm. Second, the patient who has been admitted into the sick role is legitimately exempted from certain role obligations and social responsibilities (the degree of exemption varies with the severity of the illness). Third, in return, the patient has the obligation to cooperate with the physician and treatment plan. She or he must seek competent help and comply with any recommended treatment. Fourth, the patient has to want to get well. The patient has to accept the assumption that the state of illness is undesirable, and that it carries with it the obligation to become well (see Figure 2).

Several major assumptions underlie this conceptualization of the sick role. These need to be made explicit to understand the alterations taking place under the influence of the new model. The assumptions examined in this section include the view of illness as deviance, the physician as gatekeeper, the physician's absolution function, secondary gains in illness, the parent-child structure of the physician-patient relationship, and the distinguishing characteristics of the physician's role.

Illness as Deviance

Parsons basically viewed illness as a form of deviance which is partially legitimate. Parsons and Fox regarded illness as both a psychological disturbance and a deviant social role (Parsons and Fox, 1958). Sickness is seen as disturbing the family unit, overtaxing its equilibrium. The presence of illness in a family also poses the danger of sociogenic "infection"; the secondary gains accruing to individuals are seen as too attractive to resist.

In addition to the burden illness places on the family, Parsons saw illness as dysfunctional to the society as a whole. Thus, society must minimize the amount of illness for the social system to continue to function productively. Since illness is dysfunctional, the patient is accorded a clearly subordinate status, especially in relation to the physician who maintains the functional requirements of the system.

Many of the rights accorded to the individual through the sick role are also seen in this model as functional for the individual. The main organizing force behind medicalization, one often forgotten in the recent attacks on the medicalization process, is that the sick role did have humanitarian consequences. Once deviance moved from control by the institutions of religion and law to regulation by the institution of medicine, the medical model minimized the guilt and stigma attached to deviant behavior.

Physician as Gatekeeper

The physician legitimates the conditional deviance. Thus the physician functions in a disciplinary, social control capacity on behalf of the larger society. This prevents malingering or excessive contagion within the family, and more illness than the productive capacity of a society could tolerate. Thus, although Parsons views the physician as an agent of social control, this control is seen as necessary and functional for the society.

As the Wolinskys write, the ill person does not become a bona fide occupant of the sick role until the physician legitimizes his or her patient status (Wolinsky and Wolinsky, 1981:231). They go on to describe some of the ways the physician may confer sick role legitimation, such as the common route of prescribing a medication (ibid:232).

Physician's Absolution Function

The physician essentially absolves the patient from responsibility in causing the illness. This absolution function benefits the individual and his or her family by removing much of the stigma attached to the deviant role. The humanistic consequences of viewing illness as caused by organisms beyond the patient's control are most obvious when compared to views of illness causation as retribution for personal sin. By granting entrance into the sick role, the physician legitimates the patient's claim and absolves him or her from guilt and blame.

Secondary Gains/Malingering

Responsibility for illness varies by models. Parsons' model explicitly recognized the secondary gains accruing from illness. The freedom from role responsibilities such as work was seen as so desirable that physicians needed to enforce the gatekeeping function. Although Parsons describes the patient as avoiding the everyday pressures of life through illness, he sees this as an *unconscious* choice of the individual. The underlying influence of the psychoanalytic approach is apparent throughout Parsons' model.

Parent-Child Relationship

In Parsons' model the physician has the primary authority and status within the relationship with the patient. This authority is based on expertise, the imbalance of knowledge and skills she or he possesses relative to the goals of cure. The patient is obligated to comply with the physician's plan; thus, she or he is seen as relatively passive in the medical interaction. This view fully accepts the legitimate authority of the physician, as it does the authority of the parent over the child (the multitude of compliance studies carried out by physicians or social scientists is based on this assumption). The view of the physician as the parent figure again derives from Freudian views (Parsons and Fox, 1958).[21]

Role of the Physician

Parsons described the role of the physician in terms of five additional characteristics. Besides describing the social role of the physician as *achieved*, his pattern variable analysis includes these four dimensions. First, the role is *universalistic*. The physician treats all patients in the same manner, without prejudice in terms of criteria such as age, social class, or race. Second, it is *functionally specific*, versus diffuse. In other words, the interaction is limited to activities clearly defined as medical. Activities defined as magical or religious, as well as socially oriented, should not be included in medical encounters. Third, the role is *affectively neutral*. The physician should not become involved in the patient's situation. This protective barrier or distance is assumed to be functional in terms of safeguarding professional objectivity, and it offers protective functions for both doctors and patients. Fourth, the role is *collectivity oriented*, that is, it should transcend self-interest, working toward the society's best interests.

Critiques of the Sick Role Concept

The many critiques of the sick role concept can be divided into four major groups. These will be touched on very briefly. First, most researchers in medical sociology feel the sick role concept applies more to limited, acute illness than to chronic illness, handicapping conditions, or death. Many feel that the number of exceptions limits its usefulness. Second, the concept has a strong upper middle class, urban bias. It appears to be most applicable to urban, middle class, intact nuclear families. Its usefulness is less appropriate when applied to subcultural variations. Third, the sick role conceptualization portrays the role as both specific and circumscribed. While that may be useful for analysis, illness is never that simple, and the variance between cases is problematic. In other words, the concept does not portray the subtleties and variations in behavior. It also does not allow for the conflict and negotiation that most contemporary sociologists feel routinely take place within sick role interactions. Other sociologists postulate multiple sick roles; for instance, Mechanic's conceptualization of illness behavior allows for significantly more complexity and diversity (Mechanic, 1962). Siegler and Osmond believe the ideal typical sequence occurs only rarely, and develop variations of the model that they see as accounting for more of the diversity and variation (Siegler and Osmond, 1973; 1974). Fourth, some critics charge that the concept sees sickness as concrete, while actual illness and diagnosis are considerably more complex and problematic. It assumes that the definition of "illness" is objective and nonproblematic.

Additional critiques stem from the underlying structural-functionalist approach of Parsons' theories. For instance, Marxists such as Waitzkin believe that capitalism has a vested interest in more illness because of its safety valve function (Waitzkin and Waterman, 1974). Empirical data, however, do not seem to indicate that there is more illness in capitalist societies. Freidson argues that medicine is more a function of organization than of values (Freidson, 1973). In this study, the focus is on changes in meanings and values and the consequences of those shifts when the structure of medical care (private practice office) remains constant.

Numerous empirical studies also challenge various aspects of Parsons' sick role concept. For example, research demonstrates that some degree of guilt always coexists with the exemption from responsibility for the illness (Davis, 1963; Siegler and Osmond, 1973; Zola, 1978). The mere fact that illness is defined as deviance leads to blame. Another example is that empirical studies show that people tend to leave the sick role too soon. In other words, noncompliance is in the direction of early resumption of activities, rather than malingering.

As for the role of the physician, there are numerous empirical studies demonstrating that, while the universalistic aspect of the role may be a goal, actual treatment of patients reflects the value system and prejudices of the larger society. Sudnow's work remains a classic in demonstrating the differential treatment of patients in emergency rooms, based on perceived social value (Sudnow, 1967). Freidson also critiques Parsons as describing how physicians should behave, rather than their actual behavior. His work demonstrates how strongly physician behavior reflects their self-interest as a profession (Freidson, 1970a,b). Another major part of Friedson's critique is that the sick role conceptualization ignores the patient's perspective in favor of that of the physician and the society.

Despite these critiques, the sick role concept remains a powerful explanatory model. It continues to be seen as an ideal type in acute illness situations in American upper middle class intact families. It has stimulated over thirty years of research, functioning as the orienting force in the field. Additionally, it continues to point to issues that require further research, highlighting issues like the moral component of illness. Like Twaddle, I see the sick role as most useful as a starting point for analysis (Twaddle, 1972:162). It provides a theoretically useful framework from which to analyze the interactional consequences of the shift toward the new model.

The Alterations in the Sick Role

This section presents an overview of the major modifications in the sick role within the holistic model, as observed in the settings I have studied. It must be emphasized that, while changes will be highlighted in contrast with the more traditional model, in general they represent only shifts within areas that remain well defined. At various points in the overview, the shifts will be related not only to the more traditional model, but also to the ideological pronouncements and problematic aspects of the holistic one.

Parsons' conceptualization of the sick role was portrayed above as more applicable to acute disease trajectories in upper middle class, urban populations. It must be remembered that, although the patient population in the settings I studied is primarily middle and upper middle class and urban, the majority of health problems seen in these settings represented less acute illness and chronic conditions.

Meaning of Illness and the Sick Role

The meaning of illness in the new model affects the sick role in fundamental ways. The beliefs and meanings around health and illness alter several aspects of the structure of the physician-patient relationship.

In some interesting ways, Parsons' views of the meaning of illness are much closer to those of the new holistic model than to those of traditional medicine. Not only does the holistic model encompass the social and interactional aspects most often ignored by traditional allopathic physicians (for example, family and work situation), but it defines the underlying causes of illness in closely parallel ways. For instance, Parsons is usually interpreted as describing the sick role as exempting the patient from everyday responsibility. Yet Parsons and Fox write:

> Illness, so far as it is motivated, is a form of deviant behavior, and as such, may be subjected to a standard sociological analysis of deviance. Compared with other types of non-conformist behavior, sickness characteristically entails passive withdrawal from normal activities and responsibilities. . . . For (illness) is an escape from the pressures of ordinary life (Parsons and Fox, 1958:235–236).

This underlying view, derived from a psychoanalytic base, closely approximates the views in the holistic model that illness is a response to *dis-ease* in some part of the individual's life. Both views assume a choice or volitional component, although they usually interpret the choice as unconscious.

The primary area of divergence in the two approaches has to do with the source of the solution. Parsons sees the functional need for social control at the institutional level to limit this type of deviance. In the holistic model, the individual is seen as holding the responsibility to choose to want to get well. In both these views, however, if the patient does not show the desire to get well, he or she is not carrying out his or her obligation.

From my observations, it seems that these physicians and nurses at the Mar Vista Clinic and other holistic settings have somewhat more acceptance and compassion for a patient when they sense he or she does not want to get well than would more traditional health professionals. However, those situations still seem to evoke frustration in the staff. Most of the providers in the setting (this includes the sample of holistically oriented physicians, nurses, and psychologists interviewed) preferred working with patients who were motivated to work on either recovery or improved health. In other words, they often found the social control functions of their role frustrating and removed from their goals as health professionals and healers. Malingering presents a similar problem to holistic and traditionally oriented physicians and nurses.

On the other hand, there are some definite points of divergence in the two views. First, the holistically oriented model delegates more control to the patient, and treatment is often moved from institutional settings such as hospitals into the home. These views would definitely be interpreted as dysfunctional according to Parsons' conceptualization. Parsons would see the family as only further reinforcing the patient's dependence, rather than maintaining limits on the deviant behavior. Additionally, the secondary gains may be seen as so attractive that a process of social contagion would be initiated within the family unit.

A second area of divergence derives from the beliefs of causation in illness. Siegler and Osmond (1973:42) interpret Parsons' conceptualization of the sick role as implying that the patient does not enter the sick role until he is convinced that the source of his illness lies outside of himself. If this is the case, there is *theoretically no sick role* in the new model, since the client views the illness as integral to his or her self and a direct derivative of his or her way of life.

Yet, paradoxically, while there should theoretically no longer be a sick role (and, if there is one, physicians should not function in as much of a gatekeeping capacity), these physicians continue to admit patients to the role. The small group of patients who come to this setting to get validation when other physicians have refused to legitimate their claims to sick role status indicates that this process still occurs.

Illness as Deviance

It is difficult to delineate the many subtle changes around the views of illness as deviance. Illness and health are seen as less separate in the holistic model; thus, illness is seen as less deviant and stigmatized. Stigma is also lessened once illness comes to be seen as a potential for growth, rather than misfortune. Although this appears to hold true in minor or chronic illness, it remains questionable whether patients actually view acute, debilitating disease as a positive learning experience in their lives (at least until the acute phase has passed).

As definitions of illness move in directions implying less deviance, the patient maintains his or her status despite the illness. On the other hand, as illness comes to be seen as under the individual's control, the stigma attached to illness increases. These conflictual assumptions lead to problematic consequences in terms of patient stigmatization. Because of the complexity in this ambivalent stance, this area of responsibility for illness will be developed and analyzed at length as the focus of Chapter VI.

The Healing Process

In the holistic model healing occurs, or at least is facilitated, through love and caring. The healing encounter itself, along with a healing environment, is seen as triggering changes in an individual's level of health-illness. In other words, having a place where one is recognized and respected as a unique individual is seen as promoting both health and healing.

The concept of healing in a holistic model differs in another fundamental way. In the traditional conceptualization, the physician acts on and manipulates parts of the patient to stimulate healing. The patient becomes well due to these interventions, and the objective physician or nurse is untouched by them. In the holistic model, giving and receiving are the same, and all interaction proceeds bidirectionally. Thus there are as many effects on providers as on clients deriving from a given interaction between them. This reinforces views of collaboration and a decreased status differential.

Role of the Physician

One way to illuminate the shifts in the sick role is to examine the modifications in *Parsons' pattern variables*. Three of the pattern variables remain relatively close to the original conception. The role of the physician is still seen as *achieved, universalistic*, and *collectivity oriented*. Those aspects of the physician role continue to be highly valued, and holistic physicians see them as closely allied to their spiritual commitment (those aspects are supported by the constellation of values in their underlying world view). Still, it can be argued that their self-interest is served when their patients are primarily upper middle class, rather than ghetto patients.

Two other pattern variables diverge from the traditional pattern, although again this represents a shift rather than a total alteration. The physician's role shifts from being *functionally specific* in the direction of becoming *more diffuse*. In the setting, there was far less of Parsons' specificity. The relationship between staff and patient extends beyond illness concerns to very personal and social parts of their lives. As mentioned earlier, professional and social exchanges are less separate here. The shifts in the meaning of illness also designate wide areas of the individual's life as part of the healer's legitimate concern. What becomes a "medical matter" or "health matter" encompasses most of the individual's life. In addition, once they become seen as integrally related to an individual's level of health, spiritual and mystical areas are no longer so rigidly excluded from medical concern.

Second, the physician's role shifts somewhat from the stance of *affective neutrality*. Again, this represents a shift. A protective barrier is still there, although it becomes most visible in extreme cases. While relationships observed in the setting seemed to incorporate various degrees of affective involvement, and while providers and patients are at times friends, there were definite limits on this. Rose, for example, said she would never date a patient from the clinic. And with a small number of patients who were defined by staff as extremely "needy," staff were observed to invoke more traditional types of barriers of professionalism to maintain limits to their involvement.

The healing interaction also involves *more expressive functions* in these settings. The relationship incorporates more of the expressive components of caring and nurturing (this is closer to traditional nurse-patient interactions than those between physician and patient). Unlike earlier postulations separating care and cure functions in healing, care functions and nurturing are themselves seen as curative. The expressive, nurturing components of the healer's role are much more strongly emphasized and valued in the setting. This shift towards incorporating more affective and expressive dimensions may represent an indication of what Renee Fox terms the feminization of medicine (Fox, 1984).[22]

The Physician as Gatekeeper

Accompanying the shift towards a more egalitarian relationship between physician and patient, the physician's role as gatekeeper should decrease, with the patient assuming more of the gatekeeping function. This shift does seem to have occurred, at least partially. Patients both initiate and participate in the decision-making process, and more negotiation is possible. This should provide an avenue for testing whether the social control functions of the institution of medicine are actually necessary. The final chapter will return to an examination of this issue.

The Modified Practitioner-Client Relationship

The practitioner-client relationship has definitely changed in a more egalitarian direction in the new model. The traditional relationship saw the physician with the imbalance of both authority and status within the relationship. There was a definite power differential. The physician's legitimate authority was based on his or her expertise. The new partnership implies two individuals bringing their different sources of knowledge together to solve a problem.

The patient's choices definitely assume more importance in the new model. The patient's perceptions, experience, and definitions of the situation are taken far more seriously than in the traditional medical model. Discomfort, for example, is seen as valid according to the patient's definition, rather than the physician or nurse's assessment. As everyday experience and daily activities come to be seen as equally central to events at the physiological level, the patient comes to have a greater proportion of knowledge of the dimensions relevant to the medical encounter. Thus the physician no longer has as great an imbalance of knowledge and skills to legitimate his authority.

This shift seems to be supported by the more equal access to information documented earlier in the chapter, as well as by patients initiating and at times controlling the interaction. The use of first names in talking to staff is another symbol of the shift. However, the actual degree of this shift and its outcomes remain considerably more complex than it initially appears.

The Shift in Personal Responsibility for Illness and Cure

This shift derives from the changed view of the patient in the provider-client relationship. Rather than viewing the patient as a child who requires an authority-figure to make decisions and maintain responsibility for him, the patient becomes a responsible party to the interaction. In other words, the patient is now seen as an adult capable of making responsible decisions.

The relationship itself seems to move from one representing a parent-child dyad, to one representing a consumer-oriented client collaborating with a provider. The staff see themselves, and patients in these settings either see staff initially or come to see them, as consultants and teachers as well as healers. There is more equal distribution of knowledge and responsibility between physician and layman. The more egalitarian interactions between providers and clients are echoed in the intra-staff interactions as well.

The physician's absolution function in the traditional model absolved the patient from responsibility, thus removing much of the stigma from being sick. Holding the patient responsible could increase the stigma attached to illness, yet this proves to be a much more confusing issue than it first appears.

Despite the consistent ideology putting forth a drastic shift in attribution of responsibility to the individual, the interactional data presented a much more ambiguous picture. In this chapter I have shown how the stigma attached to illness is both lessened and increased by the many subtle changes around the views of illness as deviance. In Chapter VI I will demonstrate more definitively that these holistic practitioners often grant entrance into the sick role and continue to absolve patients, using a variety of "theoretical outs." Simultaneously, many patients are receiving blame from the wider society and some more traditional physicians with the spread of simplistic beliefs of mind-body continuity. These issues of absolution, stigma, and the responsibility for illness become increasingly complex and problematic, especially when simultaneously examining the dual levels of ideology and concrete behavior.

Summary

Differences have been examined in relation to the meaning of illness, illness as deviance, the healing process, and the role of the physician. While the physician's role remains both universalistic and collectivity oriented, it shifts from being functionally specific towards becoming more diffuse. In addition, the stance of affective neutrality moves towards more highly valuing the affective dimensions of the relationship. The physician's role as gatekeeper decreases with the more egalitarian relationship between physician and patient. The practitioner-client relationship seems to have changed in a more egalitarian direction in the new model. Similarly, there seems to have been a shift in the attribution of personal responsibility for illness.

Although this section has outlined the major alterations in the sick role enactment with the emergence of the new model, a detailed analysis of each component would require a much more prolonged and extensive research project. Instead, this analysis will now focus on the two most crucial areas of change. These last two shifts, those of the *practitioner-client relationship* and the *attribution of responsibility*, are the most critical and also the most complex of the modifications occurring to the sick role. Data bearing on the subtle details of those shifts will be more extensively analyzed in the following two chapters.

5

The Modified Practitioner-Patient Relationship

The relationship between the practitioner and the patient is probably the most pivotal aspect of implementing the new model. The structure of that relationship determines more than any other single variable whether the process and outcome actually constitute allopathic or holistic medical care. A great deal has been written on the emerging shifts in the physician-patient relationship; however, only sparse empirical documentation exists to support those contentions (Bloom and Wilson, 1979; Reeder, 1978; Lopata, 1979; Haug, 1981, 1983). For instance, Eric Cassell contends that patients frequently see themselves as "active partners" in their care (Cassell, 1986:196). Similarly, Renée Fox described this shift over a decade ago:

> There is still another change in the health-illness medicine area. . . . This is the movement toward effecting greater equality, collegiality, and accountability in the relationship of physicians to patients and their families, to other medical professionals, and to the lay public. Attempts to reduce the hierarchical dimension in the physician's role, as well as the increased insistence on patients' rights . . . are all part of this movement. There is reason to believe that, as a consequence of pressure from both outside and inside the medical profession, the doctor will become less "dominant" and "autonomous," and will be subject to more controls (Fox, 1977:20–21).

Fox continues by stating that, despite this change in the direction of greater egalitarianism, it remains unlikely that all elements of hierarchy will be eliminated from the physician's role.

Chapter IV presented an overview of the shifts actually taking place in the ways interactions are structured between providers and clients in Mar Vista Clinic. Now a more in-depth analysis of the most significant of these shifts is necessary, because it influences both the attributions around individual responsibility for illness and the enactment of the sick role as a whole. The central focus here will be on the shift towards a more egalitarian relationship between the two parties. Despite this primary analytical focus, the other major changes in the relationship must be kept in mind to gain any meaningful understanding of the shifts. The three aspects of the relationship that were shown to be most changed in the new model are the parameters of *affective neutrality*, *specificity*, and *hierarchical status and authority*.

Affective Neutrality

One of the pivotal shifts in the relationship between physicians and patients in holistic settings is the decrease in affective neutrality. It is replaced by an expressive ethic where affective components of physician-patient interaction are highly valued as well as obviously visible.[1]

The ideals of spending more time, familiarity, caring, and a higher degree of involvement with patients were articulated by both providers and patients. When patients in the holistic clinic described the communication as being different, they portrayed those differences in terms like more understanding, empathy, caring, and warmth. Frequently heard descriptions included, "They really talk to you here," or "They really listen." One of the physicians, Dr. B, described components of his philosophy of caring for patients: "I need to really listen. And I use touch. It doesn't matter if it's through acupuncture or something more traditional like using a stethoscope. The touch is important to healing." In other words, patients feel, and physicians agree, that they have a right to caring and compassion in this setting. It is seen as a central part of the physician-patient contract.

When caring, nurturing components have been present in interactions between providers and clients in the traditional medical model, these were frequently defined as "less professional" or seen as tangential to the professional health provider role. In fact, because expressive components are so prevalent in nursing roles, these roles have often been defined as "less professional" than that of the physician, which focuses heavily on instrumental functions.

In holistic health, caring and nurturing become explicitly instrumental in terms of the system goals of cure, rather than an augmenting set of functions. The caring components of the relationship between practitioner and patient are seen as triggering the healing process within the patient.

One issue must be examined here. A cynical argument can be made that these caring, nurturing approaches represent "front work" (Douglas, 1976:55–82). In other words, the staff may convey "ersatz affability" or phony warmth, designed to exploit the emotional vulnerabilities of lonely people. I am convinced that in the Mar Vista Clinic the observed warmth not only is not front work, but it is based on deep commitment on the part of staff members involving convictions of dedication and service. The nine-month period of ethnographic study in the clinic allowed me to observe staff extensively in both frontstage and backstage areas. Near the end of the field work I came to be accepted as a partial insider, and got to know several staff members fairly well. During this period I observed much backstage behavior.

One additional piece of evidence denies such exploitative interpretations. Several staff members, but especially Dave (Dr. A) and Rose (Nurse A) in Mar Vista Clinic, and Dr. G in the dental office, made comments indicating their concern that I might not be seeing the "negative" parts of their practice. For instance, both Dave and Rose separately approached me with their concern that I was seeing the "successes" in the clinic, but that the patients who aren't satisfied leave. Similarly, when I commented to both Dr. A and Dr. G on approaches they used which I knew they defined as positive, they both made comments to the effect of "I try to do that, but I don't succeed as often as I'd like." Their stance of humility was again part of their larger world view, and contradicts the cynical interpretations.

Specificity

The interactions between providers and patient/clients in Mar Vista Clinic demonstrate far less specificity than in the traditional model. In the traditional medical model, the boundary between personal and professional concerns is relatively impermeable. The specificity Parsons described in the physician-patient relationship expands in the holistic model to cover much broader segments of the client's everyday life (Parsons 1951, 1958). Practitioners, whether physicians, nurses, psychologists, or body workers, have legitimate involvement in far wider arenas of the patient's life, and this involvement is seen as necessary to reach the goals of improved health or cure.

Parsons' sick role emphasizes the constraints placed on the appropriate focal areas of the physician-patient encounter. In contrast, in the Mar Vista Clinic the providers consider a far broader set of variables, because they define them as central to health and illness. Stress, nutrition, family relationships, feelings about work, spiritual beliefs and practices, leisure activities, and even attitudes towards life are seen as directly affecting whether one remains healthy or becomes ill.

Thus the practitioner has greater involvement in wider arenas of the patient's life. The pathogenic sphere is so far expanded, in fact, that it would be fair to call it the "medicalization of lifestyle" (see Freund 1982; Arney and Bergen 1984; Conrad 1984 for other references to this shift).

Status Differential

The relationship between physician and patient in the holistic setting has also shifted toward a more egalitarian stance. That is, the patient has more authority and control within the interaction than in the traditional allopathic model. Rather than the physician and patient relating like parent and child, interaction proceeds reciprocally, as between two adults of comparable status. This decreased status differential between providers and clients is also reflected in the minimal hierarchy of authority among staff members.

This aspect of the relationship shift is far more complex and problematic than it initially appears, and it is the least documented. This chapter will therefore focus empirically and analytically on this shift towards a more egalitarian relationship.

On careful analysis of everyday behavior in the holistic office, is the practitioner-client relationship actually more egalitarian? If the relationship is more egalitarian in practice, what alterations in language use and symbols accompany this shift?

In earlier chapters I concentrated on the emphasis on deprofessionalization and de-expertization in the holistic health movement as deriving from the democratic preoccupation of the 1960s; this was linked to the broader context of the consumer movement. There is a tension between the democratic, humanistic concerns and the need for expertise in a highly technological society. Egalitarian ideology does not necessarily remove the situational authority and dependency within a physician-patient relationship. Can there be a truly egalitarian relationship between a holistic health physician and a patient when the former retains the preponderance of knowledge and skills, or is it a matter of degree? Furthermore, if the hierarchical relationship is functional for both the individual and society, as Parsons hypothesized, what are the consequences of such a shift?

For instance, are there any limits on the egalitarianism increasingly demonstrated between providers and patients? Does the patient give up all dependence on the caregivers? And does this more equal division of power and authority within the relationship mean that the physician no longer functions as a gatekeeper to admit patients to the sick role? In the next chapter these questions will be extended to explore whether the physician continues to absolve the patient from blame and guilt for the illness itself.

Do patients have trouble with the shift? Do they want to maintain the physician as an authority figure? Do physicians have difficulty giving up their authority? These questions derive from larger questions of how authority and divergent role expectations are negotiated within the relationship under the new holistic model.

The Decreased Status Differential

The doctor-patient relationship in the traditional medical model includes a definite status differential. Cockerham sums up this imbalance:

> The role of the physician is based upon an imbalance of power
> and technical expertise favorable exclusively to the physician.
> The doctor exercises leverage through professional prestige,
> situational authority, and situational dependency of the patient
> (Cockerham, 1986:132).

Parsons' concept of the sick role assumes that medicine is an institution of social control of deviant behavior; he also explicitly presents this as functional (Parsons and Fox, 1958). Carlson, Zola, and Ehrenreich agree with this portrayal of medicine, although they see the social control function as less positive (Carlson, 1975; Zola, 1978; Ehrenreich, 1978). As Ehrenreich writes, "The doctor-patient relationship is a direct relationship of personal support, of domination—even, in some cases, of physical exploitation" (Ehrenreich, 1978:18). Freidson concurs in stating that entering the sick role entails entering a state of subordination in which the physician is professionally dominant (Freidson, 1970a:46). Furthermore, empirical data, such as that derived by Davis on the use of "functional" uncertainty in patient management, support this position (Davis, 1972).

Szasz and Hollender present a more diverse model of the doctor-patient relationship. They view three possible ways to structure the interaction: activity-passivity, guidance-cooperation, or mutual participation.

They assert that the three models are appropriate for different clinical applications (Szasz and Hollender, 1978:100–107). Their model of guidance-cooperation, which postulates a parent-child relationship, most closely approximates the conception common to the other authors. This may be because most physician-patient contacts studied by sociologists consist of acute, episodic illness.

In this form of the physician-patient relationship, the patient is seen as a relatively passive recipient of interventions suggested by the active physician, who possesses the many kinds of complex skills and inaccessible knowledge necessary to affect the desired change. Essentially, "the doctor knows best," and it is considered inappropriate for the patient to question the professional (Haug and Lavin, 1981).

On the other hand, Szasz and Hollender view the mutual participation model as most appropriate for chronic illness. This model also most closely approximates the model implicit in a holistic health paradigm. It appears to be more functional to have more egalitarian practitioner-patient relationships in holistic health, where the primary foci are on health and chronic disease concerns. Additionally, the upper middle class, well-educated clientele may be forcing this shift towards egalitarian relationships. An inherent dilemma remains: can the practitioner relate to the client as an equal when the physician continues to possess the predominance of available knowledge and skills?[2]

How Far Has the Authority Actually Shifted?

So far, I have focused on whether the status differential, where the physician maintains an imbalance of power within the relationship, has shifted towards a more egalitarian relationship. Some observers and advocates of the holistic model believe that an even more radical transformation has occurred, leaving the patient with the preponderance of power (Fink, 1976; Shapiro and Shapiro, 1979).

Has the shift in status differential moved to the point where the patient now maintains control within the relationship, or is it a partial shift where both parties collaborate? Donald Fink argues that in holistic practice the patient has assumed control within the interaction. After discussing the three models in Szasz and Hollender's classification, Fink contends that in holistic health there is movement to a fourth model where the balance of authority rests with the client:

> While many holistic health advocates have supported the notion
> of a mutual participation relationship, particularly in ambu-

latory care, another type of relationship is becoming more explicitly identified. In this relationship, the center of responsibility clearly lies within the "patient," who is indeed recognized as the healer. The provider or physician is the assistant, providing counsel and technical assistance; however, the responsibility and decision rests with the primary provider. In essence, this approach begins to recognize the patient as the primary provider" (Fink, 1976:25–26).

In Fink's fourth level, the client becomes the primary provider, with the health professional acting as a consultant. Shapiro and Shapiro support that view, arguing, "Ironically, we have come full circle to the notion of omnipotence in health care, only this time around it is not the physician who is omnipotent but the patient" (Shapiro and Shapiro, 1979:212).

In actual practice, it has *not* gone that far, despite the prevalent ideology and rhetoric. The interactions observed throughout the fieldwork, as well as the data from the interviews, consistently portrayed a different picture. The relationship at the behavioral, interactional level most closely approximates the mutual participation model.

Mutual Participation with Shared Authority

The interactions observed in this study fit a collegial, team relationship where the practitioner and patient share authority, and the participants approach equal status. Thus the process is one of partnership and collaboration. Still, the patient comes to the physician because of the latter's expertise, and the physician continues to maintain the imbalance of authority. The physician or nurse acts as an advisor, explaining the situation and presenting options. The patient gives input, and after joint discussion, a decision is made on the course of treatment. The data thus support both Mattson's and Gordon's contentions that staff and clients in holistic settings review the factors contributing to illness and jointly plan a program to mitigate those factors (Gordon, 1980b:473; Mattson, 1982:45–47).

The role of the physician is thus closer to that of an advisor or consultant, although it includes many components of more traditional physician roles, and of teacher and confidant as well. As one of the psychologists described the way he and the physicians he worked with relate with patients, "The doctor is really an advisor. He orchestrates, not directs, the health care." Both participants, however, take active roles in the interaction. In other words, neither the physician nor the patient maintains a passive stance while the other makes decisions. Although the physician often acts as a consultant, she or he also presents input as to the advantages of various decisions from her knowledge base, and most often those considerations are at least seriously considered, if not always followed.[3]

Although Dr. A often functions as a consultant, he actively directs and participates in decisions of both identifying problems and deciding on solutions. During the initial two visits to assess the problems and plan an approach, Dr. A has the definite bulk of authority within the relationship. Throughout the interactions, he speaks in a gentle, calm, and knowledgeable manner which could be described as authoritative, but not authoritarian. He asks for much more information about both the patient's health problems and other parts of his or her life. In other words, the diagnostic interview is much more heavily contextualized. Similarly, he elicits and encourages the patient's interpretations, perceptions, and experience. He explains far more, and he encourages more questions and input from the patient than the traditional model predicts. The addition of more information and substantial explanations and educational input also increase the actual time spent with patients in these two visits (an hour with Dr. A is scheduled for the initial visit; the second visit usually takes thirty to forty-five minutes; this does not include patient time spent with nurses and other staff before and after the meeting). At various points a more collegial mutual discussion occurs, where interaction flows up and back. Thus, although the relationship is more egalitarian, and involves a greater level of patient participation, Dr. A still directs the interaction.

The tone or texture of the interaction is never paternalistic, as it often is in more traditional medical settings. *Decreased levels of both formality and paternalism* seem to be key elements patients perceive in their definitions of a decreased status differential in the setting.

Patients have a more active participatory role in subsequent visits to the clinic, whether for treatment or for further assessment. Dr. A may dominate the initial interactions to a greater degree simply because of the amount of information he tries to obtain and impart. It also seems that with many patients it takes some time to socialize them into the new expectations. I observed many situations in the planning interviews where Dr. A tried encouraging patient input but patients appeared hesitant. The group of patients who already have been socialized to the new normative patterns seem to move into a more reciprocal relationship with Dr. A more quickly.

Is It a Consumerist Model?

Many of the descriptions of the shift in the physician-patient relationship depict the structure of interaction within the new model as consumerist (Fox, 1977; Reeder, 1978; Haug and Lavin, 1981; Haug and Lavin, 1983; Cassell, 1986). In this model, a client essentially negotiates with the physician in a businesslike relationship. Haug and Lavin's "bargaining model" is the most prominent example of this model in the literature. These authors equate the consumerist stance with a decreased status imbalance, or possibly a status reversal. As they write:

A consumerist stance clearly constitutes a challenge to physician authority. It focuses on purchaser's (patient's) rights and seller's (physician's) obligations, rather than on physician rights (to direct) and patient obligations (to follow directions). Caveat emptor, "let the buyer beware," rather than trust in the seller's goodwill, characterizes the transaction. In a consumer relationship, the seller has no particular authority; if anything, legitimated power rests in the buyer, who can make the decision to buy or not to buy, as he or she sees fit.

Patient consumerism, furthermore, implies at least a belief in a narrowed competence gap between the sick person and the care-giver. . . . In short, consumerism is incompatible with the sick-role model of the dependent patient and the doctor authority figure (Haug and Lavin, 1981:213).

Haug and Lavin found that 60 percent of their public sample indicated a propensity to adopt a consumerist perspective in medical encounters. Similarly, 81 percent of physicians adopted a consumerist perspective which questions physician authority (Haug and Lavin, 1981: 217). Yet when it came to self-reports of actual behavior, less than half of their public sample described behavior challenging physicians (ibid: 217). If the behavior was observed, rather than self-reported, the percentage within their sample would probably drop still lower.

Initially, it appears that the consumerist model Haug and Lavin portray corresponds to the shift discussed here. The primary point of agreement is the incorporation of a decreased status differential. However, there are some problems in their analysis. The first problem relates to their oversimplification of both models. First, Parsons' sick role never focused only on physician rights and patient obligations. Such an oversimplification ignores the reality of patients having both rights and responsibilities. They portray the patient as totally powerless in the traditional sick role. However, while the physician may have had the imbalance of power and authority, the patient's rights were always clearly spelled out. Patients have always had a variety of means of negotiating, certainly within the structure of private practice where switching physicians always remained an option.

Similarly, Haug and Lavin explicitly state that in the new consumer relationship, "the seller has no particular authority" (ibid.:213). However, when the "buyer" is acutely ill, the option of making a decision "to buy or not to buy" is much more complex. An additional argument is that the physician never had the total dominance portrayed by Haug and Lavin. Although patients do not customarily discuss it with their physicians, most patients have tried home remedies and often alternative practices and practitioners before, or at times simultaneously with, visits to allopathic physicians (Kronenfeld and Wasner, 1982; Svarstad, 1986). It also remains difficult to ascertain how much of the described shift to a "bargaining" model actually reflects that shift in participant behavior, and how much reflects a shift in sociologists' paradigms which more recently have come to incorporate views of interaction as always conflictual and negotiated.

Both physicians and patients have always had resources, and these have been formalized in the role expectations surrounding the sick role. Physicians in the new model continue to use their knowledge and experience, as well as their institutionalized role of gatekeeper, as resources. Similarly, patients continue to use their ability to seek help elsewhere as bargaining leverage. Patients also have the option of non-compliance, which all studies indicate is extremely high.

A second departure from Haug and Lavin's consumerist portrayal relates to their contention of the patient's mistrust within the transaction. Such mistrust of the physician's authority in general definitely existed and was frequently articulated by the group of patients I observed. However, no matter how cynical they were towards traditional medicine, they established a definite relationship of trust with these physicians. That subtle relationship of trust in the physician's goodwill continued to characterize the transaction as strongly as in any traditional medical encounter.[4]

This consumerist model also does not capture the entire essence of the relationship observed in the holistic settings, because it is *too commercialistic* and *devoid of affective involvement*. Thus it distorts the subjective experience of illness. The business stance, with its emphasis on efficient exchange, stands in opposition to the spiritual commitment of the majority of practitioners in the holistic model. Business transactions do not involve the nurturing, affective component so highly valued by both practitioners and patients. Another piece missing in the bargaining model is that the mutuality extends to a sharing of "selves." The two-way interaction is seen as profoundly affecting both parties in the relationship in a way not totally accounted for in the consumerist model.

One indication of these gaps in the consumerist model is that practitioners and patients in holistic settings rarely use the terms "provider" or "client." Health policy experts and social scientists are the ones who consistently utilize those terms. For example, Ardell describes the practitioner-patient relationship within the new model as consumerist. In a section titled, "It's Better to Be a Client than a Patient," he argues the advantages of the linguistics of a consumerist perspective (Ardell, 1977:53–54).

Initially, I tried ascertaining whether these practitioners saw patients as "patients" or "clients." It turned out that neither was correct; they saw "people" they worked with. Most of these providers and patients reacted somewhat negatively to the word "patient," but also reacted similarly to the word "client." Both the metaphors of "clients" and "people" connote more equal status within the relationship than the terms of a professional physician and a lay patient; however, there are subtle connotations distinguishing the two terms. The metaphor of the consumer/client denies affective involvement, and it also confines the interaction in terms of specificity as much as that of the patient.

There is another dimension of the relationship which clearly differentiates the holistic from the consumerist model. In discussing the status equality of patients and practitioners in holistic health, Mattson writes that medical knowledge in most healing systems is considered the sacred knowledge of a privileged group (Mattson, 1982:45–46). Fink also discusses the quasi-religious image of the medical provider in most societies (Fink, 1976:27).

This same type of process continues to have applicability to the practitioner-patient relationship in these holistic settings. It seems especially visible when Dr. A uses acupuncture. Although he encourages patients to read about traditional acupuncture as a way of eliciting their participation and involvement (the patient is therefore less passive and submissive), aspects of an esoteric and quasi-religious healing ability reside in him as the healer. Healing may come from within the patient; however, that healing process is triggered through the relationship with the healer. The subtle, implicit healing process between physician and patient remains an essential component of the relationship.

For instance, early during the field research, Dr. A expressed his concern about my observing him using acupuncture with patients. He described acupuncture as one of many holistic systems, the one that works for him. Part of the experience, according to him, is at deep inter-actional levels between the physician and patient. Similarly, a patient in the setting tried describing the differences in the way Dr. B related to her:

> Well. . . . it's not just a matter of medical knowledge, it's the way of relating. . . . he really cares! It's love! It's spiri-tual! . . . .But it's not just what you see, what he says. [The researcher agreed and asked how she could describe it. She thought for a while, and then said with much feeling:] . . . when most doctors touch you, it's just a physical touch . . . like that [mechanically, briefly touched one arm with the other hand]. When he does [pause], it's like a blessing.

These descriptions allude to the quasi-religious, healing components of the relationship which again distinguish it from a purely bargaining rela-tionship. The traditional allopathic medical model has had different sym-bols implying similar attributes.

In summary, the consumerist model differs dramatically from the enactment of the sick role in the holistic model. Charting the major di-mensions of the practitioner-patient relationship in the allopathic, the consumerist, and the holistic models can more dramatically highlight the similarities and differences between them (see Figure 3).

The grid demonstrates that, of the five variables discussed, the only correspondence between the consumerist and the holistic model is the decreased status differential. The provider-client relationship in the two models differs in the dimensions of affectivity, specificity, placebo sa-lience, and trust. Most of the other differences in the models have been discussed in the preceeding text; however, clarification of two dimensions is needed.

"Placebo salience" is a term designed to represent the sacred, quasi-religious dimension in the relationship between the healer and patient.[5] As discussed earlier in this chapter, that dimension markedly differs in the consumerist and holistic models. While the market orientation of the consumerist model rejects such notions, the holistic model specifically and explicitly values and highlights those components of the relationship.

The place of placebo salience in the traditional medical model is more ambiguous. From the perception of traditional physicians, elements of such sacred dimensions are excluded from the role, or are at best re-

The Practitioner-Patient Relationship in Three Models

	Status differential	Affective	Specific	Placebo salience	Trust
Allopathic	yes	no	yes	yes/no	yes
Consumerist	no	no	yes	no	no
Holistic	no	yes	no	yes	yes

Figure 3

sidual. Parsons also excludes this dimension from his sick role concept when discussing the pattern variable of specificity (Parsons, 1951). On the other hand, numerous social scientists and health professionals have alluded to the fact that this dimension has always been part of healing interactions (Balint, 1960; Frank, 1974; Fink, 1976; Moerman, 1980; Frank 1981; Mattson, 1982:45–46). The dimension of placebo salience could thus be seen as residual in the allopathic model (it exists, but should not), but active in the holistic model.

The dimension of trust in the physician's goodwill has also been excluded in the consumerist model. While trust remains in both the allopathic and holistic models, it may have subtle differences. Some would argue that trust in the allopathic model is necessary solely for instrumental purposes; in other words, that trust is functional to insure patient compliance. Others would argue that trust facilitates healing in the allopathic model as much as in the holistic, thus again making that component of trust residual. On the other hand, trust in the holistic model explicitly becomes the basis of healing. Another difference is that the trust within the allopathic relationship is more confined, due to the specificity of the relationship, while it extends throughout all aspects of the holistic physician-patient relationship.

Limits to Egalitarianism

Although this chapter clearly documents the decreased status differential between providers and patients in the holistic model, there are definite limits to the more egalitarian relationship. It must be remembered again that the changes flowing from the new model represent shifts along an existing continuum, not the establishment of a new one.

Both parties have power within the interaction, and movement occurs between the authority of the two participants. Still, if the patient refuses to heed any of the "advice" of the physician, one of the two parties would end the relationship. This is not so different than the situation in a traditional physician-patient relationship; however, there is a shift in the balance of authority and concomitant level of egalitarianism. This indicates that maintaining a certain degree of professionalism, both in terms of professional distance and status inequality, may be a necessary functional condition of practice, at least within this society.

The physician continues to maintain a considerable amount of professional prestige and status in the larger society, although it can be argued that this status will diminish somewhat during the next decade. The physician also continues to maintain some situational authority in medical care settings. This is most marked again in cases of acute illness. In episodes of acute illness, attention becomes focused back on the physiological level, thus giving the physician a more major imbalance of knowledge and skill. The patient then becomes more critically dependent on the physician's expertise.

Thus this critique does not deny that a shift has taken place in the relative authority of the physician and patient, but it is careful to view it as a shift rather than a total restructuring of the relationship. There is, in fact, an erosion of physician authority, but not as radical and total a shift as most authors maintain. Instead, it represents movement within a range, as in Szasz and Hollender's description.

Documenting the Extent of the Shift

Four types of empirical data which I secured document the shift towards a more egalitarian practitioner-patient relationship. These are: (1) verbal reports, (2) symbolic terms of reference and address, (3) access to information, and (4) sociolinguistic data. Taken together, the indications of the modified status differential within the relationship were very strong.

Verbal Reports of Participants

Both the ethnographic work and interviews uncovered numerous instances where both parties to the interactions verbalized directly or alluded to their perceptions of a more egalitarian relationship between physician, or other practitioner in the setting, and patient. It can be argued that this data is subjective and can represent a shift strictly at the ideological level rather than practice; however, when corroborated by additional data, it becomes more powerful.

In both Chapter IV and earlier portions of the present chapter, various quotes of practitioners and patients demonstrated their perceptions that there was a decreased status differential between the holistic practitioners and patients. Often the examples patients gave emphasized that the physician "really listens" or "really talks to you."

Auxiliary staff in Dr. A's office also commented on how differently he relates to both staff and patients, as compared to previous work settings. For example, Suzie, the office receptionist, contrasted the physicians in this office with physicians she worked with previously:

> Shall I give you something for your notes to tell you all about doctors? [The researcher joked back that it was just what she needed.] Not here, I mean. Dave and John are really different. [pause] I'm thinking how to say it right. . . . they [other doctors] keep themselves on a pedestal. I know . . . I've worked in some other offices.

During an informal interview with Ann, one of the body workers, she commented: "That's one other thing Dave does differently. He's never. . . . well patronizing to patients. He accepts them where they are. I think all of us here do."

A parallel set of comments by patients indicated that many of them used to view physicians "with awe" and were afraid to question them. As a woman with ulcerative colitis in her fifties stated, "I was much more meek and mild when I was young. Like with doctors. Now I don't look at doctors with awe. (laughing) In fact, it's more on the leery side . . . like 'you prove it to me.' "

Patients also frequently verbalized observations that Dr. A and B treated them with respect, or respected their knowledge. As Laurie, a twenty-nine-year-old patient who had seen Dave for several months, volunteered, "He's really human—not any of this 'I'm better than you.' " A parallel theme was practitioners' talk of their need for humility. Similarly, the physicians' ability to share with patients the limits of their knowledge made it more difficult for patients to see them in a lofty God-like status.

Patients also reported perceptions that these physicians and nurses did not convey the types of subtle moral judgments they had received from other practitioners. For instance, Fran, a jovial and very articulate woman in her late fifties, described past negative experiences with the traditional medical system:

I've run the gamut. I've had it with medical doctors! . . .I don't know what I'd have done if it hadn't been for my friend who told me about Dr. B.

She then related, accompanied by much laughing, that when she first had an appointment with Dr. B, she decided that she would tell him, "If you just see me as a middle age, overweight lady, let's just forget it right now!" She said that of course she never said it. When I asked why, she paused and said: "I didn't have to. The vibes were so different with him."

Another patient in the office made a similar comment: "That's another thing, I think when Dr. B looks at you, he doesn't see you as fat or short or anything. A lot of doctors prejudge on those things." Still another patient, Judy, described similar perceptions:

I feel like other doctors make a lot of judgments. I was depressed . . . really a wreck. You take out the food I'm allergic to, and now I'm a new person. He didn't judge me. [I asked whether other physicians had made judgments.] Yes, I think so. They didn't care. [I asked whether she could give me some examples] Well [long pause], I guess it was the aura or demeanor. Some of it's body language. They stand up a lot, and then they're looking down at you. Dr. B sits and talks to you. I saw most of the other doctors in the examining room without clothes. Here I saw him first sitting in his office with clothes on. Then he examined me, and then I could get dressed, and we talked in his office about what he's found. It's like there's some equality there that makes you feel you're not a specimen.

Another patient, Sue, was undergoing allergy testing in the same room, and both were talking to me. Sue interrupted Judy:

I can give you an example. . . . And then that same doctor would send me two page reports on what was wrong with me. In language only another doctor could understand. Even with my medical background, it didn't make sense. I was angry. These fellows would never do that. The more I try to think about it, the more I think of them sitting and really talking to me. Most physicians won't really talk to you. They just stand there in their white jacket!

Sue's metaphor of the white jacket was especially interesting because both physicians in this setting also wear white jackets. Yet, she still uses that symbol to denote the distant authoritarianism. Her strong reaction to receiving a technically-worded medical report was based on the meaning she ascribed to it, that it demonstrated the physician's superior position. Other patients, however, who welcome the traditional medical model, would interpret that report as evidence of the physician's exemplary qualifications, as well as the justification for his authority. So the same symbol that inspires faith and confidence in the traditional system comes to be interpreted as authoritarian here.

Self-reports also indicated that there were definite limits to how far the authority had shifted, again indicating that the modified status differential remained only a partial shift. For instance, Dr. B spoke of some of the conflicts he went through in trying to implement the holistic model after receiving his medical education in a highly research-oriented program:

I was really an idealist then. I believed I could just be a teacher, and I'd pick which approach will serve them best. Sometimes I'll tell them what the problem is and sometimes I'll tell them the conventional approach and what other approaches I see, and then I'll weight the alternatives. But then I realized I was taking the responsibility. Every time I would weigh the alternatives, I was really making the choice for them. . . .I'll sometimes have to tell them my procedures. Like if the patient has a plus three in situ (cervical pap results indicating early cancer), and there's an obvious medical treatment, I'm not even going to give her a choice of herbals or acupuncture. You may think that I don't believe in prescriptions, but I do.

[He then gave an example of a patient in his former practice who refused to take an antibiotic for a bladder infection that was backing up into his kidneys.] He wouldn't take the antibiotic, because he wouldn't put anything in his body that wasn't "natural." But that was the treatment of choice. So it got to the point where I had to repackage it for him. I explained that penicillin was a natural herbal, although it had come to be manufactured by pharmacological companies. That shows how hard I'll push to get what I believe in. At the end, he begged me for an antibiotic. I'll really push to get what I believe as much as any other physician.

That example not only demonstrates the limits of the shift in authority within the physician-patient relationship, but it exemplifies the type of remedial ideological work analyzed by Bennett Berger (Berger, 1981: 113–126). In this case, the physician was aware of the ideological work he needed to "repackage" a drug for a patient. In fact, his voice was full of self-condemnation as he described this.

Symbolic Terms of Reference and Address

The second category of data documenting the shift involved language use and symbols, particularly symbolic terms of reference and address. One of the major forms was the frequent use of first names for physicians, as well as for both other practitioners and patients in the settings. More notable than the consistent use of Dr. A and B's first names by staff was their use by many patients (this was not universal, however). Most staff seemed to feel more comfortable when addressed by first name in both front and back stage areas. For instance, I observed a patient in his thirties leave Dr. A's office, departing with a "See ya, Dave." Both verbal and nonverbal aspects of the fragment of the interaction I picked up revealed a more egalitarian, informal, collegial relationship than the more paternalistic traditional medical interaction.

A second indication provided by terms of reference involved the frequent use of "person" rather than "patient" or "client." During a formal interview with Mike, one of the clinic psychologists, I asked whether he saw his patients as patients or clients. He answered that he did not work with either patients or clients, he worked with people. At a later stage, when I analyzed the interview transcripts for the terms practitioners used while referring to patients, I was struck by the contrast in our terminology. For example, my questions and comments throughout the interviews continually used the word "patient," and they consistently used "person" or "someone I was working with." Both parties continued without noticing the other's use.[6]

Third, Dr. A's vocabulary use seemed to contribute to patients' perception of a decreased status differential. Although he frequently used medical and technical terms, he alternated such use with explanations using a more informal vocabulary. The use of medical terminology in the traditional physician-patient encounter has served as a symbolic reminder of the physician's status and authority within the relationship.

A closely related tactic was the frequent use of low-keyed humor. For instance, in this segment of interaction Dr. A had just finished inserting acupuncture needles:

Pt: You didn't put any in my chest? [questioningly]

Dr: This is different than last time. [pause] This one is from a classical book . . . 3000 years old.

Pt: Good . . . I want an old one . . . with lots of power.

Dr: This one has lots of power [gently, smiling]

Pt: Good [smiling]

Dr: Now . . . you're a certified porcupine. [both laugh quietly]

The same use of informal, at times slang, vocabulary combined with humor is also apparent in this segment of another interaction, where the patient had just jumped noticeably after the insertion of an acupuncture needle:

Dr: Tender one?

Pt: I haven't experienced one like that for a long time. [smiling]

Dr: I've been going too easy on you, huh? [both smile] Okay, breathe in and let it out slowly. [inserts needle] Feel that one?

Pt: Yes, but not as painful as the other. I don't mean that I want you to keep trying 'til it is! [both laughing]

Dr: That's not the idea. [feels both pulses again]

This type of use of humor, along with the accompanying shift from medical terminology to a casual, everyday vocabulary contributes to the perceptions of status equality.

While some of the language use and symbols demonstrated a shift towards a more egalitarian relationship between physician and patient, other instances of the language used demonstrate that ideas from the traditional medical model still maintain a pervasive hold. For instance, when I asked Nurse A how a patient was responding to a still controversial procedure, she replied that the patient had shown little improvement, "so Dr. A decided" he won't continue it at home. There were many such subtle indications that decisions were not totally mutual, despite the patient's input. Again, this demonstrates that the changes in authority only represent a shift, rather than a radical relocation of the locus of power.

Access to Information

Both providers and patient/clients shifted their expectations to wanting more equal access to information than would be expected in most traditional medical settings. The patient had freer and wider access to both general and specific medical information in the setting. First, many patients in the clinic came with considerably more knowledge about various aspects of health and illness than one would expect. Second, patients sought out from the practitioners information and rationale behind explanations frequently. Third, all the practitioners attempted to provide information, explanations, and rationale to clients on a continuing basis.

Not only did patients bring and receive more information in terms of explanations, but results of a variety of tests, whether blood pressure readings or the results of laboratory tests, were routinely made available and explained to patients. The one exception I noted was the foods being tested during allergy testing (the nurse doing the procedure explained that she could not reveal which foods she was testing until the reactions were noted, to eliminate any possible effects of expectation).

The instances where I observed three patients reading their medical charts were the most noticeable examples of increased information access (patient access to medical records remains a definite taboo in traditional allopathic settings). One patient, in describing what she valued in this clinic, gave me the example of viewing her chart:

> On my second visit Rose showed me my chart. . . . I want to be treated as what I am. . . . an intelligent, astute person. I hate it when a nurse takes your temperature and blood pressure, and you ask what it is and she just tells you she can't tell and you'd better ask the doctor! It gets me furious! Treating me like a child. It's like a parent-child relationship, and I resent that. That's not for me!

Similarly, during an allergy testing session, when Gail left the room, one patient, and then the other, picked up their charts and were reading them when she returned. She calmly answered their questions, and appeared to see no problem in their access to the information.

One additional sign of more equal access to information was that both parties to the interaction have access to a portion of the necessary information. Although it was assumed that physicians and nurses had greater knowledge at the physiological level, it was also assumed that patients had more knowledge about their patterns of daily living, their resources, their needs and priorities, and the latter was valued as being more closely equivalent to the physiological information. Thus the patient's perspective and experience of a problem was seen as more important in the setting.

Sociolinguistic Data (Micro-Level)

Additional data at the interactional and sociolinguistic level further documented the shift. The patient's increased status and authority within the interaction was reflected in a less submissive stance. *Patients* observed in the setting *more frequently initiated, questioned, expressed feelings, and contradicted physicians* during interactions than one would expect in a traditional allopathic medical setting.[7]

This was more noticeable in patients who had seen Dr. A or Dr. G over a period of time, as opposed to patients who were new in the setting. Perhaps they initially tested carefully, and on finding that more assertive, participatory responses were not only tolerated but welcomed, increased their active participation.

During instances where patients initiated, questioned, or contradicted, the input was responded to as though it came from a status equal. In other words, patients were not "put down," "given guilt trips," or subtly made to feel that they had violated any of the expectations in the setting. The tone of such interactional exchanges most closely approximated that between a physician and a consultant physician discussing a medical problem. Each side might legitimately disagree because of their difference in perspective, and lack of knowledge on the part of one would be seen as expected because of his limited area of expertise.

For example a male in his late thirties with multiple sclerosis was waiting in Dr. A's office. When Dr. A entered, Jack immediately asked him a question before he even had a chance to sit down: "Do beets color your urine?" Rather than in any way indicate annoyance or impatience with what is frequently considered a breach, Dr. A nodded affirmatively and smiled while saying, "You found that out. . . . Where are you in the food testing now?" Jack described where he was, showing Dr. A the records he'd been keeping.

An example of a patient questioning occurred when Dr. A brought up a new compound he wanted that patient to try for multiple sclerosis. He asked Jack if he had heard of it:

Pt: No . . .

Dr: It's a new compound that's in the process of testing. It provides building blocks for myelin sheaths . . . this particular compound is a precursor to prostaglandin. It's actually primrose oil.

Pt: I never heard of it.

Dr: It's definitely something I want you to be on for six months. It's very expensive—but it's probably the most important supplement for you—the one that will directly affect the MS.

Pt: *Do you have any of the research reports?*

Dr: No. The research won't be complete for years. But, since it doesn't have any negative side effects, we should try it now. [pause] Do you have any questions?

When a patient introduced a new subject, the physicians and nurses almost uniformly followed through on that concern. During one interaction with a man in his thirties, the patient switched topics to his loneliness. Dr. A discussed it briefly, then he switched away to the treatment plan and applied acupuncture. Two or three minutes later, Dr. A returned to the loneliness. Dr. A maintained control of the topic; yet, he followed through on the patient's concern.

Dr: Let's take you off the minerals. How long have you been on them?

Pt: Two months.

Dr: Two months. You shouldn't need any more. If you get too much more, you'll start to mineralize. [both laughing]

Pt: I noticed changes when I had some house guests. I felt better, but then my friend left and it really made a difference.

Dr: I know [sympathetically]. You need to see it as a blessing though—you knew it wouldn't work.

Pt: It's hard when someone is living with you for a long time and leaves. I don't mean the sleeping together part. It helped having my friend and this older relative over. Just having someone there in the morning is what I miss. I'm looking for a roommate now, so that should help.

Dr: [nods] It could be your system's too acid. We should get you to eat more alkaline foods . . . like salad and fresh vegetables. [feels patient's pulses and inserts acupuncture needles] It sounds like you're still feeling very lonely. Do you feel you have a way of dealing with this?

Pt: [nods yes]

Dr: Because this is the problem keeping you at this plateau.

Pt: [nods again]

Dr: If you don't, we have people here you can talk to.

Pt: [this time patient shakes his head indicating a no answer]

That type of switching away from a patient concern by the physician is common in traditional medical interactions; however, it is rare in this setting. Even in that example, Dr. A later returned to the patient's topic.

An extension of this use of patient authority included sporadic instances where patients initiated changes in medical treatment regimes before consulting with the physician. A woman taking prescription medication for a thyroid problem came in for a six-week check. She reported that she had "upped" her dose of thyroid medication, giving her rationale and stating that her skin was not so dry now. Dr. A asked detailed questions about symptoms, and finally decided to try maintaining the dosage for several more weeks, before cutting it down. I was struck by the fact that most patients would not so casually bring up a self-initiated dosage change.

Patients' verbal accounts of their health problems and progress were not only sought out, but were taken very seriously. This emphasis in holistic health settings on the *validity of the patient's existential experience* and definitions is another indication of the shift in the power balance within the relationship. This was also consistently carried out in practice. Even when the physician clearly controlled the interaction, he frequently used eye contact, asked whether the patient understood or had any questions, and paused so that the patient could bring concerns up. For example, after telling a patient about dietary modifications he needed, Dr. A asked, "Will that be too much of an adjustment?"

Another type of interaction at the micro-sociological level which indicated a more egalitarian relationship was the situation where patients were "noncompliant." As Mattson observes, it remains common for patients in the traditional allopathic medical system to hide their use of alternative or marginal systems from their physician (Mattson, 1982:33). I observed several instances where patients appeared to be extremely open about instances of their non-compliance or about alternative healing techniques they were using simultaneously. When I commented on this to Dr. A at one point, he told me that most patients try home remedies and alternative techniques; however, he believes his patients are comfortable bringing that up with him and knowing he will not condemn it.

A last indication of the decreased status differential at the interactional level was the more frequent two-way sharing of personal information. Although this was not frequent, I observed more in this setting than one would expect from more traditional physicians. One example of this was the two-way sharing of information about family. Similarly, in an instance where an engineer, Bob, was describing how much stress he was experiencing, he mentioned that he had been flying a great deal on business. Dave responded by saying that he'd just flown to two out-of-town conferences, and he spoke of how disorienting it was.

Negotiation of Differences

Any description of the decreased status differential in the physician-patient relationship must also examine how differences are negotiated within the interaction. Clinical situations where the physician and patient disagree provide an opportunity to observe how egalitarian the division of authority and control within the relationship actually is. Because the practitioners in the holistic clinic are attempting to combine and integrate the traditional allopathic medical model with the newer holistic model, there are many points of potential conflict in implementation.

When the differences between the practitioner and patient are major, the mismatch may cause the patient to leave and seek health care in a different setting. Dr. A felt that a small number of patients who come to the holistic clinic define health and illness concerns so differently that they don't return.

Two situations were occasionally visible to a researcher observing clinic interactions. In the first, the physician was more holistic in his orientation than the patient. In the second, this situation was reversed, so that the physician was more traditional than the patient. This section will briefly sketch an overview of how such negotiations are handled. Then a case study of a single interaction of the primary physician in the setting with a patient will be presented to more clearly portray the process of negotiation.

Case 1: Physician More Holistic

In this situation the physician is more holistic in orientation than the patient he's working with. The worst case scenario would postulate a client seeking out a holistic practitioner for cure (for example, a broken finger), and the practitioner remaining more concerned with health promotion. No conflicts even approaching this magnitude occurred in the setting; however, there were situations where patients remained in a fairly traditional medical orientation. In almost all cases of this type, the practitioner maintained the traditional symbols, language, and practices the patient was comfortable with. Slowly and gently they attempted to socialize the patient into the new model. Very little pressure was applied to these patients.

This situation occured fairly frequently in Dr. A's practice. Although the majority of patients sought out that particular clinic because they already had a commitment to a more preventive, holistic approach to health care, a fairly large group of patients came after recommendations from friends who told them that, at this office, their health problem or chronic condition could be helped. Dr. A was extremely sensitive to the discomfort such patients might feel about trying a new type of system, and he moved cautiously, maintaining more traditional interactional forms.

For instance, he introduced himself as "Dr. A," and used a slightly more formal approach as opposed to the more casual interactional style he used with patients he knew were comfortable with it. This more formal style contrasted markedly with that he assumed with patients who had been regular clients over time, or newer patients whom he sensed were already committed to the holistic model. His language forms and the areas Dr. A focused on also differed to varying degrees in his interactions with the two groups of patients.

For example, while applying acupuncture on a man in his late thirties (this man was an engineer whose appearance in terms of haircut and suit appeared very "straight"), he began to discuss how this man had been reacting to the change in seasons. They discussed this in terminology of traditional acupuncture, using concepts such as fire and water that he did not use with most patients. This patient had not only seen him several times, but he had been treated with traditional acupuncture in the past and had sought Dr. A out because of his expertise in this area.

A similar way of handling this situation was apparent in Dr. G's office. He rarely appeared frustrated with patients who were not interested in preventive approaches or did not want to make the actual decisions about the form of treatment. He attempted to assess their readiness, and then related with them in terms of the style they appeared comfortable with. One example in that office was that Dr. G routinely offered a mirror for patients to watch the oral cavity while he explained problems and treatment rationale. When patients did not want to use the mirror, he usually went into much shorter explanations of the problem. He explained to me that those patients did not want to know everything that was going on. He explicitly described dealing with those patients more traditionally, both by being more directive and explaining less. He said that he would then occasionally try introducing preventive and teaching issues to assess their readiness in the future.

Thus some patients do have the trouble Fink (1976:27) describes with accepting the authority shift (this is rarer in Mar Vista Clinic, however, as most patients seek out this practice setting for its holistic approach). These patients want to maintain the physician as authority. Both practitioners expressed to me feelings that these patients needed to "be where they were at." In these cases, Drs. A and G were slightly more structured and directive, and less collegial and collaborative, than with the largest group of patients. Still, even then, their behavior was slightly less directive and more egalitarian than one would expect in traditional medical settings.

Case 2: Physician More Traditional

In this situation, a patient was seen who was "further out" holistically than the providers. The worst case scenario would postulate a client coming for a general health promotion program, when the practitioner was concerned with an acute medical problem such as extremely elevated blood pressure or a broken finger. I saw no instances approximating such extremes with Dr. A, Dr. B, or Dr. G; however, less major variations which required some negotiation occurred occasionally. Most patients who were committed to an extreme version of holistic health would not choose these practitioners.

I observed only one instance in Dr. G's dental office that both he and I defined as extreme (none of this magnitude were observed during observations at Mar Vista Clinic). A patient was referred by another local holistic health clinic. He refused diagnostic x-rays, because they "cause cancer." This young man also talked about waiting for his hair and several teeth he had lost to "grow back" through visualization exercises. Dr.

G very gently explained the level of radiation dosage in the x-ray and the reason having an x-ray would help him assess the problem. When this patient remained firm, Dr. G dropped it and continued to do the work based on the patient's priorities. This man had very limited funds, and his priority was to do the work that made the most cosmetic difference. Dr. G was concerned with work that would prevent further damage to several teeth in danger of being lost. He tried explaining the long term effects. The patient, equally calmly, yet assertively, explained that he wanted the cosmetic work. Finally, Dr. G did the work the patient had requested, with only minor work that he saw as priority. He appeared calm, and did not continue any form of pressure; however, later he described being extremely frustrated.[8]

A Case Study of Negotiation

The examples given throughout this chapter and Chapter IV present various aspects of the interactions occurring between providers and patients. In this section I present lengthier portions of one interaction to give more of the flavor of the manner in which such interactions proceed. It illustrates the processes of mutual participation, collaboration, and negotiation that typically take place in these settings.

George was a man in his late thirties. He had been seeing Dr. A for several months, and had come for a scheduled acupuncture treatment. At two points, George and Dr. A disagreed on the approach to a particular problem. Dr. A presented information and the rationale for his choice. When George did not agree, Dr. A did not place any moral pressure on him, but looked for the best approach that would remain within George's framework. Dr. A's use of humor and his gentle, warm manner were also typical of his interactions with patients.

When Dr. A and I came in, George, who was lying supine on an acupuncture table, commented that he felt cold. Dave, as George called him, said, "Let's see if we can warm it up a little." He often begins with this type of light joking or social comments.

Dr: Let's see if we can warm it up a little. [laughing]

Pt: [smiling] Yeah, warm up the needles.

Dr: [smiling] No . . . you and the energy. How's Joan?

[After talking about George's wife, Dr. A asks questions like, "How's spring treating you?" George brings up a pain in his knee that had persisted for two weeks after doing a yoga exercise. Dr. A asks questions about duration, intensity, etc., then asks, "Do you run into stairs often?" These types of joking comments are frequently interspersed in the interaction, so that much joking, smiling, laughing is apparent.]

Dr: How's your energy been?

Pt: Okay . . . but I still get tired after lunch.

Dr: Weekends too . . . or only when you're working? [It occurs on work days; they discuss the importance of environment, feelings about work]

Dr: How 'bout enough exercise? And your diet?

Pt: My weight's finally stabilized. [George is extremely thin]

Dr: Have you gained more than five pounds?

Pt: No . . . about that . . . five.

[Other questions Dave asks are, "Any abdominal problems?" "The kids are all doing okay?" Then George brings up a knee problem, just before Dave started the acupuncture.]

Pt: Can you work on the knee today too?

Dr: Are you doing anything for it at home?

Pt: Yeah . . . I'm using that DMSO.

Dr: I'm not really impressed with that [said very low-key, matter-of-factly; no nonverbal condemnation]

Pt: No?

Dr: Not really.

Pt: [after pause] It really seemed to work for me.

Dr: What preparation are you using? Is it 100 percent pure?

Pt: 99.9 percent pure—so it must be okay.

Dr: Uhhh . . . not really. I worry that many of the preparations use heavy metals as binders. It's not regulated since it's not for use on humans. If you're going to use it, get the ointment we have here or make sure it's 100 percent DMSO.

Pt: You're not too impressed, huh?

Dr: Not really. If you tell me it works on your knee, fine, but I haven't seen a lot of impressive results here.

Pt: Can it hurt?

Dr: It shouldn't—as long as it doesn't have any heavy metals added. [pause] Take a breath in and out now.

Pt: [huge breath in and out]

Dr: That was a big one! [laughing] I have you worried.

Pt: It didn't hurt as much as I thought it would.

Dr: As long as you don't move . . . it's hard to hit a moving patient. [both smiling] [Inserted another needle, and George reacts more nonverbally than any patient I'd watched] Still with me?

Pt: [laughing] Yeaaaah!

Dr: June's going to think this hurts! [all three of us laughing]

Pt: Yeaaaaah.

Dr: This point's going to bite a little.

Pt: [Contracting legs up and grimacing when needle is inserted] Ahhhh! [I've never seen a patient who evidenced discomfort of this magnitude, but Dr. A treats his reaction very matter-of-factly]

Dr: That one is for the after lunch thing. [fatigue] I only have two requirements—that you don't move and that you don't kick me. [laughing] [checking knee again, palpating and asking whether George experiences pain, and putting it through several motions] You probably pulled this ligament here [shows him where and uses the medical term]. It's fairly stable . . . minor. I'd use a castor oil pack for a week. An hour a night.

Pt: Can I move around on it?

Dr: Sure.

Pt: What about something for this area (points to rough area of skin on his shin)?

Dr: What have you tried?

Pt: Aloe.

Dr: You could use homeopathic ointment. But medically the best thing to clear that up is a cortisone cream.

Pt: That's too dangerous. I'd rather live with it than mess with that kind of thing.

Dr: Well, you can use some zinc oxide. Try to moisturize it first. You have tried aloe?

Pt: I've done all that stuff.

Dr: Okay. I think you can go for four more weeks.

Several differences from interaction in a traditional allopathic setting are visible in this interaction. First, Dr. A is aware that people use home remedies. He wants to know what George has already tried, for both the knee and the skin problem. He knows that many of his patients use various alternative remedies, and he has fairly accurate knowledge of which patients use what system most, and what approaches they're receptive to, as he did in this situation. When a patient uses something like DMSO, he or she feels comfortable bringing it up. Even when Dr. A does not feel it is therapeutically effective, he does not subtly put the patient down, making him or her feel either guilty or unknowledgeable. He reacts in a way which indicates he is aware of the treatment, tried it with some receptive patients, and has not seen much response. He gives information, but he leaves the choice up to the patient. George feels comfortable enough to push Dave on his answer that he was unimpressed with DMSO. So the patient is more apt to share first-step home and marginal remedies.

Another example of negotiation is where Dave tells George what the treatment of choice is for the skin problem. George does not want to use even a local steroid, so Dr. A gives him alternatives, although acknowledging that they are not the most effective. Again, he acts as a consultant to the patient, and he supports the patient in his choice.

It could be argued that in this interaction, the patient ultimately maintained complete control. That could also be claimed in traditional medical encounters, where the patient may appear submissive in the office, but may never follow the prescribed treatment plan. A comparative study of the degree of noncompliance would be necessary to locate more exact magnitudes of control by patients in both types of settings. Similarly, because the physician structured so much of the direction of the interaction, it could be argued that he maintained near complete control.

Actually, although authority shifted during various parts of the interaction, it was closely balanced. Dr. A maintained a position as organizer or leader of the interaction. He did more initiating and controlled the turn-taking within the interaction, although both sides actively initiated areas of concern.

Summary

The ethnographic data indicate that the shift in authority toward a more egalitarian relationship between physician and patient extends beyond ideology. The everyday behavioral interactions between providers and clients in these holistic settings are more egalitarian than in traditional medical encounters, and they more closely approximate a cooperative interaction between two parties with nearly equal status. Decreased levels of both formality and paternalism are major components of patients' perceptions of the decreased status differential.

The shifts in the practitioner-patient relationship extend to the empirical level, so that the modified relationship is more affective, less specific in focus, and more egalitarian. The two parties share control and authority, with each having the balance of authority in different parts of the relationship. Still, it appears that the physician retains the control required to structure and lead interactions. Even in instances where the patient actively negotiates, the patient does not direct the relationship. Thus, despite the loosening of formal constraints, the relationship still falls back on an expert-client differential. In other words, the modification towards a more egalitarian relationship represents a shift, rather than a radical restructuring of the authority basis of the relationship.

Despite the close approximation to the consumerist model of the physician-patient relationship in terms of the decreased status differential, the interactions seen in these settings departed from that model in several significant ways. The physician-patient relationship in this setting was characterized by continuing trust of these practitioners on the part of patients, even when their faith in the taken for granted goodwill of other physicians and the medical system as a whole had been seriously eroded. The expressive, affective components of the interactions also go beyond the expectations of both parties in the more commercialistic consumer model. In fact, of the five variables of the physician-patient relationship analyzed, the only correspondence between the consumerist and the holistic model is the decreased status differential. The provider-client relationship in the two models differs in the dimensions of affectivity, specificity, placebo salience, and trust. The question raised by this finding is whether these holistic practices differ significantly from a more consumerist type of practice evolving simultaneously with the holistic type of practice, or whether the pure form of the consumerist model is actually carried out at the behavioral level in clinical settings.

The decreased status differential within the relationship closely overlaps with the shifts of responsibility in the new holistic model. Neither can be fully understood without examining the other. I will now begin to analyze those modifications in the attribution of responsibility for health, illness, and cure.

6

The Shift in Attribution of Responsibility

This chapter analyzes the complexities of the shift in the attribution of responsibility to the individual for health, illness, and cure. The problematic issues of absolution, stigma, and responsibility have already been raised in an exploratory fashion. Here the analysis will be extended, contrasting the numerous ambiguities and paradoxes between ideological pronouncements and actual behavior in clinical encounters.

The assumptions of illness as stigma and the attribution of blame are subtle and problematic in both the medical and holistic health models. Siegler and Osmond contrast two basic models dealing with this issue. In the traditional medical model, illness is assumed to derive from natural causes. In the moral model, however, the sick person is seen as "bad" or the process of becoming ill is blamed on his "badness," thus assuming a moral component of illness (Siegler and Osmond, 1973:42). Mechanic also specifies the two most influential perspectives used in evaluations of deviant behavior as the "health-illness" and "goodness-badness" perspectives (Mechanic, 1968:49). Mechanic then elaborates the perspective of the medical model:

> Most physical illnesses (deviations from medically derived standards of normal functioning) fall within definitions of "sickness" rather than "badness." We rarely hold people responsible or accountable for their physical illness, and although persons might not always take necessary precautions to avoid the risks of illness, we assume that illness is an event that happens to people and that it is not motivated (ibid:50).

Lee concurs from the policy perspective, writing that for scientific, Western medicine, illness results from mechanical failure rather than any "spiritual shortcoming" (Lee, 1976:23).[1]

Thus medicine exempts the individual from responsibility. The consequence of this exemption from responsibility is that the ill are subject to treatment rather than punishment.

Despite an initial acquiescence to this perspective, much of the literature presents a more problematic picture. Siegler and Osmond go on to assert that both the medical and moral views always seem to be present "even in illnesses where one would expect the medical model to hold clear title" (Siegler and Osmond, 1973:42). As mentioned earlier, they also interpret Parsons' model as implying that the patient is not in the sick role until he or she is convinced the source of the illness lies outside of the self (ibid:42). If this is the case, there is theoretically no sick role in holistic health, since the client does view his or her illness as integral to the self.

Parsons is usually interpreted as describing the sick role as exempting the patient from causal responsibility. Yet he explicitly states, "For it (illness) is an escape from the pressures of ordinary life" (Parsons and Fox, 1958:236). For Parsons, the benefits of secondary gains were constituted at the unconscious level.

Both Davis and Zola look at the moral implications and accompanying guilt more explicitly. Fred Davis, in his study of family coping following childhood polio, noted a common guilt-prone interpretive pattern in both the children's and parents' evaluation of their responsibility for the illness. On the other hand, the medical practitioners he observed attempted to assuage the families' feelings of guilt and responsibility, bringing them closer to the interpretations congruent with the medical model (Davis, 1962).

A decade ago, Zola argued that the issue of individual responsibility was reasserting itself within the medical model:

[It is] . . . not clear that the issues of morality and individual responsibility have been fully banished from the etiological scene itself. At the same time as the label "illness" is being used to attribute "diminished responsibility" to a whole host of phenomena, the issue of "personal responsibility" seems to be re-emerging within medicine itself. . . . [The concepts of stress and psychosomatics] bring man, not bacteria, to the cen-

ter of the stage and lead thereby to a re-examination of the
individual's role in his own demise, disability and even recovery (Zola, 1978:84).

Crawford also raised that concern, linking individual blame and a "strident moralism" to the burgeoning health emphasis (Crawford, 1980: 378–398).

This same notion of personal responsibility, so central to the holistic health movement, then explicitly holds the patient responsible for his or her illness. Thus, within the holistic health model, illness has the potential of being criminal and immoral. In other words, illness could again constitute a deviant act for which people would be held accountable.[2] This potential for moral condemnation may be neutralized by the opposing view of illness as a potential for growth; however, it is difficult to predict the social and psychological consequences of these views.

For example, many patients reject Carl Simonton's treatment of cancer through guided imagery because of the direct implication that they bear responsibility for the development of the disease. On the other hand, devotees of this approach see the responsibility as accompanied by the power to exert control over the disease. As Scarf writes, however, "People who are told they are responsible for their own cancers—and who do not succeed in curing them—may be devastated by guilt" (Scarf, 1980:45). Furthermore, on a more general level, society may withdraw resources for the ill if they are seen as actively responsible for their disease. This raises questions of why so many people are willing to accept that self-blame.

Consequences of This Shift

The shift in the attribution of responsibility in the holistic model has major potential implications at the institutional, interactional, and individual levels. While the primary focus of this research remains at the interactional and individual levels, it is important to outline the major impact of such a shift at the broader societal level as well. This section presents the anticipated consequences. Although some of these processes are already clearly evident, others remain speculative at this point. In later portions of the chapter, data will be presented to document those consequences which are already visible.

Institutional Level

The consequences of the shift in attribution of responsibility for illness at the institutional level have important implications for national health policy. These can be considered to fall under a rubric of "blame the victim." Society may withdraw a variety of resources for the ill if they come to be seen as actively responsible for their disease state.

The first set of related consequences revolve around economics. The single major projected consequence of such a shift is cost containment. Advocates of a self-responsibility approach continually bring up the projected savings that can accrue from a more preventive health approach emphasizing individual responsibility for lifestyle changes.

Beyond the generally perceived benefits of cost containment, other derivative effects of the responsibility shift are potentially more dangerous. If the public comes to view cancer and other illnesses as self-caused, it may lead to moral indignation towards the ill. Economic overtones combine with the shift in moral judgment to create a feeling of "Why should I pay for someone else's disease?"

Institutional incentives, such as those making up the insurance structure, could be changed to reward what has become defined as "responsible" behavior. Thus, for example, non-smokers would be eligible for lower health insurance rates (several insurance companies already offer this and similar incentives).[3] In time an elaborate structure may develop around a self-responsibility paradigm, so that each insurance applicant might be rated on a variety of categories including smoking, nutritional patterns, exercise, and stress level. This might also include a personality profile measuring coping resources, social support, and possibly "mental health status." Such a direction involves a general societal reconstitution of concrete support at an economic level, and reflects an underlying punitive approach rather than one aimed at treatment.

This argument, which is based on the shift in personal responsibility for one's health/illness state, can be further extended as a rationale to withdraw medical resources to poverty groups. The client comes to be seen as bearing responsibility for his or her own decisions, and thus resultant health, even in ghetto areas. This same process would apply to coal miners and similar groups in occupations with high levels of occupationally induced illness. Ironically, these ideologically motivated cost containment measures, when applied to preventive health, would further undermine this group's resources for taking responsibility for their health (one example is the recent cuts in federal funding for immunization programs for children).

Beyond the economic realm, this type of withdrawal of support is beginning to appear in other institutional settings. For instance, health care workers could increasingly feel that efforts in behalf of patients they see as inflicting illness on themselves, thus "choosing their illness," do not merit the same attempts in their behalf. Thus the differential quality of treatment offered to groups such as alcoholics on moral grounds in the past could be extended to broader categories (Sudnow, 1967; Roth, 1972). For instance, patients with lung cancer who smoked might evoke responses of "Why should I try to help him when he chose this?" Cardiac patients would be judged similarly because of the role of stress, nutrition, and exercise as contributing factors in the disease process. The worst case scenario derives from the total acceptance of "self-responsibility": all illness becomes a moral choice with intent, and health providers no longer have a responsibility to provide compassionate care.

If the public comes to view cancer and other illnesses as self-caused, it may lead to generalized moral indignation, or at least therapeutic indifference, towards the ill. Those who do not exercise regularly or meditate may come to be seen and subtly criticized as morally inferior. Both lifestyle and illness become culpable, and processes of societal censure and institutional control become justified.

In this process, self-responsibility can assume such a pivotal role that other etiological influences are ignored. By ignoring the cultural role in creating lifestyle itself, as well as illness, society itself is "let off the hook." For example, patterns of food consumption are heavily determined by childhood experiences and the symbolic meanings that come to be attached to specific foods, as well as to the process of eating itself. Other effects on nutritional patterns over the course of one's life include the role of advertising and the mass media, peer influence, and the more general effects of culture and fads. There is a similar cultural role in an individual's decision to begin smoking. If a high stress level makes it even more difficult for an individual to modify food or smoking patterns, is that stress level also a "simple individual choice," or do societal factors contribute?

It can be similarly argued that there is a major cultural role in creating illness itself. Beyond the sociologists and health policy experts who see society itself, advanced technology, or the capitalist system as the root cause of illness, many apolitical experts from a variety of fields increasingly stress the role of pollution and occupational hazards as contributory to a multitude of disease states.

The medical model itself argues that many diseases have at least a partial genetic etiologic component. Two people with sedentary lifestyles, both under constant stress and eating high cholesteral diets, are under differential risks for contracting coronary disease based on their hereditary disposition.

The shift in attribution of responsibility, by negating these contributing causes, would ultimately withdraw support for research and intervention programs aimed at decreasing the effects of these risks. While this strategy would initially reduce costs, it would ultimately increase the expenditure on disease which might have been alleviated by implementing preventive approaches.

Interactional Level

Since the interactional level is the primary focus of the remainder of the chapter, the projected consequences of a shift in responsibility will be only briefly outlined here. These themes will be more fully developed and critically analyzed through the empirical data, which is presented further in this chapter.

The most important interactional consequence is that physicians would no longer absolve patients from guilt and blame. Two additional interactional modifications derive directly from this shift. First, the physician-patient interaction becomes more equal with the shift in responsibility. Second, the physician is no longer as responsible or accountable for the changes taking place in the patient's health-illness status. This absolves the physician from responsibility when a patient's condition deteriorates. The obvious inherent danger here is that of creating a cover for medical incompetence, with weakened controls over the quality of care.

Beyond the consequences affecting provider-patient interactions, the shift has an impact on the everyday encounters the ill have outside of health care settings. Family members, friends, co-workers, and even strangers may withdraw emotional and social support from patients because of the moral censure implicated in the shift towards personal responsibility. Interactions characterized to various degrees by stigma and labelling may become normative in physical illness, just as they were in mental illness in the past (and sometimes still continue to be). The visibility of many forms of illness and of lifestyle "failures" (examples include obesity and smoking) invite processes similar to those studied between handicapped and "normals."

Individual Level

The major personal consequence of a shift in responsibility is that the individual experiences guilt for becoming sick, or for an inability to get well. Eventually everyone must die; however, death itself could come to be seen as a personal moral failure. The individual may come to feel responsible even for problems beyond his or her control, such as in an obvious case involving environmental pollutants and cancer.

Beyond the case of diagnosed illness, the individual is likely to experience guilt for lifestyle patterns currently defined as less than optimal, despite the cultural role in establishing and maintaining these patterns. The person who has the knowledge of "healthy" behaviors, yet is unable to change (or does not choose to, according to the self-responsibility paradigm), may be overwhelmed with guilt, shame, and self condemnation for his or her moral failure. Thus the individual may experience a sense of personal moral failure based on either illness or lifestyle.

There are many instances where a model postulating individual control and responsibility puts the individual in a double bind. For example, an executive working under highly stressful conditions might drink, smoke, or overeat to cope with the stress; in this case, the person is seen as "choosing" self-destructive, illness producing behaviors. On the other hand, if that person "chooses" to give up smoking, he or she may be exposing himself or herself to even higher levels of maladaptive stress. If that individual chooses a third alternative, to quit the job for a less stressful position, he or she might increase his or her familial stress level due to the resultant drastic cut in salary. Although these are simplistic scenarios, they show how much more complex and culturally embedded "personal choice" is than this model postulates.

A further danger deriving from the responsibility shift postulates that patients may not have enough knowledge to make informed choices about treatment. Ironically, though the patient's knowledge may be inadequate, the patient would continue to bear both the responsibility and the blame. Patients may thus bear the moral burdens of either inadequate or excessive available information.

Early Warnings in the Literature

At the same time that one group is advocating increasing self-responsibility, another vocal group is beginning to warn of the consequences. Considerable concern about the more dangerous consequences

Consequences of Shift in Attribution of Responsibility
Institutional level
cost containment
economic overtones: "Why should I pay for someone else's choice?"
society withdraws economic support for illness (i.e. insurance incentives, payment)
moral crusade/mass condemnation based on lifestyle (both lifestyle and illness become stigmatized)
withdrawal of medical resources from poverty groups
ignores cultural role in creating lifestyle (smoking, food), illness (pollution)

Interactional level
physicians no longer absolve patients from blame
physician-patient interaction more equal
physicians no longer as accountable, responsible
health professionals withdraw compassion
friends, family, others in social networks withdraw emotional, material support
further stigma, labeling in illness, disability
stigma, labeling for lifestyle lapses

Individual level
individual experiences guilt, moral failure for becoming sick, or not curing self
individual experiences guilt for lifestyle lapses (smoking, stress, poor diet, lack of exercise, poor health habits)
individual experiences further stigmatization for disability, handicaps
patients may not have enough knowledge, or access to knowledge, to make informed choices on treatment
patients may have moral burdens of excessive available information

Figure 4

has already been generated and has been reflected in the literature during the past decade. These warnings span the range of social science, health policy, and medicine. While many reflect a commitment to the medical model, others are derived from a critical or political economy perspective.

The growing chorus of warnings of the dangers of imputing blame, inherent in the views of self-responsibility deriving from the new model, is most often focused on cancer patients. This probably derives from the high public visibility of the Simonton approach as an adjunct to cancer treatment. Articles and books by social scientists, physicians, and journalists have increasingly highlighted the inherent dangers of this approach.

Maggie Scarf was one of the first to explicitly warn of these major dangers for cancer patients in her 1980 article in *Psychology Today*. As she writes:

> If there is one aspect of the method that seems to stick in people's craws more than any other, it is the notion of the cancer patient as the guilty, responsible party, the person who has "participated" in the development of the malignancy. The game here, so Simonton's appalled critics assert, should be called "Blame the Patient." . . . To Jimmie Holland, the Sloan-Kettering psychiatrist, the Simonton method is a "cruel hoax" that is being perpetrated upon frantic and desperately ill people. "Cancer patients," said Holland, "are often filled with self-blame and are therefore very vulnerable to suggestions that they've brought their illnesses on themselves merely by virtue of being who they are. . . . Many tend to believe the cancer is punishment for some past sin. The guilt associated with something that threatens your life is enormous" (Scarf, 1980:45).

Phyllis Mattson's book describing the holistic health movement from a medical anthropological perspective also warns explictly of this potential, expressing concern that a self-responsibility stance can result in blaming the victim (Mattson, 1982: 39–43,144).

A related critique commonly documented in the literature is that the self-responsibility approach "lets society off the hook." Samuel Epstein, M.D. typifies this argument in raising his concern that self-responsibility obscures the need to focus on social responsibility. Using cancer as a model, he describes the disease as an expression of past exposure to pollutants (he views cancer as an environmental disease, caused essentially by sunlight, smoking, foods, and the petrochemical industry). He sees the lifestyle approach as focusing blame on the individual when the society needs to focus on the petrochemical industries instead (Epstein, 1982).

More general cautions of those same dangers of blame and guilt, as applied to all people experiencing illness, appear less frequently and prominently than those focusing exclusively on cancer patients. An early explicit warning was contained in a letter to the editor, published in the *New England Journal of Medicine*. Shapiro and Shapiro warn of the dangers of the emphasis on self-responsibility inherent in what they call "holistic medicine." They describe our lifestyle as culturally learned and socialized, and discuss the "massive investment in marketing bad health in this country" (Shapiro and Shapiro, 1979:211). They envision the worst-case scenario as the total abandonment of our sick and dying:

> The most likely outcome of this strategy will not be self-responsibility but only self-incrimination. . . . The approach produces guilt feelings about failure of will power, and also guilt feelings about what becomes, by definition, a basically self-destructive impulse. This philosophy provokes a sense of abandonment and self-condemnation. Patients are isolated, left to their own resources (ibid.:211).

Kopelman and Moskop echo these criticisms in their attack on the part of the holistic health movement which they see as abandoning a commitment to the scientific method. They argue that holistic health incorporates a series of moral injunctions, and warn of the dire consequences deriving from a switch in that direction: "The extreme view cavalierly assigns blame for illness and seems to re-establish the ancient notion that misery, sickness and death are linked with moral failure and sin (Kopelman and Moskop, 1981:224).[4] These authors also emphasize that the sick poor would be the major victims of any reduction in illness care, while that same group has the least control over factors conducive to illness (ibid:228). This danger of using the new model as an excuse to lower care to the poor and already underserved groups is also being raised within social science and health policy circles (Crawford, 1977; Berliner and Salmon, 1980a; Taylor, 1982; Zola, 1983; Conrad, 1984; Salmon, 1984). For example, Crawford argues that the shift towards personal responsibility for health is being used to justify cutbacks for public health programs (Crawford, 1977:668).

Guttmacher extends this line of analysis, raising the further criticism that this shift "reinforces the medical system's already strong tendency to deal with disorders chiefly at the personal level and largely to the exclusion of attacking other levels, such as economic or social organization" (Guttmacher, 1979:16). Crawford similarly argues that this shift moves the focus of intervention strategies towards private, individual solutions (Crawford, 1980:385). This critique is echoed by a range of social scientists concerned with the profound implications of such a policy shift (Taylor, 1982, 1984; Zola, 1983; Salmon, 1984; Conrad, 1984; Tesh, 1988).

In addition, there are rare references to the danger of using this new approach to remove physicians' accountability. This argument is primarily raised by proponents of the traditional medical model, and portrays the danger as applying strictly to the new holistic physicians. It is ideologically based, however, as it has not examined the ways this danger may imply a reduction in accountability within the entire practice of medicine.

How is Responsibility Actually Generated?

Despite the clear-cut ideological pronouncements, the way responsibility is actually generated, both within and outside of clinical settings, remains considerably more problematic. In this section, I will move from outlining the explicit ideological view of responsibility in holistic health to analyzing the actual genesis of responsibility through the empirical data. The holistic physicians I studied, in fact, continue to absolve patients to a significant degree, as in the more traditional medical model. Self-condemnation and guilt, as experienced by patients, appears to come primarily from outside sources. In examining the ambivalence around the actual assumption of responsibility, I shall focus on the questions of why practitioners want this shift in attribution of responsibility, and why patients are willing to accept it. Throughout this discussion, the discrepancies between ideologically motivated rhetoric and actual behavior will remain a central concern of the analysis.

Punitive sanctions cannot exist without first socially establishing moral responsibility. It is unjust to punish someone unless they are responsible for their actions. Lemert writes that, "deviations are not significant until they are organized subjectively and transformed into active roles and become the social criteria for assigning status" (Lemert, 1951:75). In this view the reactions of others to assigned deviance creates moral problems, which lead to processes such as stigmatization. This chapter focuses on how patients are becoming increasingly defined as "deviant" in these moral terms.

The "Ideology of Choice"

The ideological route to blame moves from views of body-mind continuity and responsibility to a paradigm of choice. The implicit attributes of such choice are that it is *individual, conscious* and *intentional*. The resultant view, that each person chooses their level of health and illness, and also chooses cure versus death, extends the stigma that was previously attached to a small number of diseases defined as "psychosomatic" to all instances of illness, whether a minor cold or terminal cancer. At times this assumption of intent and choice also extends to personal responsibility for accidents, murder, and other events usually defined in our society as being unequivocally beyond the individual's control. Genetic, social, and environmental limits to personal choice are often overlooked in these pronouncements.[5]

This paradigm of choice and responsibility derives from a phenomenological, existential stance, and can be interpreted as an extreme derivative of the writings of both Sartre and the radical existentialists. In many ways, this view of choice closely parallels an ethnomethodological view, although it ignores any social component in the creation of reality (ethnomethodology acknowledges the interactional aspects of the process). The individual is seen as continually engaged in a process of creating reality by filtering perceptions through the expectations in her mind. Thus reality derives from our mind rather than any given "truth" which is external to the individual. A sign prominently posted in the restroom of one of the secondary holistic health clinics, where I conducted three interviews, typified the assumptions underlying this approach: "If you want to know how tomorrow will be, look at your attitude today."

Mild version. In the milder, more cautious version of the "ideology of choice," elements of choice are implicit within statements of responsibility, but the condemnation attached to illness is relatively subtle. This view comes out continually in pronouncements of a variety of health policy spokespersons, as well as many physicians and nurses incorporating holistic or preventive health approaches.

This implicit version of choice is exemplified in the frequently reiterated quote by John Knowles, past president of the AMA: "The next major advances in the health of the American people will be determined by what the individual is willing to do for himself and for society at large. If he is willing to follow reasonable rules for healthy living, he can extend his life . . ." (Knowles, 1977a: 1103). Although this common approach to preventive health assumes that the individual controls his conditions of living, the component of "choice to become ill" is not as explicit or immediate as in the more extreme forms.

Dennis Jaffe, Ph.D., extends that view in an article on "The Holistic Perspective," writing about the courses of action available to patients. He advises the patient to make his body receptive to healing. He goes on to advocate that the reader should ask himself why he became sick, simultaneously warning of the need for a desire to recover (Jaffe, 1980).

Radical version. The stronger version of the "ideology of choice" is typified by Gerald Jampolsky, M.D., in his writing and lectures, which are derived from the "Course in Miracles." In these pronouncements, the importance of thoughts in determining disease states, healing, and death are explictly linked. Concepts such as "will to live" are extended to "choosing to get well" or "choosing a particular disease state." This radical view, with its assumptions that patients have a wide latitude of control, usually ignores genetic, social, and environmental constraints on individual choice. Scarf sees this more extreme view as following from Arnold Hutschnecker's 1951 book *The Will to Live*, quoting him as saying, "We ourselves choose the time of illness, the kind of illness, the course of illness, and its gravity" (Scarf, 1980: 33).

Jim Polidora, Ph.D., an Associate Professor at the University of California, Davis School of Medicine, occasionally presents the more radical views. At one Association of Holistic Health conference, he explictly stated that we all create our own reality, and that "We create our health and feelings. The world is mind, and we create our reality with our mind." He continued by discussing how we can change our health and feelings by changing our minds (Polidora, 1977). At the same conference, Joseph Spear, D.O., spoke about how our beliefs, attitudes, thoughts, and conscious intent control what happens to us. After advocating modifying belief systems to decrease physical problems, he talked of our "need to damage our bodies for goals we believe we can't reach any other way" (Spear, 1977). The concept of "intentional" secondary gains continually arises in these views.

William Glasser, M.D., also espouses this radical version of responsibility. In a conference presentation, he presented an example of a man who "believes he's depressed" because his wife left him. Glasser explained that the man was actually "choosing to depress." His concept of choice also implies intent, through a process of learning to depress when life gets difficult. The therapist's role, according to Glasser, is to help the client "choose much better," as well as to help people see that they choose these miserable feelings to control others. Thus even guilt and depression are discussed as conscious, volitional choices. He does leave a small "out" for the intentional aspects when he says that people are not "aware" that they are making a choice, because it has become automatic (Glasser, 1982).

Jampolsky is probably the most widely recognized of those espousing the more radical version of the ideology of choice. A sampling of direct quotes from Jampolsky's public talks and his book *Love is Letting Go of Fear*, include:

> I am responsible for all I see and experience.
> We are what we believe.
> We're responsible: everything I am, I asked for (Jampolsky, 1981)
> I am not the victim of the world I see (Jampolsky, 1979:91)

Jampolsky also advocates "deciding" whether you want to be happy or right: "When you feel angry, does it bring you peace of mind? If not, choose again" (Jampolsky, 1981). One minute he describes the individual as making such choices out of fear; yet, the next minute he goes back to talking about how you "should choose to be well," as if it were a fairly simple volitional choice.

This more explicitly radical view is also highly visible in relation to recent approaches to cancer treatment, pioneered by Carl O. Simonton, M.D. In these views, malignancy is seen as a bodily manifestation of despair. Commonly both patients and providers talk of the patient "choosing cancer" as an "out" from responsibility. Closely linked are the theories blaming cancer on personality type. The resultant talk implies an element of conscious choice underlying that personality configuration. Even when patients believe that their depression or high stress levels triggered the malignancy, the underlying implication is that they bear responsibility for becoming ill.

Scarf describes the Simontons' view of the genesis of malignancy: ". . . none of us gets cancer; we reach a point at which our deepest need and wish is to withdraw from life, and we therefore "choose" to develop cancer" (Scarf, 1980:37). Thus dying from cancer (this can be extended to any illness) is the equivalent of suicide. The patient sees no other escape, whether the ultimate vehicle towards death is a self-inflicted gun wound or cancer.

The most extreme views of the "ideology of choice" see intentional choice going still further. A child is seen as spiritually "choosing" to be born into a particular family to work out specific spiritual tasks. Thus child abuse becomes defined as "self chosen," as does childhood cancer, accidents, poverty, or even murder. Extending this view negates any genetic, social, or environmental effect, since the individual "chose" the particular situation. For instance, I asked a nurse in one of the interviews how she saw a child and responsibility for health and disease. She replied, "Both the parent and child are involved together. The child chose to incarnate to that family." [6]

These Holistic Health Practitioners *Do* Absolve

Despite the fairly unambiguous ideological picture, the actual behavior of holistic practitioners contrasted sharply with the standard rhetoric. Among the group of physicians, nurses, and psychologists I studied, I found that these holistic practitioners continued to absolve patients from responsibility, using the same processes traditional practitioners have used. Not only did they continue to absolve patients from direct responsibility in creating their disease state, but they often warned me about the dangers in attribution of blame and guilt inherent in the new model, informing me of the "pitfall" of going overboard on self responsibility.

I had anticipated that this group, although highly idealistic, would demonstrate the side-effects of the new model in this area. However, it became increasingly apparent that the rights and responsibilities of patients were not that different from those hypothesized by Parsons and carried out in more traditional allopathic medical settings. In particular, the absolution function of the practitioner remained intact.

Initially, the ideological pronouncements and modalities appeared very different from more traditional practices. Yet the actual interactional processes remained fairly close. For instance in a holistic setting a patient might not carry out a recommended exercise or diet plan. This would be analogous to a patient not taking a prescribed medication (in both cases, it might be for hypertension). In either case, moral condemnation would be attached to not following the practitioner's treatment regime; yet, there was, if anything, *less* condemnation and guilt inducing among these practitioners than in the more traditional case of "non-compliance." [7]

Not only were these practitioners more aware of the danger of assigning blame, but many of the patients felt freer to admit that they had not carried out the regime than in a traditional office, where evasion is more commonly the practice. Concomitantly, many of these practitioners were aware of the high degree of "non compliance" and, although it appeared to frustrate them, attached less moral overtones to it.

In acute episodes, the interactional model followed almost exactly that within traditional medical settings, although the modalities of treatment sometimes differed. Even in the instances involving chronic illness or preventive health concerns, a similar form of the process of absolution occurred. One practitioner contrasted the way he saw the different approaches in acute versus health concerns:

> It depends on their presenting problems and priorities. If it's a crisis type of thing, we take quite a bit of responsibility in that you know, if they have to be hospitalized or if it's a situation that's serious, we feel like the traditional doctor model is somewhat good. . . . some people come in and they might need an antibiotic and they don't want to take it, and if we don't tell them take it, something serious could happen.

At an early phase of the field study, I met with a physician who had recently joined Mar Vista Clinic. In the last chapter, I relayed how Dr. B realized that in weighting the alternative treatment approaches for patients, he was actually taking more responsibility than he first realized. His example of repackaging the idea of taking an antibiotic for an unreceptive patient also illustrated that responsibility is most often taken in acute disease. When I later formally interviewed this same physician, I asked him how much responsibility he takes for his patients' health and disease. He replied, "More than I ever let them know."

During four hours of intensively interviewing the primary physician in the holistic clinic, I asked whether he felt he was taking less responsibility than most physicians:

> Dr: Actually, I think I'm taking more.
>
> Me: Taking more? How?
>
> Dr: Because I'm taking, I'm basically taking in people into my practice to work with . . . medically unresponsive disease states, in which most physicians usually end up saying "There's nothing I can do about this," and after they're told that by several physicians they come to me and I'm saying, "There is something we can do about it," so that's in a sense . . . I see that as a bigger responsibility.

A recent graduate of a family practitioner residency felt she was taking more responsibility now than during her work in the university family practice clinic:

> And in that other kind of situation, it was easier to say "Well, I've done everything for you that is possible, I've given you the right antibiotic." . . . and now my responsibility is so much expanded because a person comes with their illness and I can see that it's multi-factorial and I need to help them in the areas not only of just treating the organic symptom with the appropriate pharmaceutical drug, but talk to them about diet, exercise, stress, their spiritual well being, their emotional well being, and that all that is part of my role too, to be working on them with.

One of the last interviews I conducted came after the completion of the clinic field study. This interview was with one of the leading physicians in the national holistic movement. When the issue of responsibility came up, he immediately said that it was no different from that in the traditional model, despite all the talk of the differences. This was consistent with everything I had already observed and concluded.

During the interviews, almost every practitioner I spoke with mentioned the dangers of assigning responsibility in the new model. Physicians, nurses, and psychologists usually brought up the problematic aspects long before I got to the portion of the interview where I planned to focus on the issues surrounding responsibility. I had structured the interviews so that I first raised general questions about what they saw as differences in the ways they now interacted with patients, and later moved to more specific questions, including those centering on responsibility. I rarely got that far, however, before they would begin warning me of the possible dangers and misinterpretations of responsibility. Many of these practitioners also mentioned spontaneously that they "went through stages" in developing their current views on self-responsibility (they described some of their earlier interpretations as involving more of an element of blame). It was clear that at least this group of highly respected practitioners was aware of the dangers of simplistic interpretations and attempted to guard against them.

At an early point in the field setting I spoke to one of the psychologists while he waited for a patient. I briefly mentioned my interest in the switch towards more self-responsibility, and he said that he felt that was vastly overrated. He continued by saying he thinks the pendulum is swinging too far towards responsibility and that we need to find a point somewhere closer to the middle.

Further into the field study, I went for lunch with one of the two massage therapists. I talked informally to Ann about the work she did, and then casually asked her whether the emphasis on self-responsibility affected her work.

> That's the one part of holistic health I'm completely against! Everyone talks about self-responsibility as if people make a conscious choice to be ill. It doesn't work that way. They have blocks and problems they can't work out. . . . Maybe it's because of the problems I had [a whiplash injury]. I remember how depressed I was with the pain, and at that point there was nothing I could do. I felt desperate and I worried I'd be that way all my life. So I know people aren't consciously choosing to be there!

> [In a later interview I asked this staff member if she could elaborate on her strong reaction to the term self-responsibility] Well, particularly in Southern California. You have EST and holistic health. People tell someone when they're sick, it's their problem. They caused it. Or it's only in your mind. They're saying it's not real. But by the time a problem is somaticized, it's no longer just in the mind. And you can't decide to just get well. . . . The goal isn't guilt. The guilt fits with Christianity . . . really it's the whole Judeo-Christian thing of punishment for one's sins. I never talk about how they created their problem when I work with a patient.

During the interviews, one of the psychologists in the setting reacted strongly when I asked him how he saw the meaning of illness:

> So, [pause] I think that sometimes one of the problems that I have with holistic health . . . and it happens in this clinic too, is that there's too much blaming the victim, that there's too much saying that the person is ill because it's their own karma and it's taken to mean it's their own fault. And almost regardless of the difficulty, it's their own fault and that's absolutely untrue. I don't see it that way at all. It's untrue in that the person was conscious of what was going on, that planted the seeds for

their present illness. It is untrue that all of the factors that led to the illness were within their control even if they were conscious of it, such as genetic factors. There's also, it relates a lot to your question about responsibility. What is responsibility? How can we take responsibility for ourselves? Can we take responsibility for ourselves, for example, if we're not conscious of certain factors about ourselves? Is that responsibility? I don't think so. I don't think it's possible to take responsibility unless you have enough ego-strength and awareness of what all the factors are involved in a situation and make a conscious choice to deal with that situation. Otherwise it's more like not responsibility or somehow the issue of responsibility doesn't even arise at that level.

The primary physician in the clinic reacted similarly as soon as the word responsibility was mentioned:

I feel that responsibility is a very, very tricky area to deal with and most holistic practitioners do it very poorly, and responsibility usually ends up being guilt, and I don't usually, I never lay that on people. And I've seen this happen too many times . . .

One of the nurses in the clinic implied a similar orientation during our interview. After reacting to the ways responsibility is misinterpreted, she described going through a stage where she "laid guilt trips" around illness, and talked of the process she went through in changing her views:

I did go through a stage where being sick was a failure. There was something in your life you had not dealt with and so that is why you became sick. Now I have even grown through that, and now I see it differently. My favorite quotation about illness is, "Illness is an invitation to change." I see it that way now. I don't see it as something you need to feel guilty about or something that points out the fact that you don't have your life together or whatever.

The dentist whose office I studied also warned me repeatedly of the problems consequent to guilt. During the actual formal interview, he said, "I think the price of the guilt is perhaps greater than the potential control gained through biofeedback or meditation or some other relaxation procedure."

One could argue that, despite their knowledge of the dangers of the "ideology of choice," their explanations may not reflect actual behavior. The pilot field study in the holistic dental office and the more extensive ethnography in the preventive medical clinic provided considerable data to analyze for attribution of responsibility and blame. There were almost no instances that could be interpreted as implying blame, and those rare instances where it occurred at a subtle level were primarily confined to two specific individuals within one of the practices.

One nurse used the ideology of choice fairly freely, without always checking carefully to assess the meanings it might have to specific patients. She did not appear to be as aware as other staff in the setting of the potential problems her words might cause. Although the difference was usually subtle, I sensed she "wrote patients off" just a little more easily than the other practitioners. In one instance, three patients were discussing the importance of nutrition and health habits. A friend accompanying one patient said, "If you could just get them (people who don't understand) on a week's program of eating right and they'd see!" Nurse B responded with, "People pick and choose what level of illness they want." All of us in the room nodded, but I wondered how the new patient with multiple sclerosis interpreted that. Did she see herself as picking and consciously choosing to develop multiple sclerosis?

In another instance, Nurse B expressed similar views with another new patient, an older Italian male, who was very sociable and articulate.

> Tony pretty much monopolized the conversation, telling us he had had a cardiac by-pass, but that "if I had known about all this thirty years ago . . . it's too late now." He then expounded on the need to educate children when there was still a chance to help them. Gail interrupted: "I believe that at any time in your life you can choose to move to a new level of wellness. It's never too late. To say you give up is locking yourself into a pattern."

There was a definite limit to the absolution function, but that limit was a variant of that found in the traditional model. When the patient has all the information and has seen results due to lifestyle changes, practitioners start pointing out increasingly to the patient that it is now his or her choice and responsibility. This situation closely parallels that where the physician has prescribed a medication, and the patient comes up with "excuses" for why she or he doesn't take it (for example, the side effects may be more disruptive than the problems it was prescribed for). Practitioners, after trying to motivate the patient, no longer feel the non-compliance is their responsibility. Practitioners have never defined "non-compliance" as their failure within the traditional medical model.

Both the dentist and the family practitioner whom I studied intensively essentially take responsibility when they assess that patients are not ready, or do not want, to take full responsibility. They both explicitly described this, and I observed it in both settings at the behavioral level as well. Thus they extend, rather than restrict, absolution from responsibility.

Two qualifiers need to be added here. First, those patients in Mar Vista Clinic who may have felt pressure from attribution of blame probably left the practice and sought out another physician, so that I might not have observed them. On the other hand, I did not observe any instance where Dr. A presented information or interacted in a way that implied patient guilt. Only one patient, when interviewed outside the setting, mentioned a situation where she felt that had occurred with Dr. A. Second, Dr. A mentioned in our interview, when I commented that I had not seen much of that, that although he tries to be very aware of the dangers, he does not always manage to live up to the level he strives for, and that he is sure he misses that sometimes and unintentionally comes across in ways that induce guilt in patients.

Theoretical "Outs" That Avoid Attribution of Blame

An elaborate analysis of both the ethnographic and interview data demonstrated seven theoretical "outs" these practitioners used to avoid blaming patients for their illness. If one or more of these beliefs was integrated into the model, a "blame the victim" stance did not result from the views of body-mind continuity and responsibility. These beliefs revolved around. *intent*, *unconscious processes*, *learned processes*, *social dimensions of reality construction*, *body-mind continuity*, *health as a relative value*, and *karmic acceptance*.

Dividing these beliefs into categories is of course an artificial process of conceptualization. For instance, one recurring problem involves the situation where traditional medicine refuses to admit a patient to the sick role (no observable cause is found), saying "It's all in your mind." It is not only body-mind continuity that is at issue here, but the problem

of mind and beliefs about intent. Moral and legal responsibility in a culture rest on views of volition and control. So one returns to whether
patients become ill for conscious versus unconscious reasons.

Thus, most of the responses from practitioners, as well as their observed behavior, did not fall neatly into the categories. For instance,
when asked how she dealt with the problems around guilt, one of the
psychologists in the clinic replied:

> Oh . . . well . . . my general posture is always to have people
> see whatever's going on inside of them as being natural. That
> it's normal. Even if . . . what that does is it allows people to
> have a healthier relationship to whatever they are. And to stop
> their blaming and the guilt producing. Essentially saying, lis-
> ten, you know, it's understandable, you know, . . . your mother
> had arthritis and your grandfather had arthritis, why wouldn't
> you have arthritis? You have tension, well look at what you've
> been living with for the last fifty years. It's natural that you
> would have tension. It's unfortunate that you didn't have some
> tools to deal with this a long time ago. But, you know, we have
> to work with where we are now.

An internist also looked at the broad picture, encompassing many of
the categories. At one point in the interview he stated:

> The whole thing is that the concept I have is that we are a
> response to everything. That is the genetic influence, prenatal
> influence, the family that we had around us, the environ-
> ment . . . external and internal, the foods, the chemicals that
> we're exposed to. Everything. Now, what happens to us is a
> sum total of that.

Both these responses encompass several of the categories.

(1) Ideas of intent and volition. The idea of intent is crucial to assigning responsibility. Practitioners who see a patient's illness as intentionally induced attach quite different moral connotations to it than those
who feel, whether due to intervening theories of unconscious motivation
or lack of knowledge, that the person did not purposely attempt to become ill. Holistic practitioners who see people becoming ill when they
see "no other outs," do not necessarily see illness as an intentional
choice. An obvious illustration is that we view a person who became ill
and died of food poisoning while eating at a restaurant very differently

than a case where a person added poison to his own food before eating it, in an attempt to kill himself. Very different moral meanings are assigned to the act of ingesting poisoned food in the two situations.

For example, a psychologist in the clinic described his outlook on intent:

> What I'll say is, well, obviously you weren't aware before and what you have now may be the result of a lifetime of habits of doing things that you didn't *know* would lead you to this, or things that were biologically caused which obviously were out of your control. You couldn't control what you were doing if you didn't *know* it was gonna lead you to this.

A similar sentiment was expressed by a board-certified physician in internal medicine, who combined homeopathic medicine with his practice: "Other doctors talk about noncompliant patients . . . noncompliance is not because the patient doesn't want to . . . the patient can't!"

And the other psychologist in the clinic, when asked how she deals with the guilt and self-blame some patients feel, answered:

> When you were five years old, did you decide that your parents would treat you in this way or that way? Was it your choice that your father died when you were five? Of course not. Well, it's pretty clear though from research that the pattern for an individual's response to the overall use of the immune system is set by the age of six. Did you decide that? No, you didn't, of course you didn't!

Thus intent and volition emerge as a primary consideration once body-mind continuity is accepted. If, for example, a link is found at the biochemical level between depression and lowered immunological function, does that become interpreted as the patient "causing" the disease, with all the connotations of intentional causation? Did the person intentionally "cause" the disease? Or did they purposefully "cause" the depression that made them vulnerable to the disease?

(2) Belief in unconscious processes. Practitioners who believe in unconscious processes do not apply the same moral meanings of intent to choice and responsibility in creating illness. Jampolsky talks of fear as keeping people from loving and peace, but fear is not "intentionally chosen," certainly not at a conscious level. Fear derives from a notion of

unconscious processes and defenses; this paradigm prevents assigning blame. The analytic conceptualization of "needs" also provides exemption from blame.

Historically, the notion of unconscious processes came to exempt the "insane" from responsibility. With the spread of mind-body continuity research, the same notion can at times exempt the physically ill from moral blame. There have been major humanistic consequences from the process of medicalization, which has increasingly added formerly stigmatized groups such as the mentally ill, or alcoholics, to the cases exempted from responsibility through the medical model (Conrad and Schneider, 1980). As mentioned earlier, however, the more recent trend towards demedicalization may not only have the effects of re-stigmatizing formerly outcast groups, but also stigmatizing the physically ill themselves.

A participant in a class on holistic health modalities asked the instructor how she explains to people that they have "chosen illness" as a way to deal with their problems or whether she makes that explicit to her clients. The psychologist instructor replied that she tells people whom she feels are ready to hear it, but she tells them the problem is "unconscious." She elaborated: "The subconscious mind directs you from old patterns."

Midway through the field study, I approached one of the nurses during a quiet period. I reminded her of a young woman undergoing testing for ulcerative colitis, and how this patient talked about how previous doctors told her it was "all in her mind." Out of hearing, I had expressed to this nurse how angry I feel when physicians use that response with patients when they cannot find a physical cause. She had replied, "But then, June, it *is* all in the mind!" I had nodded, assuming I understood her meaning. Now I told her that I knew enough about the meanings that there was a danger of my assuming something incorrectly, and that I wanted to be sure of what she actually meant by that comment. She thought a while before replying:

> There's a mental, psychological, and spiritual component to each illness. I truly feel [stated slowly, carefully] there's an imbalance, a need in the mind-heart-spirit before someone becomes ill. That's not to say people deliberately become ill. If we were perfect, we wouldn't become ill. When we become sick, our bodies protect and relieve us—they help us avoid danger. [I asked what she meant by that.] In two ways. It's both a message from your body and also the body's doing you a favor

by helping you avoid situations. I don't mean it like the Christian Scientists. They say you create all your illness. How can you explain that to a kid without making him feel guilty? And adults too. I like the way Haas says it. He says illness is an invitation to change. That doesn't say it's your fault.

[I asked her how she presents this concept in her work with patients] How much I explain to a patient depends on their readiness. Some people see themself as the victim. Others see it as their fault. . .that's not responsibility. I tell them they weren't at a stage where they could handle it better. Like my aunt. I told you she had all these illnesses after her daughter married, and then she got the breast cancer. I talked to her about how people often get cancer after a loss they couldn't handle. [I asked whether her aunt experienced guilt] Yes, but I explained that it wasn't her fault. I should tell you though, June, I didn't always see it this way. I've gone through lots of stages to get here! I went through all sorts of phases. As a young nurse I hated psychiatric nursing. [laughing] Then I said that yes, it's a person's responsibility but also your fault. Now I see responsibility and fault as separate. [I asked how she explains the difference between fault and responsibility] The unconscious. It's not consciously, deliberately choosing to get ill.

So Nurse A distinguishes between fault and responsibility, using the concept of the unconscious to exempt the patient from blame. An internist interpreted the situation similarly:

Me: One comment I hear a lot and I would like your reaction to it is, "We choose our level of health and illness at each moment."

Dr: I think that basically goes along with responsibility and the essence of it is true. It is just that that statement is open to many interpretations and the interpretation that most people who are naive in the field would understand is that there is "consciously" between "we" and "choose." That is what is interpreted by the individual and I think basically we do choose, but we don't do it on a conscious level.

(3) Belief in learned processes. Another theoretical "out" postulates restriction of individual control through past learned behavior patterns.

For instance, Emmett Miller, M.D., talks of children learning metaphors and "building a map of reality." He sees our lives as adults as run by these childhood metaphors and images (Miller, 1982). Similarly, William Glasser talks of people "choosing" to depress, while he explains at other points that "depressing" may be a learned pattern of coping from childhood. Many lifestyle patterns, feelings, and behaviors are learned socially. Can an individual be truly responsible for them?

A related view, derived from a belief in learned processes, implies that people cannot be held accountable for something they don't know. Thus most of us, while living in a highly stressful society, have never learned techniques to decrease the effects of stress. When people learn that feelings may decrease their resistance to disease, they feel they should be able to control their feelings; however, they have no knowledge or techniques to accomplish this. In fact, many would argue that most attempts to control or mask feelings would cause more problems, according to this same paradigm.

A holistic internist, when asked how he deals with the self-condemnation he sees in patients who have read about pain control techniques but find they are unable to use them, replied:

> I just tell people, what you are saying is the same thing as if you read a book on how to play piano and you couldn't play Beethoven in two days, and you're a failure. It's the same thing.

(4) Personal versus social construction of reality. A view which incorporates the social and cultural dimensions of reality construction also avoids the pitfalls of assigning moral responsibility for illness. When the cultural and interactional aspects of lifestyle are accounted for, there is less of a "blame the victim" stance. There are always social constraints on individual reality construction. In fact, when social constraints are not perceived and acted on, a person is defined as schizophrenic (it could be argued that even the most severely delusional schizophrenic takes interactional considerations into account, including within the delusions themselves).

Beliefs develop within a specific cultural and temporal milieu. For example, a generation ago, most nutritionally informed people in the United States believed that eating large quantities of red meat produced health; that has changed, or is at least under dispute, one generation later. At the interactional level, if a patient believes her or his actions directly caused the illness and the physician does not (of course, the reverse could also occur), a negotiation between them takes place over time.

When Jampolsky tells people, "I am responsible for all I see and experience," it is interpreted to mean that each individual creates reality in her mind in isolation. This variant of the "ideology of choice" can be interpreted as both over-psychologized and radically individualistic. It ignores the definite constraints on the reality we create, deriving both from the physical world and our interactions with others. Reality is created socially, both interactionally and within social constraints. These social constraints derive both from the existing social structure and from early cultural socialization.

The ecological variant of this argument is typified in Samuel S. Epstein, M.D.'s book, *The Politics of Cancer*. Epstein sees personal responsibility as overemphasized in relation to social responsibility. He stresses the limits of an individual constructionist approach when confronted with environmental pollution and the resources of the pharmaceutical industry (he views the chemical and medical industries as suppressing the information people need to make responsible choices) (Epstein, 1978).

(5) Body-mind continuity. Misunderstandings abound in attempts to apply the concept of body-mind continuity. Simplistic interpretations of the concept see it in terms of a one-way causal relationship: mind influences body. The more sophisticated holistic conception sees the direction of causation moving both ways, with such a high degree of interrelationship that no single causal point can be demonstrated. Most misinterpretations ignore the causal relationship from body to mind. Thus, once a person experiences physical illness, it initiates changes in feelings and cognition (for example, the depression so often linked with cancer may be a result, rather than a cause of the disease process). Similarly, any genetic predispositions towards specific illness are ignored in the simplistic views of mind-body continuity.

Holistic health advocates believe that it is difficult to comprehend body-mind continuity within a Western world view. They argue that our language does not have the appropriate words: the basic Cartesian duality is so taken-for-granted that we have no images for the concept. Cartesian duality similarly accounts for the constant search for cause vs. effect. There are no ways to conceptualize stress and disease process as a mutual feedback loop, continually interacting and in process. Even when changes can be measured, only correlations can be demonstrated because of the complex interrelationships.[8]

In contrast, holistic health participants believe that an Eastern view conceptualizes this area as integrated. For example, Dr. A saw his acupuncture training as the major factor in changing his thinking about body-mind continuity:

My acupuncture training, that's one of the biggest impacts I
have being that there is no, in Chinese thought, that mind-body
is written together as a hyphen, not as two separate words, and
if you'd like, it should be mind-body-spirit with two hyphens
rather than three separate concepts. . . . I think what has happened basically is that we've gone from a set of "it's all in your
mind" through "all in your body" to a set of "it's all in your
mind," and we have failed to see that the body causes mind
disturbances, as well as the mind causes body disturbances. . . .
And I would never have gotten that if it wasn't for my acupuncture training . . . It does not lay the seed of disease in terms of
mental processes. It says they're together and the imbalance in
your chi energy will manifest physically or mentally depending
on circumstantial things. . . . So, the key is the equation that
moves in both directions.

Misinterpretations and over simplifications are continually apparent
in this area. For instance, a woman in her early forties was interviewed
outside the primary setting. Janice had problems with recurring bladder
infections and had been placed on a tightly restricted diet which also
excluded alcohol. During a period where she was under intense stress she
had a glass of wine with friends one evening, then developed another
bladder infection. She reproached herself for her "self-destructive act,"
defining it as a moral failure. But the social use of wine in small amounts
may also decrease stress and increase sociability. Within a holistic framework of true mind-body continuity, this would be seen as improving her
attitude, thus having the potential to improve her physical state. Similarly, any self-condemnation would be seen as detrimental to emotional,
and thus derivatively, physical health.

Earlier I discussed how the label "psychosomatic" has implied "it's
all in your mind" within allopathic medicine. The use of "psychosomatic" has been a definite pejorative label implying personal responsibility with moral weakness.

One of the few moral judgments I saw made in the clinic was one I
would expect in a more traditional medical office, and it concerned the
implications of psychosomatic illness. A young man had discussed his
past history of "severe diarrhea" with me, and told of the dramatic improvement following his eliminating cow's milk. During a lull in the office I decided to take a quick look at Brian's chart, and I was surprised to
see the diagnosis of ulcerative colitis. That label has somatic connotations
that are considerably more severe and life-threatening than diarrhea; in

addition, it has connoted a specific emotional configuration as an established "psychosomatic" disease (individuals with ulcerative colitis are characterized as displaying a characteristic compulsive/dependent personality style). When Nurse B came by, I casually commented that Brian seemed "very controlled," wondering if her response would reflect the subtle moral connotations. She replied offhandedly, "Well, you know, he has ulcerative colitis." The same labels are taken-for-granted by most physicians and nurses in more traditional settings. According to the more complex view of mind-body continuity, all diseases have an emotional, stress, attitudinal component; however, one of the dangers is to subtly stigmatize patients as she did.

(6) Health as a relative value. Assigning moral blame to the individual for illness assumes that health is an absolute, ultimate value taking precedence over all other values. Practitioners who did not impute moral blame were aware that patients were continually making choices which balanced a complex multiplicity of values.

Dr. A, in talking about how hard it was to motivate patients to make lifestyle changes, even with knowledge, stated that he often puts people with suspected food allergies on a modified food fast for a week. He said that if allergies are the primary problem, they feel so much better at the end of the week, it becomes an immediately attainable goal, rather than an abstract, future-related motivator. This same physician was aware of factors such as the importance of eating out, the social implications of eating, and the time constraints working women faced.

A patient in the setting (a male dentist in his late forties), talked to me at length of the problems he had experienced in controlling his asthma symptoms. These difficulties reflected his attempts to balance conflicting values. He described improvements in his condition after eliminating smoking and certain foods that triggered problems. He then discussed the ways he tried to balance his need for sociability with the asthma management:

> I know what seems to bring on the symptoms too . . . cigarette smoke. And beer too. I know I shouldn't have it. But sometimes I cheat and one doesn't seem to hurt. But then I have two, and everyone's smoking around me while I'm having the beer. And then it starts. I'm never sure how much is the beer and how much the smoke. But it's really hard to change my life completely so that I won't ever go into a bar. I know I shouldn't, but all my friends are there. It's not the beer so much as seeing them.

(7) Karmic acceptance. Many of these practitioners were able to accept the individual's responsibility for illness without moral condemnation because of their belief in an Eastern philosophical, spiritual framework. In many ways this view closely parallels the "outs" provided by the unconscious paradigm. The assumptions underlying both the unconscious and a karmic acceptance of destiny mediate views of volitional choice.[9]

One of the two holistic obstetricians I interviewed discussed the dangers of guilt, and how they could be avoided by self-acceptance:

> The general principles of self-love are accepting yourself for . . . as someone who's really doing the best you can with what the situation is at the moment. If you could do better, you would. Or do differently, you would. And to try to help the patient to rid themselves, as I do myself, of shoulds in life. By self-love. . . . we have to have the ability to be kind to ourselves and laugh at ourselves and to know that we're subject to frailties . . . it doesn't help in any way to berate oneself.

Another physician, who had also been personally immersed in Eastern spiritual practices, although his practice in an internal medicine specialty initially appeared fairly traditional, tried to explain how he avoided the guilt or blame many patients feel when they are exposed to the idea of responsibility for their illness:

> Well, I avoid that to a great degree by not broaching the subject of responsibility directly. By doing it in a circuitous fashion. By using metaphors and things of that sort. . . . I attempt to get them to understand that responsibility and blame are two separate things. It is a very difficult concept for people to understand. That responsibility indicates a positive action that one has control over what happens. Blame is a negative action by which a person says that they are a bad person. Responsibility is merely a force. It is neither good or bad. It is a force just like any other force or energy. Whereas, blame is a value judgment. The whole purpose as I see it in life is to understand the forces and work with them and forget about value judgments. Value judgments are always detrimental.

Since this last category of karmic acceptance, along with beliefs in unconscious motivation, was the major pattern used to maintain the medical function of "absolution" seen in this group, it will be further elaborated and developed at the end of this chapter and in the concluding chapter. Once again, it must be emphasized that any combination of these "theoretical outs" can prevent these holistic practitioners from blaming their patients.

Is There Actually a Shift in Attribution of Blame?

The next question that arises is whether any blame is actually being attributed to patients due to the new model. This chapter has already established that there is an "ideology of choice" that explicitly holds the individual responsible for both their level of health or illness and ultimate cure versus death. Yet, despite the elaborate rhetoric emphasizing this responsibility for illness, holistic practitioners in this study almost always continued to absolve patients from blame for illness at the interactional level.

While these holistic health practitioners continue to absolve their patients, the patients do experience diffuse stigmatization within the general societal arena. Lay people, and many traditional physicians and health care providers, are interpreting mind-body continuity and responsibility in terms of personal blame and moral failure. In other words, the plethora of warnings apply to actual beginning shifts in the level of attribution of blame and condemnation; however, the moral condemnation is primarily coming from outside these holistic settings. This "ideology of choice" is apparently being extended to attribution throughout the spectrum of health and illness.

Holistic health and the "ideology of choice" become a *secularized version of salvation and predestination*. In this new version, everyday actions act as visible symbols of salvation and predestination, just as in Calvinistic theology. Eating cake, for instance, becomes a visible index of nonelection and symbolizes a lack of grace. Scarf implies a similar analogy in relation to cancer:

> Many cancer specialists consider the Simonton method a form of medical evangelism in which old-fashioned sin is replaced by depression, repression, and denial, and redemption requires confession and an altered lifestyle. The metaphors used by Simonton—personality change and rebirth into health—do in fact resemble the metaphors of religion (Scarf, 1980:45).

Similarly, in the area of health, the appearance of vigorous health, physical fitness, and low weight visibly signal the state of grace. On the other hand, both illness and lifestyle lapses indicate personal moral failure.

My data here depend on the much broader interpretation of the concept of "field" in ethnographic research. The explicit condemnation of patients had to be documented from broader cultural materials, as well as from comments and interview data of both participants and practitioners within the confines of my smaller field study.

Data at the Cultural Level

The first source of data includes a wide variety of sources at the cultural level. The mass of people buying books and attending conferences where the "ideology of choice" is elaborated in detail attests to the popularity and visibility of this shift in meanings. The tremendous commercial success of a huge number of books, typified by Jampolsky's *Love is Letting Go of Fear*, Le Shan's *You Can Fight For Your Life*, and the Simontons' *Getting Well Again* demonstrate the popularity of the approach (Jampolsky, 1979; Le Shan, 1977; Simonton and Simonton, 1978).

Articles expounding this approach pervade the mass media, as well. A broad audience is exposed to the new ideology through newspaper and magazine articles and television pieces emphasizing patient choice and responsibility in health and illness (these include the range of versions from mild to radical). For instance, Barbara Taub, R.N., described a documentary on CBS reporting on the Taubs' work. It featured the case of a twenty-year-old girl with aplastic anemia. The program ends with the reporter saying, "Next time your Doctor tells you it's all in your mind, tell him he's right!" (Taub, 1982).

Again, the more radical views are most visible in relation to cancer therapy and visual imagery approaches to treatment, stemming from the Simontons' work. An example of the articles in the popular media is Jonathan Kirsch's article, "Can Your Mind Cure Cancer?" (Kirsch, 1977). At the time Kirsch wrote the article in early 1977, the Simontons were receiving as many as 300 patient inquiries a week at their clinic in Fort Worth. In describing Simonton's use of visualization as an adjunct to cancer therapy, Kirsch writes:

> (Simonton) insists that his patients answer the underlying question: "Why did I need my cancer in the first place?" And he suggests that the "secondary gains" of the disease—sympathy and attention from family and friends, relief from job stress and day-to-day chores—might account for the patient's need to surrender to cancer (Kirsch, 1977:43).

Courses for cancer patients based on this approach are also highly visible. They further disseminate these ideas, as well as attracting those already imbued by them. One cancer patient I spoke with outside the primary setting took a university-based extension course offered by a local psychologist, who used mental imagery based on the Simonton approach. He was angry at the psychologist at the point we spoke. Three of the course participants had since died, and he saw the entire approach as quackery, offering patients false hope and then letting them down.

At an interdisiplinary program on grief, offered through the Western Behavioral Science Institute in 1982, I asked two of the panelists, both conducting research in the fields of terminal illness and bereavement, whether the patients and families they worked with were experiencing this type of moral condemnation. The psychiatrist studying bereavement after death from heart attack replied that many of his patients were receiving such messages from friends and relatives. These included comments such as, "He chose to die." The psychologist working with terminally ill children also acknowledged seeing a fair amount of that phenomenon. He spoke of the damage "unintentionally" done by people like Jampolsky, stating that parents often received comments like, "You know, she could get well if she wanted to." He discussed how much anguish these comments evoked in the parents.

The range of mild to radical versions of the "ideology of choice" also appears in the popular media focused on "preventive health." Various programs for health enhancement, from holistic centers to traditional medical centers, are frequently featured in both print and television media reports. While most articles and publicity for programs aimed at "preventive health" and "health enhancement" subtly emphasize the individual's responsibility for health, some explictly convey the radical version. For example, an advertisement for Loma Linda's preventive health program, featured prominently in the *Los Angeles Times*, pictured a middle-aged man holding a gun to his head. The large, accompanying caption read: "DON'T COMMIT LIFESTYLE SUICIDE!"

The increasing institutionalization of similar concepts are reflected in the recent restructuring of insurance plans. For example, a San Diego CBS affiliate news program recently reported on a life insurance plan offered by ITT Life in Omaha. Rate reductions of 50 percent for life insurance were being offered for "non-smoking runners." The story went on to detail other risk factors ITT Life was computing to reach individualized rates; these included height/weight ratios, blood pressure readings, and driving habits.

Another reflection of this cultural sentiment is the strong public re-

DON'T COMMIT LIFESTYLE SUICIDE!

The Surgeon General warns, "We are killing ourselves by our own careless habits." *

To help you avoid this hazard, Loma Linda University announces its COMPREHENSIVE HEALTH PROMOTION PROGRAM. This is your chance to get away from it all for one week and assess your life priorities.

The place – RANCHO LOMA LINDA, a live-in health promotion center in a quiet country setting near San Diego.

The program — a comprehensive medical evaluation including treadmill testing plus vigorous exercise, proper nutrition, and instruction in lifestyle modification.

The price – $1,020.

A LOMA LINDA UNIVERSITY PROGRAM

* *Healthy People*, p. viii.

This coupon will get you our free brochure. So will a phone call –
(714) 463-0211

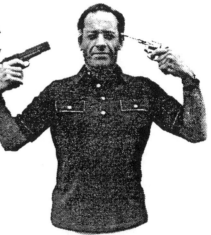

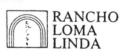
Figure 5 (*Los Angeles Times*, October 19, 1981: Part V, p. 8)

action protesting the insanity defense, following the innocent verdict for John W. Hinckley Jr.'s assassination attempt. During the following year, the American Medical Association recommended the insanity plea be legally abolished. This represents a definite shift of the medical establishment towards demedicalizing an area that has been held exempt from moral censure. Basically the shift from supporting treatment to punishment reflects a return to views of emphasizing the volitional elements of choice.

Still another institutional indication of this shift is the 1988 Supreme Court decision allowing the federal government to exclude alcoholics from some benefit programs (Savage, 1988:1). The decision upheld the Veteran Administration's policy of classifying alcoholism as "willful misconduct." This again represents a shift away from the established disease conception of alcoholism towards earlier views holding the individual morally responsible for the problem.

Data from Interviews

The practitioners who brought up the dangers inherent in "self-responsibility" detailed similar instances where patients were receiving those messages from others. The interviews documented the prevalence of the "ideology of choice" in both patients and health providers.

Dr. A discussed how many patients came into his office already experiencing that guilt. He found that many patients had gone through programs such as EST training, and came out feeling they were "responsible for everything." He described frequently having to work to "undo the guilt."

Two physicians with teaching responsibilities at a research-oriented university medical school discussed the prevalence of the ideology of choice among the medical students they work with. One full-time faculty member described the attitudes he saw in many of his medical students:

> I've heard students say, "I don't want to take care of anybody who smokes. I don't want to take care of anybody who drinks alcohol in excess." "If they're not willing to participate in their health care, why should I beat my head against the wall with them, why should I take care of them when they go into liver failure or whatever, you know . . . when they have their G.I. bleed or whatever it is." I've heard that; I've heard that from students. I really understand that position. Why should you beat your head against the wall? . . . and, you know, my answer is what I said earlier, "Why are you in this profession?"

A part-time clinical faculty member discussed similar concerns:

> I just did a course with the second year medical students, and
> we had a group session on whether medical care is a right.
> These are nice kids, June, I've got to say that first. But then
> we're discussing expensive machinery and whether everyone
> has a right to dialysis, and the whole group came to a decision—
> before I started putting my two cents in—that someone had no
> right to treatment if it was their fault. Like smoking or drug
> abuse or being overweight. It was scary! They meant it!

That same physician described students at a university health-services
facility as holding similar attitudes towards themselves. He spoke of students regularly coming in and giving a "standard litany," telling a story
of how their behavior caused their illness. As he described it, "They tell
me they're 'sinners'; it's all 'mea culpa'. It's always their fault that they're
sick." When asked to elaborate, this physician gave examples of student
comments such as, "I was up too late the night before" or "I wore the
wrong kind of shoes and that's why I twisted my ankle." The group of
students who come in to lose weight also see themselves as "sinners."
When this physician commented that the students were not getting those
views through student health services, I asked where they got it. He
found they read *Prevention* or they heard those views from friends. He
described having to constantly battle such views: "I have to laugh and
push the germ theory. I tell them there are real viruses, and it's not all the
'sin theory'." [10]

A patient I interviewed who had undergone extensive treatment for
chronic back pain discussed the stigmatization she experienced. She
spoke at length about how chronic pain was defined by traditional physicians, nurses, and social workers in terms of "secondary gains." Because
of her simultaneous position in the health field, Susan was acutely aware
of the judgments applied to chronic pain patients. She spoke of her attempts to *minimize the visibility* of her problems because of those judgments. For example, she described her reasons for trying DMSO: "One
of the reasons I tried the DMSO was that it hurt so much without the
collar, that I was increasing my pain medication, and I decided to try it.
The DMSO wasn't visible." When I asked Susan what this illness meant
to her, she replied, "Uuh . . . a failure. Another step in . . . I felt at the
time it was a failure, almost a thing I was perpetuating on purpose, even
though I knew that I wasn't." This same patient mentioned that, after her
third surgery, when they found widespread scar tissue in her spinal col-

umn, the surgeon apologized, saying there was a "real" physical basis for the pain.[11]

Data from the Ethnographic Setting

In my observations in the primary setting, patients who showed self-condemnatory behavior had developed those attitudes from the larger cultural arena: through reading, the media, friends and relatives, and often through other medical practitioners. This situation often arose when I was observing and talking casually with patients during the allergy testing. These patients were at the entry point of their experience in this clinic and had recently transferred from other medical settings. Self-condemnation was frequently expressed by patients, especially if they felt they had not previously been able to make lifestyle changes or control pain. They were essentially saying, "I know that I should be exercising more" or "I know I should be able to control my migraines."

Some patients had heard from other medical practitioners that their symptoms were "all in your mind." For example, a woman in her mid-twenties was undergoing testing for long-term gastrointestinal problems. Donna described having this problem since childhood. "The medication they (the doctors) gave me . . . it was unbelievable. Then, for a while, the doctors treated it as a social thing . . . all in my mind, you know."

Another patient in the clinic was a nurse in her late twenties. Laura talked of how, when physicians cannot find a physical cause they can document, they tend to locate the problem in the patient's mind.

[After having trouble with dizzy spells, she saw one of the doctors where she works, and next thing she knew, she was on the "medical revolving door circuit." She described seeing several different specialists, and everyone felt the problems stemmed from their particular specialty. All had different remedies—all prescription medication.] They make you feel if you're not buying it, then it's all in your mind. You know . . . like you're a crock or you're malingering. What really did it was when the neurologist told me the dizziness was probably small seizures, even though the EEGs were all normal. He wanted me to go on Dilantin for the rest of my life. That's when I came here.

[Laura then talked again of how easily physicians tend to think symptoms are all in the patient's mind. I asked if she ever finds herself doing this when she works as a nurse in intensive care.] Yes . . . I see a lot coming from within myself in the hospital.

When the treatment doesn't work, I find myself start to write them off. Now I think of myself, and suddenly I feel sorry for them. [I asked her to give me an example.] Well, you give someone morphine for cardiac pain, and they don't respond. And I find myself thinking it's something with them. Then, after surgery, you find out they had no right coronary artery, and then you know their pain was real. I feel so sorry for them about what all of us had thought.

This points up some interesting paradoxes in the attribution of cause in the two models, medical and holistic. The biggest critique of traditional medicine heard from patients and holistic providers is that the medical model fails to deal with the underlying cause; in other words, it only treats symptoms. At the same time, the medical model is tied to a causative paradigm. When an objective cause is found, the patient is absolved from blame, as Parsons postulates. However, when the cause is not located, the patient is subsequently blamed and accused. The physicians say it is all in their minds: this not only blames them, but devalues the mind, as well as separating it from the body. Once traditional practitioners and lay people start accepting body-mind continuity, they continue to see a simple causal relationship which implies willful causation of disease. These patients perceive a holistic physician like Dr. A as absolving them from blame more than in the traditional model; yet, even his philosophy has an ambivalent stance.

"It's all in your mind" does not have those pejorative connotations from the comprehensive holistic view. Also, it cannot be *all* in the mind, because the mind cannot be separated from the body and spirit. Yet, in cases involving food allergies, Dr. A is actually finding the cause and removing it, which is what the traditional model is supposed to do. Thus, in this case, Dr. A is practicing traditional medicine, in terms of the underlying paradigm. However, if the person's attitudes and state of mind were more positive or more "evolved," the same patient should have less problems in overreacting to those same allergens; that puts the problem back in the mind. Dr. A is aware of these ambiguities and how the model breaks down if you analyze it in too much detail from a Western perspective.

For many of these patients, holistic health defined their problems as *real illness*. Holistic practitioners basically exempted these patients from responsibility for their problem. In this type of case, the traditional medical system did not find objective symptoms and thus would not admit the patient into the legitimate sick role, with its accompanying exemption from responsibility. In this situation, alternative systems, including holistic health, were used to gain entree into the traditional sick role with the accompanying benefits. As one patient put it, finding that her problems were due to allergies made her problems "real" and acceptable to family, friends, and herself.

Another instance where attribution of blame and responsibility had come from traditional physicians was brought up by a woman in her late forties. She was talking at length to the nurse and me during preparations for an exercise EKG. Margaret asked me about my background in nursing, and I mentioned I had worked with dying patients. She responded, "My daughter died last year. You'll be interested in that. I hang all the guilt on them. Every little thing!" I told her I was not sure what she meant, although it seemed she was very angry at the doctors. She explained that her daughter had had childhood diabetes, and that she had died the year before at age twenty-three.

> It was the peer group thing. Everything had to be measured out. Every little thing. And the doctors always made you feel like you should be doing more. I was always worrying . . . you always worry you're doing the wrong thing anyway. [later] . . . I think it all stemmed from the guilt trips the doctors gave her. All that lecturing—it really changed her. [I asked Margaret if she could give me an example.] Sure. Like . . . "If you don't take your medicine, you'll go blind." "If you don't lose more weight, you'll die." I used to get so angry. I could handle it, but it really got to my daughter.

Margaret essentially described an instance of blame levied by traditional physicians.

In another situation where a patient blamed herself, it seemed interesting that she did not think of blaming the physicians. This woman, Gloria, had undergone three surgeries for Crohn's disease. She now drove more than a hundred miles to see Dr. A, because she had been searching for a physician with expertise in nutrition. Many of her comments, as she described the history of her problems, indicated self-condemnation. After she repeated something to the affect of "If only I had known more about nutrition then," three times, I finally responded:

> Me: Two or three times now, you said that if you'd known or researched this earlier, maybe you wouldn't be here now or that

things would have been different. [I told her I was interested in that because it seemed as though she was feeling guilty or blaming herelf for not knowing what she knows now about nutrition in the early sixties.] Do you feel guilty or somehow responsible?

Gloria: Yes (nodding) . . . sometimes I go into a mild depression when I think about that.

Me: During this whole period . . . where you somehow blamed yourself, did you ever think of blaming the physicians? [She looked surprised] For their not knowing about these things then? You said doctors don't know about nutrition.

Pt: I never thought of blaming the doctors.

Me: Why?

Pt: My body's my responsibility, I guess.

Me: It sounds almost like you're blaming yourself morally, like it was your failure that caused it.

Pt: [nodding] When you do something, and it's your responsibility, if something goes wrong, it's your fault.

This patient also mentioned recent studies indicating a possible viral causative agent in Crohn's disease. She described her reaction: "Now I read about viruses every once in a while. That's a new theory about Crohn's disease. That would take it all off me! It's not something I did to myself." In her perception, a viral cause would have "let her off the hook," while a stress or nutritional cause attributes the responsibility and resultant blame to her. Again, it is the traditional medical model, rather than the holistic model, that has not absolved her from blame.

Diet and nutritional change evoked the greatest amount of self-condemnation observed in this particular clinic. One attractive woman in her late thirties, who worked full-time and had school-age children, was found to have multiple food allergies. She was to eliminate those foods in an attempt to reduce the incidence and intensity of her severe headaches. The first time I observed her, Joan wanted to talk about how hard it was to give up the foods. She described herself as a "chocolate addict" who drinks all her coffee and tea with sugar. She reacts to MSG, and has been having increasingly severe problems with migraine headaches. As she said, "I eat all the taboo foods for migraine." She said that both she

and her husband "live to eat," and described that as their "main recreation." Being on this restrictive diet, even temporarily, was very disruptive to her entire life. She spoke of how eating out and having chocolate
was the only pleasure she really allowed herself, and that she could not
face giving that up. Her talk was punctuated with comments like "I know
I should be able to" and other comments indicating self-defined weakness
and failure.

Many patients expressed similar guilt when they talked of eating
"junk food" or not taking the time to exercise. Frequently women especially talked of feeling guilty about being unable to give up chocolate or
sweets. Not infrequently, this form of talk emerged spontaneously in talk
between the nurses, the receptionist, and myself. So even clinic staff
members at times engaged in similar self-recrimination.

When I asked one woman why she was seeing Dr. A, she described
migraines that had been occurring with increasing frequency and intensity. She spoke of how she had read books that described techniques for
controlling the pain. It would make sense to her at the time; however,
when she had another episode, she "couldn't handle it." I commented
that it sounded as though she were "coming down on herself" and asked
why. She told me how her friends said, and the books also stated, that
she "should" be able to control the pain, and she was defining her lack
of control as a personal moral failure. While Jean described her headaches, she commented:

> Jean: The codeine really bothers me. I want to get off it. I can't
> cope . . . I'm disappointed in myself. It's pain, and I get mad
> at myself! [said angrily with self-condemnation]
>
> Me: It sounds like you feel you should be able to control the
> pain and you feel guilty [said questioningly].
>
> Jean: [nodding] Yes, you have a tendency to come down on
> yourself. I have so many mixed emotions. Well . . . I feel like
> I should be able to cope better.
>
> Me: Why?
>
> Jean: Well. . . . I read a few articles, like on living with pain.
> Some people have to learn to live with it. Why can't I? [again
> sounded angry at herself] It's fine for me to think about learning
> to live with it when the pain's not there. But, when I get it . . .
> the pain, I can't handle it without something.

Later, during this same session, when another patient spoke of how difficult it had been for him to eliminate several foods from his diet, Jean responded, "The diet changes are really hard. I've been guilty of throwing so much junk into my body over the years! It's all in my mind though [pointing to her head and laughing]. I know I should be able to do it."

During another day in the setting, a very articulate man in his thirties was undergoing fitness testing. Gail, Dan, and I were casually talking and joking while waiting for the physician. We talked about all the technology utilized in hospitals (Dan's work as a minister involved visiting sick patients frequently), and I commented that it was becoming apparent in holistic health too, mentioning biofeedback rings and pocket-sized machines to monitor skin temperature as a measure of anxiety level. Dan said that got him upset. He described attending a dinner with five people, where everyone tried a portable machine that measured relaxation/anxiety level. Everyone else treated it "almost as a game," but Dan found it upsetting: "I was really uptight, and it bothered me for everyone to see it. Relaxing is optimum now; you 'should be' relaxed. What if I want to be angry?" Here again, the element of visibility is symbolically important.

Casual Comments

Beyond the focused data, casual comments I frequently heard from friends and colleagues pointed to the same shift in attribution of blame, coming from a diffuse societal shift towards an "ideology of choice." One frequent example was the kind of self-condemnation expressed by friends in relation to their perceived poor nutritional habits, exercise regimes, excess weight, and high stress levels. Comments such as "I know I should be able to give up smoking" echo the pressures for special non-smoking areas in public places, such as restaurants. Many of these comments follow a formula of the individual expressing that she or he has the knowledge of what she or he "should" do, but is unable to implement those lifestyle changes.[12]

The strength of these kinds of moral judgments that are usually taken-for-granted was also exemplified by several comments made by my then eleven-year-old son during the course of my research. For example, after he attended a staff beach party with me, he commented on his surprise that one of the nurses was "so fat." I was taken aback, because this woman was only slightly overweight. When I commented on my reaction, he replied that he expected more of her "because she's working in a holistic health office and she should know better." His comments reflected that he had already picked up the cultural norms around self-responsibility and choice, and that he felt moral indignation was justifiable in relation to lifestyle lapses.

Managing Lapses

I was surprised at the strength of my self-condemnation and began to ask staff (initially in the setting, and later in the formal interviews) how they handled their "lapses." I focused in on how much of the ideology they carry out and how they feel about any deviations. I found that many practitioners "came down on themselves" frequently, although many others described themselves as becoming more accepting, or already being accepting, of where they were.

Nurse A had expressed on at least two occasions how angry she gets at herself for eating so much and not losing weight. I asked Nurse B whether she "comes down on herself" the way I find myself doing for my lapses. She replied: "I used to. But now, when I start thinking that way, I just say to myself, 'Get off my back!' [laughing] It's just one more stress to deal with. So I don't let it get to me anymore."

The practitioners who seemed to be most sensitive to the complexities of the holistic model seemed to have less trouble with their lapses. As one psychologist said:

> No . . . what I always do is I always come back to it being understandable and natural. I need to nurture myself. I go and I have coffee and I love ice cream. And I'll have ice cream sometimes. I know it's not the best thing for me. But, damn it, I'm not going to be perfect! What the hell is perfect, anyway?

Another practitioner acknowledged handling the problem similarly:

> Me: Do you find you ever have trouble ridding yourself of those shoulds?
>
> Dr: Certainly. Everyday.
>
> Me: Of coming down on yourself?
>
> Dr: Everyday. That's part of being human, I think.
>
> Me: . . . unfortunately. [both laughing]
>
> Dr: . . . we have to have the ability to be kind to ourselves and laugh at ourselves and to know that we're subject to frailties and that we have to . . it doesn't help in any way to berate oneself.

Why Practitioners and Patients Want This Shift

Two crucial questions that are raised by these early signs of a broad societal shift in the attribution of blame for illness relate to the reciprocal effects of the shift. Why do practitioners want this shift in the attribution of responsibility, and why are patients willing to accept it? It is initially easier to see the advantages of the shift for practitioners than for the patients, who derive more blame along with the added responsibility. On the other hand, the more I came to understand the meanings both providers and clients attached to the shift, the more ambivalent and problematic those symbolic meanings and motivations appeared.

Meaning to Practitioners

A definite tension existed in the symbolic meanings practitioners attached to the shift. On one hand, this group of practitioners wanted to give up, or at least lessen, their responsibility for patient health and illness and direction of cure. Beyond their beliefs in the ultimate advantages of the new model for patients, two broad categories of advantages that arose pertained to practitioner self-interest. On the other hand, it turned out that practitioners were taking on additional areas of responsibility, even as they were talking of giving up the traditional areas for which they were held accountable.

In a broad range of studies on physicians, it has been found that doctors have, if anything, trouble giving up the authority and responsibility deriving from their role. Two areas cropped up in this group of physicians which contrasted sharply with those findings. While some physicians, when asked whether it was difficult for them to give up some of their responsibility in relation to the patient, described it being difficult at first, others talked of it being easy or even a "relief." The reasons behind this positive disposition towards giving up the responsibility in the relationship had one of two bases.

First, some physicians wanted to give up the responsibility because they "cared too much." These physicians experienced the burden of professional responsibility very heavily and found themselves overwhelmed by it or having difficulty handling it. The shift in responsibility inherent in the new model provided them a measure of emotional relief. It was almost as if these physicians had not been adequately socialized into developing a strong barrier of defenses, maintaining their separateness from patients. Their involvement with patients was more intense than most physicians.

One young female physician expressed surprise when I asked whether it was initially or presently difficult for her to give up her responsibility. She described it as a relief, but then immediately needed to do ideological work to reconcile her shift with her primary values of caring and involvement:

> Me: There's a very close balance between really caring and also having some protective barrier to allow yourself to keep going.
>
> Dr: Yeah. Exactly. And a little bit in there comes patient responsibility for his or her problems . . . that I finally figured out that I wasn't going to last long taking on everybody's problems and caring so much as if it were my own problem. And then that sounds a little selfish for me to pull back to that space, even that much, which wasn't very far but enough to keep a distance. And then the realization came that actually it's patients' responsibility for their own health, for their own well-being, comes in there . . that concept comes in there.

Several other physicians I interviewed described it as relatively easy or a relief, although they described many other physicians as having a more difficult time with relinquishing responsibility. On the other hand, a psychologist who worked in a large, interdisciplinary holistic clinic spoke of how hard it had been for all the doctors in that clinic to give up their responsibility and authority (he described them as not being aware of how much trouble they had).

Both the physicians who had been in practice the longest described their giving up of responsibility as relatively easy and a relief. They also had found the responsibility became increasingly emotionally draining over the years. As one physician described it:

> Me: Was it ever hard for you to give up your responsibility?
>
> Dr: Oh, it was a total pleasure . .
>
> Me: It was a pleasure? Okay . .
>
> Dr: That's why I left (traditional) medicine . . . I couldn't handle the responsibility. I couldn't handle it. It was very clear.

The other physician responded similarly:

> The other thing basically was the gradual concept or willingness on my part, or realization that it's very freeing to the physician to turn over the responsibility to the patient for their

health and well-being to the degree that they want it and are willing to accept it, and that it's very burdensome to carry that responsibility and lonesome, and that sharing it with a patient eased my mind, eased my tensions.

Besides these emotional costs of physician responsibility, a second area of self-interest was economically motivated. I was surprised when a physician I had a superficial relationship with very candidly stated in an early portion of the interview that he wanted to give up his almost total responsibility because of the escalating costs of malpractice insurance. He described how he finally decided it was "better malpractice insurance" to candidly discuss all aspects of the choices with patients. After describing how liberating it was to share his responsibility with patients, this doctor continued:

And I have several reasons for doing that that I rationalized to myself, and one was that I realized as I looked around in the field of medicine that a lot of malpractice suits came out of anger and frustration on the part of the patient . . . for not having been allowed to assume responsibility, for not being told what he or she wanted to know..to expect and to make some intelligent participation in what happened to them, but they felt that they were being treated with haughty arrogance or indifference or coldness and they were angry. And when something didn't go right, they struck back at the doctor through suing them. And I saw as I reflected on my training years, there were a couple of doctors that were just exceptionally warm and caring and not necessarily the most technically competent. And if something happened to their patients, we just knew they wouldn't . . . there was no way they were going to get sued. The patients just wouldn't sue ol' Frank or ol' Joe or whatever. But, although the fellow may be a brilliant surgeon or something, if they just didn't see him as a caring human being and something went wrong, it's much easier for them to say, "Well, what the hell, sue him!"

Basically, this physician saw shared responsibility, combined with a caring relationship based on mutual trust, as economically protective, as well as an end to itself.[13] Although only one other physician in the group discussed similar considerations, an undercurrent of economic pressure may have combined with their more humanistically-motivated concern to foster a shift towards a mutual, shared responsibility.

An almost identical comment came up in an interview with another family practitioner. I had asked whether he saw any advantages of physicians giving patients more responsibility fairly late in the interview:

Dr: Do you mean an advantage to getting people better quicker or an advantage for me?

Me: For you.

Dr: Well, that calls to mind a totally off-the-wall subject which is medical malpractice, which I think is not a symptom of an aggressive legal profession or even doctor ignorance or lack of knowledge, but is a decline in the social contract between the doctor and the patient about mutual responsibility . . . and that, in fact, the big advantage for the doctor from doing that is not to throw the ball in the patient's lap but to have a therapeutic contract between peers about getting better, each contributing what they know best and recognizing that the patient may fall down and the doctor may fall down . . . but that kind of a dialogue is the essence of a good doctor-patient relationship. And having that approach to patients has the advantage to doctors. . . . I mean, like I took care of a kid who had a hard appendix for ten days . . . two weeks . . . I missed it. If you want to call that negligence and malpractice . . . but I think the nature of the relationship I have with the family is such that everybody's glad he had his operation and got better, and I don't think they're going to sue me. But if I was uh . . . not into that kind of relationship, I'd certainly be biting my fingernails.

The economic pressures deriving from increased malpractice suits have initiated a variety of self-protective strategies by physicians. One common strategy is usually referred to as "defensive medicine," where a physician orders a variety of diagnostic tests unlikely to disclose new problems on a statistical basis. Various analysts have pointed out the protective benefits to the physician, as weighed against the economic and physically intrusive costs to patients of such strategies. This group of holistically oriented physicians would be ideologically opposed to any self-protective strategies that would maximize the use of technological tools. Developing a caring, trusting relationship, however, can minimize the risk of malpractice suits, while avoiding the costs to patients of such defensive medicine and remaining true to their primary values.

At the same time that some providers are describing feelings of relief accompanying a decrease in their responsibility for patient health and cure, it also became apparent that these same providers were not giving up as much responsibility as it initially appeared. Rather, they were shifting the areas for which they took responsibility within the provider-patient interaction. Several providers, physicians as well as psychologists and nurses, spontaneously brought this up in the interviews. It became continually apparent in both field settings as well. Not only did the process of absolving patients remain similar, as discussed earlier in the chapter, the degree of responsibility taken by practitioners remained fairly constant. Often only the content areas of responsibility actually shifted.

Thus, while practitioners felt less responsible for whether the patient followed through on what they jointly decided was the best therapeutic or preventive plan, they felt more responsible for educating the patient, for explaining the alternatives in terms understandable to that person. They also felt more responsibility for their knowledge around communication and motivation, as well as their knowledge in the areas of nutrition, exercise, and stress reduction. Another area that continually emerged was the feeling of responsibility for assessing how much responsibility the specific patient was ready to handle at a particular time, so that the degree of information and choice offered varied between patients and through time, based on practitioner assessment of patient readiness. As one physician stated:

> And then there's the additional responsibility of giving them their responsibility at the optimal rate, because I just can't, on their first visit . . . can't just say well, listen this is what's wrong with you . . . Here, it's in your lap, go do something about it. I have to judge when is the best time to hear what parts of it and when, and not overwhelm them too fast . . . not say the whole picture too fast that they might interpret it as threatening . . . like, well, in that case, I'm just a terrible person and there's no hope.

Especially for the physician, these new areas for which they experienced personal responsibility and accountability were often areas in which they had had no professional preparation. Communication skills and knowledge of nutrition are conspicuously absent in most medical school curricula. Knowledge about spiritual well-being is even further removed from their training.

One last area emerged as an important dimension of responsibility for these practitioners. This was mentioned explicitly by only a few practitioners during the intensive interviews, but it was also apparent in related comments and the field observations. Practitioners felt a responsibility to "be there one hundred percent" when interacting with a patient. An intense level of involvement and attention, as well as utilizing all the available knowledge, was part of the provider responsibility, whether a physician, psychologist, or nurse. While this derives partially from the overriding world view of this group, it also implies a similar, though modified, view of professional responsibility. As one of the physicians explained it:

> Okay . . . the responsibility I feel towards my patient's wellness or illness is to be able to maintain a sense of being there completely for the patient. Being there . . . not just in my physical being there, but being there for that patient during that hour's time and being prepared with the . . . through the experience that I have had to offer that individual help through the tools that I have. I do not feel a responsibility for that patient using those tools.

Meaning to Patients

The complex symbolic meanings to patients of the shift in responsibility and attribution remain even more subtle and ambivalent. At first glance, there are fewer reasons for patients to gain from the increased responsibility, while they stand to lose a great deal if each illness comes to be defined as an intentionally chosen state. Given that this view is like "blaming the victim," why do some kinds of people welcome it, while others react negatively? Do different kinds of people assume the blame?

There appear to be two primary reasons why patients are willing to accept this responsibility. First, the other side of responsibility and attribution in illness is *power and control*. Proponents of holistic health, both providers and clients, stress this as the most important aspect of responsibility. Many practitioners describe their goal in working with patients as to "empower" them. If a patient, for example, comes to realize that he or she "caused" his illness, he or she can then modify the parts of their life that manifested themselves physically, and thus cure the problem. So the responsibility is accompanied by the power to exert control over the disease. Furthermore, taking control in one area of their lives gives people a feeling of being in control of their life as a whole. They perceive themselves as more powerful and less the victims of fate.

Scarf raised the issue of blame with patients attending a Simonton group meeting she observed. She described the patients as objecting to this criticism:

"Blame is not the same as responsibility," a lymphoma patient
insisted tartly. "Responsibility means power, blame is helpless.
The fact is that if I actively cooperated with the disease, I gave
it to myself. And if I gave it to myself, I can make it go away.
The sense of power and control is there, you see, very strong"
(Scarf, 1980:45).

Such comments show the values placed on independence and self-
control, as well as the perceived relationship of self-responsibility with
self-worth.

One woman I observed in the practice was a business executive in
her mid forties. The previous summer her regular physician had discovered she had a blood pressure of 170/80. Already fairly ambivalent about
traditional medicine, she heard of this clinic through an older friend who
was also skeptical of doctors. As she said, "I felt I had nothing to lose,
so I tried it." Within three weeks of beginning stress-reduction techniques, she had brought her blood pressure reading down to 155/90, and
it was 124/80 when I saw her (she was still on low doses of medication).
She described feeling tremendous control following the changes, and
those feelings of power had motivated her to change her diet and begin a
mild exercise program.

The second reason patients are willing to accept this responsibility
is that it serves a protective function when they are healthy. In other
words, the "ideology of choice" gives people the *illusion of control when
they are well*. Western ways of living and thinking give rise to an obses-
sional expression of the need to be in control, and the ideology of choice
feeds into an illusion of having that control. Individuals are more willing
to take the blame when well. Although more systematic tests need to be
carried out to substantiate this, it seems that healthy people or those who
feel they are curing their problem are most willing to accept responsibility
for their health.

Being ill is almost synonomous with being out of control. Severe
illness leads to devastating feelings of powerlessness and loss of control
over one's body and the intimate details of one's everyday life. The powerlessness accompanying illness and hospitalization are difficult to deal
with in our society, and the ideology of choice seems to be an attempt to
deal with our lack of control in these areas. Thus it serves a protective,
denial function.

When well, this belief allows people to feel they are healthy by
choice, and thus they can remain healthy as long as they choose. These
omnipotent feelings of control may be adaptive during health. Unfortu-

nately, all of us must die eventually, and it is when faced with severe illness or death that this view results in the most damaging effects at the societal, interactional, and individual levels. If the price of egalitarianism and responsibility is guilt, people are more willing to put up with it when healthy.

One of the holistic internists I interviewed spontaneously brought up similar observations when I asked him how much trouble patients have taking the responsibility for their health:

> Oh, in general, once they become patients they have a tremendous amount of difficulty doing that. People who are basically healthy have an easier job. Just like most of us, when things are going good, it is easier to be happy than it is when things are going badly. When people have diseases, particularly because they have not been trained that diseases are anything else but things that come out of the blue, then it is very difficult for them to accept that responsibility.

It is as if, when healthy, the ideology of choice provides a "guarantee," an illusion of a level of control over our lives. That illusion crumbles with evidence of serious illness. One of the patients I interviewed talked of the anguish her father experienced when he developed cancer:

> My father died when he was 55 years old. He was the type who believed in taking responsibility for yourself. My father was the type who played golf two or three times a week . . . exercised. He ate very well, very nutritionally. Took vitamins, and tried all the vinegar diets. And read a lot of books. . . . Adelle Davis types of books, on keeping well and staying well. He didn't smoke. And he died when he was fifty-five of lymphosarcoma. We went to Dr. Contreras down in Tijuana for Laetrile treatments. We did not . . . he did not take them, but we investigated it, and when we were in the office that day, he looked at Dr. Contrares, and he said, "I'm the one this is not supposed to happen to. I'm the one that has done all the things that I'm supposed to do, but yet the person who smokes two packs of cigarettes a day can live forever, but I'm dying." And I think it made it much harder for him to die. Because he was the one that followed everything you were supposed to follow, and he died.

I conducted an exploratory survey on attitudes towards holistic health with a group of undergraduate students at the University of California at San Diego. The students responding were almost all in their late teens and early twenties and had no obviously visible illness or handicapping conditions. In this group of 36 students, *every* student thought that the individual should be responsible for his or her health. They invariably gave several advantages for individual responsibility for health and illness, while they did not list any disadvantages. I suspect that the same questionnaire administered to a group of terminally ill patients would get dramatically different responses.[14]

Additionally, many patients who use the rhetoric freely do not actually want to take responsibility. Besides the group who use the responsibility rhetoric when well and then want the physician to assume responsibility once they become acutely ill, the practitioners interviewed frequently mentioned that some patients who spoke of wanting to take responsibility did not actually want to or were not yet ready to assume that responsibility. For example, one physician described about two-thirds of his patients as extremely motivated in this area. In describing the other group, he said: "maybe about a third are very . . . you know, they're still coming from having someone do it for them. The magic pill now becomes the magic acupuncture needle or the magic herb."

A Caring Stance of Providers is the Mediator

The primary mediator in determining whether the "ideology of choice" was translated into blaming the patient at an interactional level is a caring stance of the provider. Those practitioners who guarded against translating talk about "responsibility" into blame or guilt were the ones who also brought up concepts of *caring, compassion and spiritual commitment* in the interviews. The practitioners who saw their work with patients as embedded in a larger spiritual commitment do not induce blame; in other words, they continue to absolve patients. They may use any combination of the theoretical outs discussed earlier to justify their continued absolution function; however, the compassion and karmic acceptance proved to be the most salient uniting aspect. On the other hand, the "less evolved" practitioners translate the responsibility issues into terms of guilt and condemnation.

Again, while almost all of these practitioners framed this compassion and spiritual commitment within Eastern terminology and concepts, it could have actually come from either an Eastern or Western monistic tradition. Besides their specific attributions to movement into Eastern spiritual disciplines, their linguistic categories reflected that derivation.

Shapiro and Shapiro's warning article on the dangers of self-responsibility summarizes the dangerous aspects of blame when they write, "Into the righteous rhetoric of the holistic health movement, we would like to inject a reminder of compassion and humility toward ourselves and others" (Shapiro and Shapiro, 1979:212). In many ways their comments were consistently echoed by the holistic practitioners I observed and interviewed, but without the Shapiros' self-righteous overtones.

For example, one of the clinic psychologists, Shirley, answered my question about her degree of personal involvement with her patients: "I think that I have a great deal of personal involvement in that I do care and I care unconditionally about those patients. And I have a great deal of compassion for the state that they're in." Later, during this same interview, Shirley spoke of people coming for help when they were ill and needing the professionals to be "compassionate," so that providers don't fall into the "trap" of blaming patients.

When I asked a physician during our interview about his reaction to more doctors and nurses questioning whether they should spend time on patients who have chosen to smoke, etc., he thought the response was fairly obvious:

Me: How do you react to that?

Dr: Very negatively! [laughs] That's . . .

Me: Why?

Dr: Well, that's . . . first of all, we don't know that for sure, so it's making some scientific . . . so-called scientific assumptions, and, secondly, it's unkind. We . . . again the same thing would come up if you were in an emergency room and somebody who was brought in who was shot while shooting someone else and you say, "Well, he brought this on himself. Let him die. He deserves it." Well, you're not in a position to make those moral judgments about people.

Me: What is it that allows you to care for people without the moral labels and derogation?

Dr: Well, nothing special. I . . . we're all human and we. . . . there isn't anything that anyone has ever done that I wouldn't be capable of doing under certain circumstances myself, so that individual is no different than I and it's . . . one's behavior is different than one's essence, one's spirit, one's soul. And I don't think we can, or should particularly, as physicians, or clerics or whatever, just discard another human being because of his behavior, however reprehensible it may seem to be. We don't know what was really happening inside that individual that produced that behavior.

Further in the interview, in talking about healing, this physician returned to "acceptance": "I think that we need to be sure that we ourselves strive toward charity and acceptance of human frailties."

Other similar comments that came up in the interviews, indicating the importance of that kind of compassionate acceptance, included:

People are human. I'm not perfect, nobody is perfect, and it's just part of their humanness that is being manifested then (Physician in secondary holistic clinic).

the basic philosophy of being in the health profession, and that is to help. It's not to reject. In very simple feeling levels, I think that's the way I see it (Physician in secondary setting).

The way I see that is going to the bottom line of the whole thing for me, which is unconditional love. I think that's something that is infinitely happening, and that's not a place you arrive at or a state that you come to . . . it's a process that we are continually in (AHH leader).

But if you come from a position of caring and a position of love, then you do what you can with a patient, and if your motives are pure, all the time, which of course is actually impossible for any of us who are human, you keep trying, you know, you don't give up the ship (Physician on medical school faculty).

One of the nurses in the primary clinic was almost a model for living this compassion and acceptance of where patients were at. During her lengthy interview at the end of the field study, I asked why she seemed much more patient with many people than most health professionals, and what allowed her to be that way. Her answer is reported in considerable detail because it illustrates the deeper level of meanings underlying the usual superficial answers:

> Nurse: I think because I have more compassion for the weaknesses of human beings. I just feel that we are not perfect, and we are all on a journey, and it doesn't mean that you are going to do everything perfectly. It doesn't mean that because you know what you are supposed to eat, you're going to. It is because of the particular place you are in your life. If you are having difficulty doing it, I can understand that it's hard. I am not condoning it, and I continue to encourage them to make the changes. If, for some reason they can't do it, I understand the weaknesses of the human condition.

> Me: And you don't have to blame them?

> Nurse: Yes, I don't blame them. I understand them.

> Me: Do you blame yourself, or do you understand yourself when you realize that you're . . .

> Nurse: Yes, I understand myself. I feel that I'm doing the best I can and that I am not totally evolved yet.

> [further in the interview, after more probing]

> Nurse: I am much more compassionate with people now and that has to do with things that have happened in my personal life.

> Me: You mean . . . as you have felt pain, you become more tuned in to pain in other people?

> Nurse: Right. I guess I basically felt that if you were a good person, you didn't make a lot of mistakes. . . . then life went great, life ran relatively smoothly. If you started making wrong choices or bad choices, whatever you want to call them, then you got punished. That's how I saw it and so I judged people that way. My life for a long time ran very smoothly and I felt I made all the right choices, and I was a "good" girl. Well, when things started happening in my life, when my life seemed to crumble a bit and when I wasn't living up to my own image of myself, then I went through this time of depression and a time of guilt and also a time of tremendous growth. Now I realize

that these crises in people's lives are growing times. So they're good. That, if you always walk what you consider the straight and narrow and never risk and never take a chance and never do something that you question the value of, then you never grow. You stay unconscious. For a lot of my life I was unconscious.

Me: When you talk about being more compassionate, many people I am talking to mean the same thing as caring. It's very hard for them to define what caring is. Isn't that related to what you were were talking about . . . being very compassionate and not judgmental?

Nurse: I think that's a part of it. Although I think I was a caring person even before in that I was very dedicated to what I was doing. Always there late and doing things for patients that maybe other people wouldn't have done. So I was caring in that way; but now, I am caring at a deeper level. I care not just about their physical comfort as I probably did before or if they were crying I would stay, but I really didn't really understand, and I couldn't get to them at any deep level. Now I feel that I can be there spiritually, and emotionally and psychologically where maybe before I was just there physically in some way, or I was there emotionally but at a very superficial level. Now I feel that I am there at a deeper level, and I think people feel that because I have had people tell me all the time that they feel that I really do care. I have a feeling my touch has changed in some way, because I get that kind of feedback too. That when you touch me, I feel you really do care.

[later in the interview we talked about other practitioners blaming patients for illness]

Nurse: In my experience it has taken a long time to make a change in a person's life. My own included . . . and maybe especially. I realize that even though I know all the basic principles about nutrition, I don't follow them. Okay. So I know that making a change in your life is difficult, and it doesn't happen maybe with just one exposure to someone giving you information about that change, or someone encouraging you to make that change, or even you yourself seeing that a particular change in someone's life has been for the good. It takes, in my experience it has taken more than one time.

Me: [discussed the problems I see when people take parts of the picture and misinterpret them] Some people are taking parts of the picture and what they immediately say is, "Ah, hah! They are not getting well if they are not trying to get well." People get a little piece of this, and it comes out, "You caused your illness" or "You don't want to get well!"

Nurse: First of all, I think you have to accept that not getting well is okay. It is as okay as getting well. So it is okay if you get well, and okay if you don't get well. I'm not saying, June, that your goal isn't that they get well. . . . your goal is that they get well.

Me: How do you mean?

Nurse: It is okay to fail. I guess that's what I'm saying. It's okay that when you try to do something, if you don't do it correctly, or you don't achieve your immediate goal . . . then that's alright. . . . I know what we see in Western society is success, and in the traditional model of course that is getting well. Death is a failure. So until you come to the point where you see death as not a failure, but just as a transition, then you are going to have that problem. So it is not that you are not giving this person all the tools that are possible to use in order to achieve this goal. You are encouraging them, and supporting them lovingly, but at the same time if they don't get well, it's okay.

Jampolsky talks of how, when you are "totally loving . . . accepting where a person is," you cannot experience anger at them or blame them (Jampolsky, 1981). At another conference, many things Jampolsky said also implied the opposite of the guilt so often attributed to his approach. He spoke of the importance of "rewarding yourself," and then continued by saying, "When you make a mistake, remember you learn more from mistakes. There's no right or wrong behavior, no right and wrong answers. All experiences are gifts, opportunities for growing" (Jampolsky, 1982). These comments, like those made by the nurse in Mar Vista Clinic, epitomize the shared philosophy of the practitioners who espouse the "ideology of choice," yet continue to provide compassionate care without blaming their patients.

Another indication from the data that this variable was crucial was the frequency with which practitioners spoke of the importance of "carefully choosing" staff for their offices. As discussed earlier, practitioners talked about the level of sensitivity, compassion, and humility of individual staff members being pivotal in carrying out their goals. Similarly, the underlying spiritual commitment of staff members was consistently emphasized (this was usually couched in Eastern terminology). In exploring what that meant, they repeatedly came up with humanistic, caring kinds of qualities.

Throughout both the interviews and the field study, a dialectic tension between patient responsibility and this caring stance of the provider emerged. As difficult as it is to abstract the qualties involved in this kind of caring, accepting relationship, deriving from a deeply spiritual commitment to service, this parameter is the crucial mediator in the attribution of blame. In the final chapter, this mediation process will be linked to the broader societal picture, while the implications of the united model will be explored.

7

Beyond Responsibility

I have already analyzed aspects of the shifts in the provider-patient relationship, along with closely related aspects of the sick role. The last chapter extended the analysis of the sick role enactment by focusing on the shift in attribution of responsibility to the individual. The data at the behavioral level in the holistic settings contrasted markedly with the "ideology of choice" voiced by movement participants. These holistic physicians continue to absolve patients in a process closely paralleling the absolution function of more traditional physicians. I outlined the mechanisms that allow these practitioners to continue to absolve patients from guilt, while emphasizing self-responsibility. I then demonstrated that patients actually do experience blame and guilt, but that it is derived from outside these settings with the diffusion of simplistic interpretations of holistic concepts of mind-body continuity and the "ideology of choice" into mainstream medicine and the larger society.

This final chapter will conclude by extending the analysis of the themes developed in those chapters. As mentioned earlier, it is tempting to continue the analytical separation of components of the model. The complexities of analyzing the meanings of responsibility alone are overwhelming, without including the interactions of the entire constellation of beliefs, meanings, and behaviors associated with the more holistic, participatory model of health care. While useful analytically, however, crucial aspects of the phenomena studied are easily overlooked through such a division into component parts. For example, the shifts in attribution of responsibility can only be completely understood when analyzed simultaneously with the shift towards a more egalitarian physician-patient relationship. Furthermore, both these shifts are related in fundamental ways to the potential for a widespread moralistic lifestyle crusade.

In what way does the dialectic tension between patient responsibility and the provider's caring stance have an impact on a broader societal level? And how can the overwhelming number of paradoxes unearthed be explained sociologically, again against the background of the broader historical context? These questions become the central focus of this final chapter.

The implications of uniting the model will be developed in terms of three major outcomes. First, the potential for a widespread moral crusade will be further examined. Second, the relationship of the holistic health model to processes of medicalization will be elucidated. Third, the interrelationship between the more egalitarian physician-patient relationship, the decreased gatekeeping function of the physician, and the shift in the attribution of responsibility and blame will be demonstrated in an explanatory construct clarifying the functional aspects of such a moral crusade.

Interpretations of the potential lifestyle crusade also need to take into account the intersection of two very different philosophical belief systems. In the next section I will describe the processes that occur at the interface of Eastern and Western world views. The effects of the diffusion of Eastern beliefs into a Western world view further explain how a humanistically based model can come to at times have antihumanistic effects.

Just as ambiguities, flux, and paradox pervade the moral reasoning of participants, my analysis requires a syncretism of theoretical approaches. I will resort to a synthesis of both radical and conservative theoretical conceptualizations in developing an explanatory theoretical framework. Once again, meaningful explanation rarely fits in the neat, constrained categories that social scientists develop to make life easier. I need to also acknowledge that portions of this analysis are somewhat more speculative than the heavily documented arguments presented on the shifts in the provider-patient relationship and self responsibility.

The Potential for a Widespread Moral Crusade

The humanistic versus individualistic contradictions underlying the attribution of responsibility at times set the stage for a kind of 1984 therapeutic tyranny, where the pursuit of health becomes an infinite quest, and moral condemnation and the withdrawal of resources accompanies evidence of illness. In this section I will explore this possibility of a moralistic social crusade against the ill and those who demonstrate lifestyle lapses. This phenomenon increasingly appears to present the major danger posed by the diffusion of the holistic, participatory model of health care throughout the society.

The focus on responsibility attribution in this concluding chapter emphasizes its nature as a public rather than a private problem. Joseph Gusfield creates a conceptual model through which to analyze public problems that acknowledges the interrelationship of their cognitive and moral dimensions. As he writes:

> As ideas and consciousness public problems have a structure which involves both a cognitive and a moral dimension. The cognitive side consists in beliefs about the facticity of the situation and events comprising the problem—our theories and empirical beliefs about [the problem]. The moral side is that which enables the situation to be viewed as painful, ignoble, immoral. . . . Without both a cognitive belief in alterability and a moral judgment of its character, a phenomenon is not at issue, not a problem. . . . The reality of a problem is often expanded or contracted in scope as cognitive or moral judgment shifts (Gusfield, 1981:9–10).

In the introductory chapter I discussed my basic underlying assumptions in the areas of deviance and social control. Here I will very briefly reiterate them. First, I assume that any examination of deviance and social control also studies moral reasoning. Morality and values come to be presented as taken-for-granted, factual, and apolitical. I also assume that medical designations are at least partially social judgments with both ethical and political bases. As Conrad and Schneider write:

> medical designations are social judgments, and the adoption of a medical model of behavior, a political decision. When such medical designations are applied to deviant behavior, they are related directly and intimately to the moral order of society (Conrad and Schneider, 1980:35).

Similarly, I view science as a social enterprise, where the claims of moral neutrality cover taken-for-granted ethical and political assumptions and values (Gusfield, 1981:19).

I am not arguing here that moral designations are so-to-speak immoral or unacceptable. Instead, I recognize that there are always moral designations implied within any cultural context, and that awareness of those assumptions is necessary for understanding social phenomena in context. I also do not personally see self-responsibility as an unacceptable concept. Instead, I want us to be aware that the role of health professionals has historically included the responsibility not to blame and inflict further pain on those already suffering. While the realities of everyday life medical practice may at times depart from that ideal, most health professionals and policy makers feel a moral obligation to maintain that stance.[1]

Medicalization

Medical sociology has a lengthy historical tradition of viewing medicine as an institution of social control. Variants of this basic assumption can be traced through the functionalist, Marxist, symbolic interactionist, and radical theoretical perspectives. In other words, varying degrees of social control by physicians characterize the range of theories, from conservative to radical.

Medicalization has come to be the concept used to describe medicine's expanding influence in defining and controlling many forms of deviance as illness. The process posits a shift from sin or crime to illness definitions in the treatment of deviant behavior. Over time, increasing areas of societal deviance have come under medical control. As Zola writes:

> medicine is becoming a major institution of social control, nudging aside, if not incorporating, the more traditional institutions of religion and law. . . . Moreover, this is not occurring through the political power physicians hold or can influence, but is largely an insidious and often undramatic phenomenon accomplished by "medicalizing" much of daily living, by making medicine and the labels "healthy" and "ill" relevant to an ever increasing part of human existence (Zola, 1978: 80).

Peter Conrad and Joseph W. Schneider have most thoroughly documented the historical development of this process in their work *Deviance and Medicalization* (Conrad and Schneider, 1980). They summarize the historical development of this trend:

> When treatment rather than punishment becomes the preferred sanction for deviance, an increasing amount of behavior is conceptualized in a medical framework as illness. As noted earlier,

this is not unexpected, since medicine has always functioned as an agent of social control, especially in attempting to "normalize" illness and return people to their functioning capacity in society. Public health and psychiatry have long been concerned with social behavior and have functioned traditionally as agents of social control (Foucault, 1965; Rosen, 1972). What is significant, however, is the expansion of this sphere where medicine functions in a social control capacity. In the wake of a general humanitarian trend, the success and prestige of modern biomedicine, the technological growth of the twentieth century, and diminution of religion as a viable agent of control, more and more deviant behavior has come into the province of medicine. In short, the particular, dominant designation of deviance has changed; much of what was badness (i.e., sinful or criminal) is now sickness (ibid.:34).

Conrad and Schneider demonstrate the process of increasing medicalization in historical perspective through specific examinations of the deviant areas of mental illness, alcoholism, child abuse, and homosexuality.

While most sociologists have recently analyzed the medicalization process in terms of what they defined as "negative" effects, the shift in attribution from sin or crime to illness has had some obviously humanistic functions. As discussed in the chapter on responsibility, the moral character of illness may be inescapable. People who become sick, as Davis found, universally tend to look for at least an element of causation in their own self or behavior, leading them to experience feelings of guilt (Davis, 1962). In this connection, physicians and nurses in this society have functioned to downplay the moral nature of illness, thus absolving sick individuals from blame. Conrad and Schneider acknowledge this humanitarian aspect of medicalization, presenting the example of medical treatment for alcoholism as therapeutically oriented, and thus more humanitarian than retributive or punitive modes of social control (Conrad

Gusfield, on the other hand, challenges this notion that medicalization and the use of therapeutic metaphors remove blame and stigma. In focusing on the case of public definitions and solutions to the problem of alcoholism, he argues that the medical approach also results in the attribution of stigma. As he writes, the imputation of being an alcoholic "entails the description of a flawed person. The offender, in this perspective, has not committed an incompetent deviant act. He is incompetent and deviant" (Gusfield, 1983:2). On the basis of his research in drinking-driving school classes, he concludes that medicalization is punitive: "Rather than absolving the self from responsibility it appears to result in a greater attack on the defendant as deviant" (ibid.:9).

I argue that Gusfield's conclusions actually illustrate that a certain degree of moral attribution is always residual in illness designations. Despite the stigma still implicit in illness metaphors, a return shift towards demedicalization would even further increase the stigmatization and attribution of blame to patients. Thus the shift towards attribution of responsibility for health, disease, and cure to the ill person is analogous to a shift back from illness to designations implying sin or crime. Punishment is again seen as justifiable in relation to actions for which one holds responsibility.

The medicalization argument can be summed up as a historical shift in deviance designations. I argue that a major component of the trend is reversing, and that one of the consequences of the return shift is in the direction of imputation of sin and moral failure.

If medicalization involves a shift from sin or crime to illness designations in the treatment of deviance, holistic health represents a reverse shift in this sense. Since I have shown that there have been some humanistic consequences to the medicalization process with its designations of sickness, a reversal in the historical process can lead to the anti-humanistic consequences portrayed in the chapter on responsibility. Thus a major paradox exists between the humanistic goals and the anti-humanistic consequences of the guilt often induced in the new model.

Holistic Health as Demedicalization or Further Medicalization?

One of the pivotal paradoxes of this shift is the dialectical tension between medicalization and demedicalization resulting from the dispersion of ideas associated with the holistic model of health. As notions such as individual responsibility, mind-body continuity, and the meaning of illness become diffused throughout the society, often in their most simplistic interpretations, the interpretations of the consequences are highly ambiguous.

While the proponents of holistic health argue ideologically for demedicalization, and a process of demedicalization does derive from the shift in responsibility towards the patient, other consequences of a holistic model actually indicate further medicalization rather than demedicalization. Before continuing, it is important to differentiate the dual components usually lumped together under the concept of "medicalization."

First, medicalization is used to refer to the process of expanding the spheres of everyday'life which come under medical control. Thus, for example, child abuse or alcoholism has historically moved to become defined as a "medical problem," one that is part of the medical province. Those problems are no longer seen as the province of the religious or criminal systems. Increasing areas of societal deviance, as well as areas of life traditionally under lay influence, have come under medical control. In this sense, holistic health actually represents a further increase in medicalization, since it places increasing areas of everyday life under medical control with its emphasis on lifestyle modification.

The second sense in which medicalization is used implies the increased social control function physicians have in relation to the individual. The physician's control was merged with the absolution function. In that sense, holistic health represents the demedicalization its proponents claim. The more egalitarian status of patients, along with the movement from institutional to individual solutions, represents decreased physician control. It is in this sphere, where the individual regains control and responsibility, that the cost can be a punitive societal trend. In this sense, holistic health's attempts at demedicalization ultimately lead to more punitive moral sanctions against individuals for illness or lifestyle lapses.

This section will briefly analyze holistic health as the *medicalization of lifestyle*. This focuses attention on the first component of medicalization. Along with the natural childbirth and death/hospice movements, holistic health explicitly attacks the pervasive medicalization in our society and seeks to reverse it. However, during the study I increasingly questioned whether the consequence of implementing beliefs deriving from the holistic health model is actually further medicalization, rather than demedicalization.[2]

As discussed in earlier chapters, patterns of exercise, rest, and nutrition become defined as health concerns and increasingly require consultation with holistic health practitioners. This attention to lifestyle, combined with the view of patient responsibility, leads to expanding medical control.

Chapter VI detailed the already visible consequences in terms of this medicalization of lifestyle. For instance, there is already pressure for increased insurance premiums and public restrictions against smokers. As the public comes to view cancer and similar illnesses as self-caused, it will increasingly lead to moral indignation towards the ill. Similarly those who do not run regularly, meditate, or eat appropriately will come to be seen and criticized as morally inferior.

The emphasis on health, rather than illness, has been discussed as central to the holistic health model earlier. Prevention and health promotion, whether advocated by practitioners of traditional allopathic medicine or holistic health, invariably focuses on life-style change. Thus it can easily evolve into a moral crusade. Despite the holistic ideological focus on demedicalization, the moral overtones of lifestyle change are placing even wider areas of everyday life under medical supervision and control.

Moral crusades have usually occurred to increase medical control. This one certainly puts increasing areas of everyday life under the jurisdiction of the medical system. Physicians increase the arena of social control if lifestyle becomes causative of illness. Once food, exercise, stress, feelings about work, family relationships, and spirituality become implicated in whether an individual becomes ill and whether he or she recovers, health workers must increasingly assess and intervene in these areas.

Additionally, these assessments and interventions become necessary at any point on a health continuum. The problem in the allopathic system was "illness." In the holistic system, even in the absence of any problems, preventive action, or at least constant surveillance, becomes imperative.

One of the most visible forms of this type of medicalization of lifestyle is the blossoming of multiple varieties of health and fitness programs. Established medical centers such as University of California, Los Angeles or Scripps Clinic are offering "total health" or "health enhancement" clinics under physician control. Health Maintenance Organizations such as Kaiser Foundation are offering programs in stress reduction, biofeedback, weight loss, smoking cessation, and similar preventive areas dealing with lifestyle. Simultaneously, increasing numbers of employers are coming to discern the economic advantages of such programs in terms of improved employee productivity. Early programs focused on preventive wellness examinations as part of "occupational health." These public health oriented programs have expanded into areas of stress reduction, wellness education, and fitness.

Thus the medicalization of lifestyle already shows signs of becoming a *subtle moral lifestyle crusade*, as documented by the cultural data presented in Chapter VI (the interactional data within the holistic settings did not demonstrate such processes). Projected into the future, this would increasingly involve condemnation, both institutionally and at an interactional level. Both deviations from the "optimal" lifestyle and evidence of illness become defined as criminal and/or sinful. Additionally, physicians and related health practitioners would increase their arena of social control if lifestyle patterns and stress come to be seen as the cause of illness.

In this way many holistic approaches can be thinly disguised versions of the old model. Practitioners can preach with different rhetorical content while continuing traditional behavior (the providers who do this can come from either the traditional or holistic ranks). Other health practitioners, both those holding traditional and those holding holistic world views, will continue to absolve patients compassionately, as did the group of holistic physicians and nurses examined in this study.

Physician rhetoric increasingly reflects elements of this lifestyle crusade. Perhaps the most often quoted example is that written by John Knowles in his editorial in *Science*; this article has been repeated and expanded in several additional sources (Knowles, 1977a). I have already presented the most frequently quoted portion. In the following segment, however, Knowles stresses the individual's responsibility with more explicitly moral overtones:

> Prevention of disease means forsaking the bad habits which many people enjoy—overeating, too much drinking, taking pills, staying up at night, *engaging in promiscuous sex*, driving too fast, and smoking cigarettes—or, put another way, it means doing things which require special effort—exercising regularly, improving nutrition, going to the dentist, *practicing contraception*, *ensuring harmonious family life*, submitting to screening examinations. . . . The cost of private excess is now a national, not an individual, responsibility. . . . I believe the idea of a "right" to health should be replaced by that of a *moral obligation* to preserve one's own health. The individual then has the "right" to expect help with information, accessible services of good quality, and minimal financial barriers (ibid.: 1103).

Even his use of language, such as "*submitting* to screening examinations," reflects a highly moralistic stance, as well as medical dominance. Issues of "promiscuous sex," speed of driving, the use of contraception, and "ensuring harmonious family life" are included in his admonitions.

This strong moralistic tone, equating specific life habits and value-laden decisions with moral failures (sin) and action destructive to the society as a whole (crime) is increasingly echoed in the popular media by physicians. An example from the editorial pages of the *Los Angeles*

Times captures the essence of this moralistic tone. Mike Oppenheim, M.D., a general practitioner with the Ross-Loos Medical Group in Los Angeles, wrote to express his annoyance that so many people blame the medical profession for the current health care crisis. He describes his day as:

> full of useless work, resulting in unnecessary expense to those I treat. It's not my fault; it's the patients'. Most of them are not even sick. . . . [after describing 20% of the patients he sees as having colds, which are untreatable, he describes several "fallacies"] Fallacy No. 3: A doctor is responsible for keeping his patients well. This is a vicious, but almost universally held, piece of nonsense. I'm not responsible for keeping anyone healthy but myself. When ill, my patients have a right to my best effort to make them well. When they're already well, my responsibilities are less. So I point out their bad habits and encourage them to get the simple screening tests I've listed. Beyond that, it's up to them. . . . Thus the solution to the high cost of medical care is simple: Laymen should stop expecting miracles when they are ailing, and they should act responsibly and sensibly when they are healthy. By doing so, they'd save lots of money and avoid lots of useless doctor visits, which would save me lots of wasted time. And, most important, everyone would be lots healthier (Oppenheim, 1978).

These "simple" lifestyle changes and habits Knowles and Oppenheim describe are considerably more difficult for individuals to implement than taking medications. Yet research has demonstrated how high the noncompliance rate is for taking prescribed medications. Individuals weigh complex sets of costs and benefits in making decisions, as Luker demonstrated in her research on contraception, and many of the symbolic meanings and values underlying those choices differ markedly from those of the health professionals interacting with them (Luker, 1975).

Many of the increasingly popular health appraisal questionnaires (computer versions are now springing up as well) are premised on such simplistic decision-making models. Most smokers are well-acquainted with the potential risk of smoking behavior; however, smoking has become a learned and reinforced habit which meets certain needs. Again, the complexity of the meanings behind mind-body continuity, volitional choice, and motivation are ignored.

Conrad and Schneider briefly mention this possibility as a potential future scenario for the trends they analyzed in medicalization. Although they do not emphasize this alternative, I argue that it already appears to be an established direction. They speculate on this phenomenon that I already see as established:

> Scenario three: Individuals are considered responsible for their illnesses; so activities that are seen as leading to medical problems become defined as deviant. Smoking, eating poorly, getting insufficient exercise, or eschewing seat belts all will be defined as deviant. Certain medical problems could be excluded from NHI coverage because they are deemed to be willfully caused [i.e. "badness"]. This final scenario takes us full circle, as we would develop the notion of "sickness as sin" (Conrad and Schneider, 1980:256).

Much of the danger posed by such a lifestyle crusade appears to come more from traditionally oriented physicians rather than holistic, although individuals in both groups can be involved. This may imply the cooptation and use of the holistic ideology for purposes related to the self-interests of medicine.

Examples of such cooptation include the adaptation of holistic, preventive health approaches by large numbers of corporations who offer stress reduction, wellness, and alcohol rehabilitation programs. Such programs invariably aim for increased employee productivity.

Kotarba's research demonstrates the emerging use of holistic health principals by medical bureaucracies to increase control over patients. He documents that those areas of lifestyle open to social control had indeed been implemented by NASA in their comprehensive health program. His data disclosed the incorporation of holistic principles into space medicine at NASA, with the explicit aim of optimizing work performance, but without any organizational commitment to the overall ideology of the holistic health movement or the use of holistic modalities (Kotarba, 1983a). He then links the social control implications of such employee health programs to work productivity issues:

> The social control implications of all these employee health programs can be seen in the trend towards defining patients'/ employees' total psychological and physiological make-up, and that of their families, as the primary cause of work problems. . . . Moreover, the comprehensive scope of holistic programs allows employers to not only learn of workers' behavior

in private life . . . , but also to intervene in those private lives, thus raising serious issues of civil liberties (ibid:25).

Another issue beyond those of social control is raised by this shift. Can physicians carry out the spiritual and emotional intervention postulated by the new model? Their education involves minimal preparation in these areas; yet, many claim to be able to deal with these concerns. This seems to call for a more interdisciplinary model, one involving nurses, psychologists, and ministers more centrally. Yet, while it initially appears that psychologists, especially those in health psychology and behavioral medicine, have the most to gain from a shift in these directions, it is already clear that traditional medicine will attempt to use the shift to extend, rather than relinquish, their arena of control.

Broader Punitive Societal Trend

The growing lifestyle crusade is closely linked to the recent societal shift towards more punitive, as opposed to therapeutic or reformative, attitudes towards criminals and other deviants. Contrary to the accepted view of most sociologists that the prototype of medicalization is the case of mental illness, recent evidence indicates a public backlash against the idea of mental illness granting exemption from individual responsibility.

The current public reaction against invocation of the insanity plea supports this claim. There are numerous indications of public demand to "lock criminals up," as well as increased support for the death penalty. For instance, in 1982 there was mass public indignation in response to the insanity verdict for John W. Hinckley Jr., after his assassination attempt on President Reagan. This indignation is highly representative of a return in public sentiment towards individual responsibility for behavior, the reversal of medicalization.

A *Los Angeles Times* editorial by George F. Will, a syndicated columnist in Washington, expressed the popular public sentiment of outrage towards the verdict:

> Did the accused know the nature of his act . . . and did he know it was wrong? Law must assign responsibility. All of psychiatry's permutations of determinism locate "responsibility" somewhere other than with an autonomous 'self'-whatever 'self' can mean after enough acts and attributes are explained in terms of a yeasty subconscious. . . . It is an old joke: A person kills his parents and demands mercy because he is an orphan. The joke is now the jurisprudence of "compas-

sion". . . . Today, Americans have an admirable but uncon-
summated desire to see the law express, through commensurate
punishment, the doctrine of individual responsibility and the
wickedness of political assassination (Will, 1982:7).

Conrad and Schneider also note this punitive shift in public reaction
(Conrad and Schneider, 1980:256). They characterize this "backlash"
as a conservative reaction against the increasing "liberalization" in deviance treatment and the progressively liberal Supreme Court decisions
providing for the rights of criminals. They describe this process as beginning about 1970, and also conclude that it may ultimately result in a
process of demedicalization:

> This swell of public reaction may be in part a response to the
> therapeutic ideology and the perceived "coddling" of deviants.
> Should this backlash and other recent public reactions such as
> California's Proposition 13 taxpayer revolt continue to gather
> strength and grow in popularity, they well may force a retreat
> from the medicalization of deviance (ibid.:256).

The recent indications in the popular mass media, along with the
trends documented by my broad cultural data on responsibility, argue that
this retreat is already well under way. In the same way that there is pressure for reversal of the insanity plea, I argue that we will increasingly
make implicit judgments that people are guilty of physical illness, despite
processes of responsibility implied in the concept of "insanity." The concepts of responsibility are closely paralleled in mental and physical illness. Just as assessments that the insane did not willfully choose their
behavior, and thus could not be held "responsible" for it are returning to
assessments assigning personal responsibility, we may be moving to a
position which will hold individuals responsible for the "behavior" expressed in their somatic illness.[3]
Since holistic health can be seen as widening the definition of mental
illness (in the radical interpretations, all somatic illness derives from attitudinal and spiritual problems), it expands the domain of psychological
intervention. If demedicalization reattaches stigma to insanity, it likewise
increasingly stigmatizes illness with somatic manifestation.

Movement from Institutional Toward Individual Solutions
One of the major functional outcomes of the moralistic lifestyle crusade is that society is "let off the hook." While this danger was docu-

mented in relation to the data on responsibility, it needs to be mentioned in the larger context of this problem. In relation to problems of health and illness, this moral crusade represents movement away from institutional solutions.

The major responsibility for solving health and illness problems becomes attached to individuals. Conrad and Schneider write that the medicalization of deviance is part of a larger phenomena: the individualization of social problems in general (this also occurred formerly under the criminologist model). They link the search for causes and solutions to complex problems targeted at the individual to the same process of "blaming the victim" analyzed in the last chapter (Conrad and Schneider, 1980:250). However, it appears that the reverse process, that of demedicalization, also results in further individualizing the problem and absolving societal institutions from blame.

Individual responsibility thus absolves the society as a whole, as well as the economic structure. Again, both the cultural and social structural role in lifestyle is ignored. As Guttmacher concludes, the focus on individual responsibility leads to interventions "that do nothing to change pathogenic aspects of the social and economic structure which placed him or her at high risk in the first place" (Guttmacher, 1979:19).

This parallels Gusfield's findings of how the problems of alcohol use came to be located in the individual alcoholic through a process of psychologizing social problems (Gusfield, 1980:viii). Crawford also argues that this individualistic solution fosters an illusion that no interventions against disease need be focused on the contributory social and economic causes (Crawford, 1980:377).

Similarly, Tesh shows that the lifestyle theory of disease, which she sees as the primary chronic disease prevention policy in the United States, obscures the primary causes of illness, thus deflecting potential social and public health interventions (Tesh, 1988). Her recent work develops the most compelling argument on the use of individualistic political ideology in determining policy approaches to disease prevention in the U.S. She analyzes crucial aspects of individualistic ideology, such as the beliefs that the individual is the ultimate arbiter of morality and that the appropriate study of social problems should concentrate on individuals. The pervasive ideology thus inhibits public health oriented preventive interventions and ultimately supports existing structural conditions (ibid.:159–161). Within this context, it is obvious why the "ideology of choice" has flourished and may continue to develop as a moralistic crusade, as the holistic health ideas become integrated into the cultural mainstream.

Additionally, once each person is viewed as the cause of illness problems, the institution of medicine is absolved. In the traditional medical model, when a physician is unable to diagnose the problem, she or he has other "outs" (for example, "science has not yet found a cure"). In this model, blame can no longer be directed at science (or its representative, the physician) or at God/religion (or its representative, the priest). Blame is placed on individuals, and they are held accountable for finding solutions.

It can of course also be argued that such conceptualizations represent the self-interest of the medical profession. At a time when physicians, and science as a whole, are increasingly under attack by the public, this absolves medicine from blame. Instead, the blame is redirected against both the ill and under-privileged. The warning in relation to a "blame the victim" approach to the underprivileged are most dominant at this point. As Guttmacher writes:

> Cost containment added to self-help provide ready rationales for limiting the provision of medical care to those who are able to pay for it . . . The socially and economically privileged can see most clearly the benefits from a holistic approach to health (Guttmacher, 1979:19).

Thus the consequences of a shift in the direction of a more holistic, participatory, preventive model of health and illness would have a highly unequal distribution throughout the society. The differential distribution crosses both continuums of wellness/illness and socioeconomic classes. Such a moral crusade would benefit those who remain well (both economically and in terms of the illusion of control), the wealthy, and the society as a whole (economically). The major costs would accrue to the ill and underprivileged groups. Both these groups would suffer economically and in terms of the withdrawal of socially supportive resources in favor of stigmatization.

The Functional Need for Moral Condemnation to Limit Illness

So far, the potential for a major moral crusade based on lifestyle considerations has focused on its derivation from the shift in responsibility for health and illness to the individual. However, to analytically understand its functional significance, relationships between various parts of the holistic model must be integrated. Although it was initially helpful to abstract and examine parts of the model relating to the sick role, with primary emphasis on the shifts in the practitioner-patient interaction and in the attribution of responsibility, these parts must be reunited for explanatory analysis.

The shift towards a more egalitarian relationship between practitioner and patient/client has already been detailed. Although the conclusion was that the physician still held the balance of authority within the interactions during the field study, there was a shift towards a more egalitarian, collegial role for patients. This shift is further amplified by the fact that increasing proportions of health and illness interactions take place with non-physician providers. Providers such as nurses and psychologists, although they assume a more pivotal role and increased power within the new holistic framework, command a lesser status differential than physicians.

Physician control has been described as serving a gatekeeping function for the society as a whole. No society can tolerate too high an incidence of illness among its members and maintain productivity. Physicians, as described in earlier chapters, have had the authority and obligation to determine who is admitted into the sick role. That gatekeeping function becomes even more crucial during a period dominated by cost constraints and the allocation of scarce health care resources.

As patients assume more equal power within the relationship, the physician's gatekeeping function becomes weakened. The factors discussed earlier, such as the consumer revolt against expertism, result in what many physicians view as the "demanding" patient (Freidson, 1973): the individual who insists on a larger part in determining whether they are legitimately sick, as well as the direction of their treatment.

A weakening of physician authority in relation to the gatekeeping function leads to a functional need for alternate means of controlling or containing the amount of illness. The combination of structural and interactional withdrawal of resources which accompanies the "ideology of choice" combats any secondary gains of illness. An atmosphere of moral condemnation functions to limit the amount of illness, thus compensating for the loss of physician gatekeeping.

While these shifts are presented here in stark terms to dramatize the modifications, it must be remembered that they represent subtle shifts rather than radical restructuring, as emphasized in the previous three chapters. However, even a small magnitude of change in the gatekeeping function of physicians can result in a higher level of illness than the society can handle. Similarly even a minor shift towards more condemnatory attitudes towards illness can swing the balance away from the previously attractive secondary gains.

The *economic context contributes* to this trend. As our society increasingly faces severe economic restrictions on the utilization of medical services and new technological advances, individuals are demanding higher levels of care and the right not only to that care, but to by-pass gatekeepers in gaining entree to that care. Again, economic considerations underlie the movement away from institutional solutions towards individual action and accountability.[4]

For example, it seems "heartless" to deny lifesaving treatment for dialysis or open heart surgery. Yet, as our technological abilities increasingly overshadow society's economic means to provide technologically intensive services in all situations, we need to do ideological work to justify the decisions of nonintervention. Seeing illness as derivative of moral weakness, sin, or voluntary choice more easily allows such a withdrawal of societal resources.

One would expect major ideological work here to rationalize economically motivated measures while denying any anti-humanistic consequences. This is supported by Guttmacher's warning, "the concept of self-help is regularly invoked to justify policy proposals that would curtail publicly financed health services in the interest of controlling costs. . . . Cost containment added to self-help provide ready rationales for limiting the provision of medical care to those who are able to pay for it" (Guttmacher, 1979:19).[5]

This ideological work assumes additional importance because of the inherent contradiction between the two major grounds supporting holistic health models—humanistic versus economic. A constant tension exists between the critiques of rising costs and dehumanization: this tension persists among both health policy experts and the public. When economic considerations must take precedence, this form of ideological work allows participants to maintain their view of themselves as acting in humanistic ways.

The Intersection of Belief Systems

So far this chapter has demonstrated relationships between the decreased gatekeeping function of physicians and the functional need for moral condemnation to limit illness in a context of economic austerity. While analyzing shifts in medicalization, responsibility, and provider-patient interactions, paradoxes and inconsistencies abound. Those problematic paradoxes themselves have structural sources, and these in turn relate to larger processes of social change.

Many of the apparent inconsistencies described derive from the intersection of two very different realities or belief systems. The interfaces and transitions between divergent ideological systems are highly problematic, and also less amenable to sociological analysis. While the discipline of sociology has increasingly recognized the highly pluralistic nature of American society and also increasingly explored the social construction of reality, these analyses are rarely fully extended to processes of social change.

Views of Social Change

Most views of social change remain somewhat simplistic. Existing paradigms account for aspects of the process but are unable to integrate the full complexity. Focusing on the intersection of these two views of reality, in terms of the shift towards a more holistic model of health, can illuminate more over-arching processes of change in our society.

Perhaps the dominant theoretical paradigm in social change is Weber's notion of the *routinization of charisma* (Gerth and Mills, 1946: 51–55). Charismatic leaders facilitate the development of a social movement; however, over time an inevitable process of routinization and bureaucratization occurs, often subverting many of the original movement goals. Gusfield describes the adoption of the Weberian perspective to analysis of the internal dynamics of social movements, writing of the normative process by which early charismatic leaders are superseded by more rigorously bureaucratized forms of coordination (Gusfield, 1978: 131). Starr supports this argument in relation to the strong pressures to impose bureaucratic organization on any new system of medical services (Starr, 1978:191).

It was mentioned in Chapter III that massive bureaucratic pressures would conflict with and subvert the organization and ideology of the holistic health movement. Examples of such developments have been presented in this work. Yet, while not denying the explanatory power of such formulations, they do not totally account for the complex phenomena I am attempting to integrate.

The second framework of analysis in the area of social movements that is taken-for-granted is that of *partial incorporation* or *cooptation*. McCarthy and Zald, for example, in speculating on the future of the social cleavage between the values of the traditional social culture and the counterculture of the sixties, wrote, "the dominant culture may react by partial incorporation, taking over some of the values and behavior of the counterculture." They continue by providing examples of normative changes which may be contributing to a deemphasis of the culture/counter-culture cleavage (McCarthy and Zald, 1973:28).

This study could be easily interpreted within such a framework. Mainstream allopathic medicine already shows strong evidence of adopting holistic, preventive, participatory trends. Some of these seem to be initiated by medicine, while others have been more strongly pushed by consumer groups and the public. Combined economic and humanistic pressures are already forcing rapid shifts in these directions.

However, the incomplete aspect of both these explanatory perspectives is that they present a one directional, linear model of change. This precludes a true interactional model. Two views of social change which more closely approximate the complexity postulated here are those used by Richard Madsen and Bennett Berger. The dimensions they represent add to those inherent in bureaucratization and incorporation frameworks.

Madsen's work illuminates the underlying processes used by the peasants of Chen village in their discourse about social morality. He analyzes their moral discourse in terms of two predominant moral paradigms which often conflict: that of utilitarian individualism versus one derived from the classic Confucian tradition (Madsen, 1984). As he summarizes:

> People who argue about moral issues often enough argue past one another. This is because there are different "paradigms" for moral discourse: different basic assumptions about human nature, the relationship between self and society, and the nature of good action; and in addition to such basic assumptions, different ways of proceeding from premises to conclusions, from basic assumptions to one's responsibilities in a concrete case. In a complex modern society, it is in fact likely that several different paradigms for moral discourse are available (Madsen, 1984:9–10).

Bennett Berger analyzed similar processes in his work, *The Survival of a Counterculture* (Berger, 1981). His descriptions of the uses of ideological work among Northern California communards documented how they needed to justify actions motivated by self-interest which were opposed to their stated ideological beliefs. In many ways his analyis is more similar to Madsen's than it initially appears. Ideological work can be seen as a universal process of attempting to reconcile conflicting aspects of belief systems held by an individual or group.

Berger and Madsen thus present views of social change which incorporate the added dimension of complexity postulated here. At a macro level, America is a highly pluralistic society. The number of coexisting world views leads to constant transitions and negotiations between alternative belief systems. On the micro sociological level of this study, the participants observed during interaction constantly engaged in behavior while balancing often divergent and conflictual assumptions from their commitments to different paradigms of health and illness.

As discussed earlier, this group of health care providers was chosen to constitute an ideal-typical group with strong commitments to *both* the traditional and holistic medical models. Patient/clients who chose the clinic shared those dual commitments to various degrees. Thus this group represented an exemplar case of what happens in the intersection of belief systems, as embodied in the two models.

Translation of Eastern Philosophy into Western Terms of Utilitarian Individualism and Calvinism

The primary interface of belief systems in this situation derives from Eastern and Western world views. The underlying phenomenon can be conceptualized as the wide diffusion and translation of Eastern philosophy into Calvinistic terms of utilitarian individualism and guilt.

In Chapter II, the ideology and belief system underlying the holistic health model were delineated in contrast to the traditional allopathic medical model. Some of those parameters will be briefly reexamined here, highlighting the crucial differences underlying Eastern and Western world views.[6] Underscoring the essential differences in world view frames the paradoxes resulting from their intersection. The holistic health model borrows heavily from an Eastern perspective and Romanticism; however, most of its adherents were socialized into and live in a society dominated by images of reality derived from Calvinism and utilitarian individualism.

One of the most prominent polarizations in these two world views relates to their images of causation and human action. The *Western view* of causation postulates unilinear processes of objects (including individuals) acting on other objects. The attribution of causation derives from a Cartesian notion of duality. This assumption is so pervasive in Western thinking that its taken-for-granted corollaries affect all our thinking. Our language does not even have the words or images that allow us to conceive of processes without a causative element.

The strong Western interventionist bias is integrally related to this view of causation as well. One person is seen as acting on another individual or object in terms of "affecting" or "effects." This combines with the strong emphasis on individuality. Both science and medicine derive from and almost epitomize the causal and interventionist stances of a Western world view. The process of scientific research explicitly assumes an inviolate separation between subject and object, as well as predictable, causal relationships between objects and events which can be discovered. Johnson thoroughly documents the centrality of the analytic-deductive mode in the Western concept of self (Johnson, 1985:113–114, 124).

Several other pivotal assumptions and values comprising *utilitarian individualism* and a Western world view derive from the views of duality and causation. The interventionist, activist bias has already been mentioned. Freedom, independence, personal achievement, and control are all highly valued in American society, and they are related to a far more individualistic perception of the world (Marsella et al., 1985; Bellah et al., 1985). For instance, Johnson, in discussing the basic qualities central to the western subjective self, writes, "The emphasis on individualism has direct and indirect effects on both the presentation of self (in public ways) and the experience of self (in private awareness)" (Johnson, 1985:121–122).

Steven Tipton summarizes the two primary interpretations of reality in America as biblical religion and utilitarian individualism (Tipton, 1982:2).[7] One of the primary ways of thinking in utilitarian individualism is the assumption that there are always evaluative consequences in terms of self-interest. As Tipton specifies, "Utilitarian individualism locates the end of human action in the subjective satisfaction of self-interest rather than in objectified obedience to God's will or compliance with rational principles" (ibid.:9). In describing the integration of the biblical tradition with utilitarian individualism, Tipton writes:

> The ideal of the Christian community in which social relations manifest the virtue of charity gives way to a collectivity of individuals whose social relations manifest the contingent fact of reciprocity (not, strictly speaking, cupidity). One gives in order to get, or because one has already gotten. One does not give in order to give (ibid.:11).

Thus utilitarian individualism is integral to the Western tradition. The maximization of individual interests and relationships based on reciprocity derive from this value.

Both Weber and Parsons described the secularizing effect of Calvinism. Parsons' description of the individualism of ascetic Protestantism relates the form of asceticism to the orientation to action:

> Ascetic Protestant activism meant that "inner-worldly" callings constituted the primary field for the individual to imple-

ment his religious commitments. The intensive activism of the general Christian commitment to regenerate (and hence upgrade) life was thereby channeled into achievement in worldly callings, among them, although by no means predominantly, business achievement. . . . This individualistic pattern bestowed the strong sanction of religious commitment on what is now often called achievement motivation and fostered the internalization of such motivation by typical individuals (Parsons, 1968:243).

A materialistic focus was thus closely related to the individualistic focus, as well as the Cartesian duality. Again, this analysis is based on a Weberian analysis of Calvinist doctrine and the relationship of belief to the accumulation of wealth (Bendix, 1968:496).

Calvinism and the American biblical tradition also clearly separate good and evil. The stress on human imperfection and sin leads to a strong emphasis in the Christian-Judaic tradition on guilt and blame. Such views result in a judgmental, evaluative stance of both oneself and others. Thus notions of an internal critic, constantly passing moral judgment on actions as extensions of our being, are pervasive.

In contrast, a world view based in *Eastern philosophy* does not separate processes into distinct cause and effect. In an all-connected universe, analytical divisions are not perceived; instead, an essential unity provides the lens through which phenomena are interpreted.[8] Similarly, instead of images of acting on objects and others, Eastern views see the individual experiencing him or herself as connected with everything. Thus the stress is on non-seeking and non-action, the opposite of a Western deterministic, interventionist, achievement-oriented approach. This implies a more passive, receptive Eastern self. As Thomas Merton writes, "Chuang Tzu's proposed secret is not the accumulation of virtue and merit . . . but the non-doing, or non-action—not intent upon results and not concerned with deliberately, consciously laid plans" (Merton, 1965:24).

Above all, an essential unity is experienced within this world view. Key terms in descriptions of Eastern philosophy include unity, monism, monistic holism, collective consciousness, and interdependence. This unity is inseparable from a transcendental awareness and emphasis on spirituality. There is less focus on the individual ego or materialism. As Merton writes, "The Tao of Ju philosophy is, in the words of Confucius, 'threading together into one the desires of the self and the desires of the other' " (Merton, 1965:21). Thus the Eastern self is far less individualistic.[9]

Relatedness and monistic holism leads directly to transpersonal love and compassion. Since the self is not set apart from others, it is not above them and thus nonjudgmental. Self-love is part of universal love, but the individual's needs and self interest are seen as part of the other's self interest, rather than in a conflictual or antagonistic relationship. Tipton summarizes this contrast between the monistic and dualistic orientations most cogently, applying the distinctions to differences between the counterculture and utilitarian culture:

> This monism constitutes the fundamental difference in cognitive orientation between the counterculture and utilitarian culture, which is predicated on philosophical realism or dualism—the view that material objects exist externally to and are independent of our experience. Utilitarianism begins with the indissoluble distinction between subject and object, self and other (Tipton, 1982:14–15).

Bellah also characterizes the belief in the unity of all being as a core meaning differentiating systems based on the Oriental religions from established American views. He summarizes, "For them ultimately there is no difference between myself and yourself, and this river and that mountain. We are all one and the conflict between us is therefore illusory" (Bellah, 1976:347).[10]

If there is no dualism, giving and receiving become the same, rather than opposites. There is less judgment of others because good and evil are not conceived of as separate. Both good and evil are part of all of us, and this recognition leads to humility and a less judgmental stance. As Tipton writes, "Monistic denial of the individual self as an independent entity undercuts the idea of better or worse selves, higher or lower status individuals" (Tipton, 1982:162).

Karma versus Determinism

The paradoxes result from the intermingling of the two world views. Both providers and patients, even those with a strong commitment to a more holistic model and world view deriving from views of Eastern monism, acceptance, and nonaction, were socialized into and continue to function within a society dominated by a highly individualistic and deterministic world view.

The concept of karma is used here to represent an Eastern view of acceptance, yielding, non-seeking, and inaction. Non-judgmental compassion and love are seen as flowing from this monistic perspective.

Determinism here represents a Western, interventionist, authoritative, activist approach personified by the scientific perspective. Authority and control are intimately related to views of sin, guilt, and moral absolutism.

The intersections between these world views provide the source of many of the paradoxes. A concept of responsibility generated from within an Eastern, karmic framework easily translates into sin and blame, of both self and others, within a deterministic belief system.[11] In that translation the individual comes to be seen as totally responsible for his or her state of health. The component of radical individualism departs from the Eastern view, which buffers individualism with the dual emphasis on discipline and a network of obligations and responsibility to others.[12]

Visible Indicators of Grace

Not only does the translation of an Eastern view of responsibility into the framework of utilitarian individualism lead to blame and guilt, but the images of sin and grace from the Calvinistic tradition become superimposed over the concepts originally derived from an Eastern framework. As stigma is increasingly attached to illness, both the individual and others around him or her come to define levels of moral rectitude in terms of health. Evidence of illness becomes a "scarlet letter A," while the athletic, trim, healthy appearing individual visibly exudes the same moral grace as a successful Puritan businessman. Again, a process of image control becomes integral to both.

Increasing examples of the importance of this visibility, beyond the data already presented in Chapter VI, are occurring. A prominent case is that of the increasing incidence of eating disorders such as bulimia and the societal obsession with weight control. Attempts to purge after eating, along with many fad diets, have unhealthy, often dangerous effects, but they maintain the individual's "trim" or "healthy" external appearance.[13]

Moral Syncretism

The translation of ideas from one embedded cultural context into another can be termed moral syncretism. Syncretic combinations blend different forms of beliefs or practices. As Richard Madsen describes the concept, it involves a lived synthesis of divergent cultural themes (Madsen, 1984). Continual examples of the paradoxes that result from such a synthesis have been presented throughout this work.

Madsen found that the peasants of Chen village were most powerfully affected by the same two paradigms of moral discourse presented here: that of utilitarian individualism and that deriving from Confucian thought. In analyzing the ways political leaders attempted to deal with moral conflicts between their moral stance and the concrete actions necessary for maintaining political power, he found they continually combined aspects of the two paradigms:

> villagers attempted to escape their (moral) predicaments by mixing paradigms of moral discourse together to form a new syncretic synthesis which would give them both current political capital and a new way of meaningfully understanding and justifying their position in the world (Madsen, 1984:20).

He continues by suggesting that it has not been a historically linear process of movement from Chinese traditional values to modern Western values, and that a "neat moral fusion" of the two has not and does not exist. Instead, he sees people in such rural villages as "play(ing) down certain themes in their traditional culture and emphasiz(ing) others that fit their contemporary social situation; and that they do the same for the modern themes of the official ideology" (ibid:20). After then discussing how traditional and modern themes become mixed into a "synthesis composed of partially integrated, partially contradictory parts," he discusses how their moral justifications involve a complex pattern of often inconsistent arguments (ibid:20).

While Madsen has demonstrated the process of moral syncretism in relation to a specific culture in a specific historical context, this study shows parallel processes in a very different situation. Instead of focusing on rural peasants in China, this study examines urbanized Americans. While Madsen focused primarily on political interactions, holistically oriented practitioners and their patients also arrive at syntheses of similar contradictory elements in their encounters.

Despite the huge cultural gaps in the two groups studied, both are attempting to reconcile the same major cultural world views. Each group was initially socialized into different dominant systems, with one system superimposed on the other over time. Interestingly, transition in either direction carries equivalent dangers of moral crusades.[14]

When social scientists and historians study cultural forms, the process of analysis and conceptualization ultimately provides an ideal typical view which emphasizes patterns and consistency. This study has also tried to discover and analyze patterns; however, the inconsistency, paradox, and flux always remained integral to the patterns. No belief system or cultural world view appears in pure form. When cultural, political, or religious doctrines are internalized by individuals, vacillations, tensions, compromises, and paradoxes are always apparent in their everyday behavior. This is especially the case in a highly pluralistic society like America, and processes of moral syncretism are even more pronounced during periods of rapid social change.

Both Tipton and Bellah found that many counterculture participants "retained aspects of the utilitarian outlook in their own behavior and attitudes even as they were repudiating it in theory" (Tipton, 1982:14). Bellah makes several allusions to the residual utilitarian views that are apparent in those who reject utilitarian individualism most strongly. He refers to the "utilitarian individualism that is latent in all the countercultural successor movements, political and religious . . ." (Bellah, 1976: 350). That utilitarian individualism is also residual within the holistic health movement.

Examples of similar contradictions from my data will be briefly reiterated here. One that was continually apparent in both office settings and throughout the interviews was the ambivalent stance towards objectivity and science. While science and technology are often attacked in favor of more "natural" approaches, holistic providers do ideological work to present themselves and their approaches as scientific. Similarly, many of the rationales for holistic treatments are carefully framed in scientific images. This is closely related to the tension over valuing intuitive and objective sources of knowledge.

Another example of the contradictions deriving from a synthesis of the two world views relates to causation. While an Eastern view opposes dualities and consequential processes, positing an integrated whole, very basic ways of Western thinking continue to permeate participants' assumptions. Thus, while some of the most committed practitioners (usually these have been most immersed in Eastern spiritual views) focus on imbalances within a patient, one of the primary criticisms within the holistic rhetoric is that traditional medicine attacks symptoms rather than actual "causes." Thus holistic approaches often present themselves as dealing with underlying causes. Even when practitioners say they can correct the imbalance by intervening in many places (modifying nutrition, emotional or spiritual counseling, or acupuncture will positively alter balance and thus increase the individual's resistance), the language is still that of "intervention" and the images continue to imply dualism and causal effects on the patient.[15]

Boundaries

When examining the phenomenon of moral syncretism, the concept of boundaries assumes importance. The degree of openness or closure of a group to the outside world affects the degree of tension experienced between opposing views. In some of the small communities Tipton studied, those who lived in more self-contained settings such as youth who spent most of their time with others in the Buddhist or Christian denomination were able to arrive at a more cohesive, stable world view. In other words, a group construction of reality was developed which was less open to continual outside challenge.

In the holistic clinic and dental office I observed, staff were chosen for a preexisting degree of philosophical congruence. Constant work together over time helped to sustain certain group versions of reality, just as they did in Berger's commune. Some of the paradoxes and tensions came to be resolved in specific ways. Once the system is open, even more paradoxes and conflicts develop. As ideas derived from Eastern and countercultural world views diffuse throughout the larger society, with all the highly diverse subcultural views, even more conflictual, paradoxical interpretations emerge.

Thus the highly committed practitioners I observed and interviewed had enough immersion in Eastern and countercultural thought to prevent the concept of responsibility from generating into a lifestyle crusade with moral overtones. Once concepts of responsibility and body-mind continuity spread through popular media in simplistic forms, without the grounding of the contextual world view from which they were derived, they come to assume new meanings with very different, often moralistic and stigmatizing overtones.

Microcosm of Change

The intersection of Eastern and Western realities and the resulting moral syncretism seen in relation to holistic health represents a microcosm of change. In other words, it reflects a larger societal transition. Both the ambiguities of moral discourse and the diffusion of Eastern cultural ideas are occurring throughout American society. The health care system exemplifies the processes that are taking place in wider societal arenas.

Phyllis Mattson, in concluding her book on holistic health, describes it as a religious movement, and sees its ultimate goal as a radical change in world view (Mattson, 1982). Instead, I see the transitions, and the process of transition, in the holistic model as reflecting a larger, but subtle, societal transition. As Eastern views popularized by the counterculture of the sixties diffuse throughout the society in diluted form, similar contradictions will continue to occur in the interface between belief systems, as people attempt to apply them to concrete situations in their everyday lives.

Conclusion

In Chapter VI it was shown that a dialectic tension between patient responsibility and a caring stance of the provider emerged as a crucial mediator in the attribution of blame. In this final chapter, this mediation process has been linked to the broader societal picture, while the implications of the united holistic model were explored. The various parts of the new holistic model were integrated, and related to the larger picture.

I have demonstrated the potential for a widespread lifestyle crusade. I showed the possibility of a therapeutic tyranny, where the pursuit of health assumes paramount importance, and moral condemnation and the withdrawal of resources accompanies evidence of either illness or lifestyle lapses.

The concept of medicalization was also described and analyzed, including contradictory elements in the ways medicalization is commonly portrayed. I examined whether a shift towards a more holistic, participatory model actually represents demedicalization or further medicalization. This confusion derives from two concepts which are used simultaneously in the discussions of medicalization in the literature. While holistic health represents further medicalization in terms of expanding the pathogenic sphere, and thus extending medicine's influence over lifestyle, it simultaneously represents a reversal in the ways medicalization has represented an absolution function in relation to deviance.

I argue that the trend towards medicalization, in that latter sense, is reversing at the societal level, and that one of the consequences of the return shift is in the direction of imputation of sin and moral failure in relation to illness. In other words, medicalization has involved a shift from sin or crime to illness designations in the treatment of deviance, and this shift has come to exempt groups from stigmatization. The diffusion of elements of the holistic model is now resulting in a shift in the opposite direction. There have been some humanistic consequences to the medicalization process, and this form of the demedicalization trend reverses those.

Yet this process of stigmatization and indications of a moral lifestyle crusade were not apparent within the holistic settings studied during the research. This contradictory finding requires explaining. There has always been a dialectic tension between holding the individual responsible for illness and the physician's absolution function. In other words, a certain degree of moral attribution is always residual in illness designations. Any shift in either direction exposes the contradictions and paradoxes.

Holistic health broadens the sphere of pathogenesis, which disturbs the delicate balance, thus making those contradictions more visible.

I have argued that the decreased gatekeeping function of the physician may set the stage for a functional need for societal moral condemnation of the ill to limit illness in a period of diminished economic resources. Thus even the slight decrease in the physician gatekeeping function, which derives from the somewhat more egalitarian physician-patient relationship, must be countered to maintain limits on the societal level of illness as a whole. Minimizing the attractiveness of the secondary gains from illness discourages too large a societal burden of illness.

Simultaneously, processes resulting from the intersection of the Eastern and Western belief systems and world views contribute to these societal trends. The wide translation of Eastern philosophy into Calvinistic terms of utilitarian individualism promotes the more dangerous views of individual guilt and blame. The tension between karma and determinism was examined, as well as the ways in which health and lifestyle become the focus of visible indicators of grace. The process of moral syncretism was shown to explain this intersection of two different world views, and how the more dangerous interpretations of responsibility as blame come to develop. That process is a microcosm of change, reflecting a far broader societal transition and illuminating processes of social change. Thus the shifts in the realm of health and illness represent broader tensions in the society as a whole.

The book has thus explored the major social consequences of a shift towards a more holistic, participatory model of medicine. The primary focus has been on the implications of the shift towards the new model on the sick role. Data from the ethnographic study and interviews were analyzed to describe what actually happens when practitioners attempt to carry out health care combining the best of both models. The practitioner-client relationship was found to be more egalitarian in the new model; however, this change represents only a partial shift within definite limits of continued physician control of the interactions. The new interactional model also does not fit the description of a "consumerist" model, because it incorporates much broader affective components and less specificity than either the traditional medical or the consumerist model postulate.

Similarly, despite the ideology purporting a drastic shift in attribution of responsibility to the individual, the interactional data presented a much more ambiguous and complex picture. These holistic practitioners continue to absolve patients, using a variety of "theoretical outs." Instead, many patients are receiving blame from the wider society and some more traditional physicians with the spread of simplistic beliefs of mind-body continuity and responsibility. The interactional data also demonstrated a strong dialectic tension between caring and responsibility. The practitioner's compassion acts as a mediator to prevent the attribution of personal, volitional blame. Thus the compassionate and caring commitment of practitioners can buffer that blame, as it did with these holistic practitioners.

As an exploratory study, the analysis raises almost as many questions as it answers. The data illustrate the strengths inherent in the new model, and the ways it meets the needs of a group of practitioners and patients who experience dissatisfaction with the traditional, allopathic medical model. Yet it also points to the potential strains deriving from the model. As component ideas associated with the more holistic, participatory model of health diffuse throughout the society, simplistic interpretations abound. Such simplistic interpretations of parts of the model, especially in the areas of responsibility and mind-body continuity, can easily translate into views of blame and guilt that are not part of the model when it remains embedded in its deeper set of meanings.

Thus, within the integrated holistic model, as it was understood by the committed practitioners who translated the model within its context of deep meanings, it was understood that "personal choice" was much more complex and culturally embedded than the simplistic "ideology of choice" postulates. These practitioners understood that the genetic, social, and environmental limits to personal choice were often overlooked in the rhetoric, and they guarded against the negative consequences of imputing moralistic judgments and blame. In this way, the absolution function of the practitioner remained intact.

These findings stress the importance of understanding the individual parts of the model as they are embedded in the context of the entire constellation of beliefs and meanings of holistic practitioners. They also demonstrate the dangers of extrapolating specific components of the model without understanding the broad context from which they derive.

The findings also warn of the need for the provider to maintain a compassionate, caring stance, not only because it mediates the tension of patient responsibility and absolution, but also because of the strong need and desire of patients to incorporate the affective, expressive dimension of care, along with treatment as a near status equal. These dimensions represent what most of those patients were seeking in these holistic settings.

The mixture or interface of the two models, especially during this period of transition, has significant consequences for the domains of individual illness, health policy, and the organization of health service. The complexities of both the ideological pronouncements and the data at the interactional level must be continually kept in mind and weighed as we search for solutions to these dilemmas.

As we move in the direction of incorporating parts of the new more holistic, participatory model, we need to be continually aware of the dangers of incorporating elements without the deep background meanings. With the pervasiveness of new model beliefs and modalities becoming integrated with more traditional forms of practice, we need to be alert for the dangers, as well as the strengths, of such syncretic combinations. Perhaps, most of all, we need to guard against the danger of simplistic interpretations of parts of the model that ignore the complex ambiguities and constant tension between caring and responsibility.

Appendix A

Interview Guide

Chapter I discussed the methodological focus of the research. Beyond the informal exchanges and interviews that continually occurred throughout the time spent in the ethnographic settings (these informal conversations and interviews also occurred during attendance at holistic courses and conferences throughout the study), I conducted twenty-five intensive interviews outside the settings. These were carried out between September 1981 and June 1983, and the respondents consisted primarily of providers and leaders in the holistic health movement in the Southern California area. Four patients were also included. These interviews lasted between twenty-five minutes and over four hours, averaging an hour and a half.

There was considerable variability between interviews, as one would expect in this kind of qualitative study. First, the sequence of the interview in relation to the time-frame of the larger study had a major effect. Initial interviews covered broad areas. The focus gradually narrowed during the period of the research, so that more specific, focused and probing questions dominated the final set of interviews. Second, the background of the respondent played a part in the directions the interview took. Obviously, the interviews focused on quite different areas when the respondent was a holistic practitioner versus a leader in the movement versus a patient. Third, the degree to which I had previously gained the respondent's trust determined both the areas covered and the timing with which more sensitive areas were broached. Even more important, because I was interested in learning participants' symbolic meanings and world views, their individual perspectives were sought out, rather than steering them into more structured, aggregate types of answers.

For each interview, I prepared a list of topic areas to introduce with open-ended questions. These were intentionally informal and open-ended, and I encouraged participants to elaborate on issues they saw as important. Before beginning the actual questions, I used informal, social talk to relax respondents. While I attempted to touch on as many of the issues I had prepared as possible, I followed up on any directions that respondents brought up in the interviews. For example, two of the physicians interviewed spontaneously brought up malpractice insurance as a factor influencing their ways of interacting with patients. In both instances I explored the meanings they attached to it at length. The interviews were also structured so that questions eliciting how practitioners viewed their clinical practice in their own terms came earlier than questions which might have alerted them to specific differences and areas I was most interested in.

Following are two sample interview guides, one for a patient and the other for a provider. They should give the interested reader a feel for the scope of topics covered.

Interview Guide—Patient

Age   Sex   Marital status
Occupation
Illness Status
How did you learn about Dr. ———?
How long have you been coming here?
Why are you here today?
Have you seen any other physician about this problem? If so, specialty,
    # visits, outcome, satisfaction
What kinds of things seem different in this office?
Do you feel that Dr. ——— relates to you differently than other doctors
    you've seen in the past? If so, how?
Can you tell me something about what caused your illness?
What treatment has Dr. ——— prescribed?
    Will that mean making any change in your lifestyle?
    If so, how difficult is that for you?
    How much have you been able to stick to the treatment plan?
    Do you have any questions or concerns?
    Are you seeing any other physician at this time for other problems?
        (If so, ask re specialty, freq. of visits, outcome, possible conflict
        between 2 approaches)
What does this illness mean to you?
    What does it mean to your family?
How has your illness affected your everyday experience?
    How has it affected your family?

How knowledgeable do you feel you are about health issues (i.e.: stress, nutrition, exercise)?

Do you exercise regularly? Do you abstain from smoking?

Do you make sure you obtain a nutritionally balanced diet?

Are you under a great deal of stress?

   Do you feel you should change your behavior in any of these areas?

   Do you ever feel that there are things you should be doing that you're not doing? (Elaborate)

Do you sometimes feel that you're getting pressure to change? (If so, from whom: family, friends, this office, professionals, media—and how often?)

   How do you handle that?

Do you feel that a person should be held responsible for their own health?

   What advantages do you see for individuals taking more responsibility for their own health?

   What disadvantages do you see for individuals taking more responsibility for their own health?

Do you ever come down on yourself, feel guilty, if you can't carry out health measures or treatment you feel you should?

How much time do you spend thinking about health and/or illness and how you feel?

   More than you used to?

How would you describe your spiritual commitment?

Interview Guide—Provider

Age

Sex

Discipline

What does holistic health mean to you?

How did you become interested in holistic health?

   Professional education, experience

How is your practice different since incorpoating HH ideas? (After answer, probe these areas):

   relationship with patient?

   degree of responsibility assumed by patient?

   meaning of illness?

   orientation towards health vs. illness?

examine family, work situation, environment?
preventive focus?
mind-body-spirit continuity?
professionalism (degree of, definition)? (formality)
personal involvement with patient
healing process
modalities (treatment)?
Why do most patients come here?
    How do they learn about the center? (ads, referrals)
Composition of your practice:
    Average age
    Gender breakdown
    Socio-economic level
    Level of knowledge/sophistication re health issues
In your practice, what proportion of patients you see are:
    Healthy vs. sick?
    Acute vs. chronic?
    Need physician vs. emotional intervention?
    Which kinds of patients do you prefer to work with?
What are the most rewarding aspects of your work?
    Least rewarding?
What are your approximate compliance rates?
    How compare to more traditional practice?
    If better, due to your approach or are patients already motivated?

Responsibility

How much responsibility do you feel/take for your patients' health/
disease?
Has it been, or is it ever now, hard for you to give up your
responsibility?
    Is it hard for other practitioners or students to give up some of their
        responsibility to the patient?
Do patients have trouble taking responsibility for their health?
    What if a patient comes wanting crisis, acute care?
    What if a patient doesn't want to take responsibility, change life style?
        Do you have trouble with that?
    Do patients come after having taken responsibility, or do you moti-
        vate them to take responsibility in your practice?
How would you handle these situations differently from most
physicians?
    patient with broken arm

patient with acute bronchitis

patient with long term severe asthma

What advantages do you see for patients of taking more responsibility?

What disadvantages?

Any difficult aspects?

Motivation?

More or less involvement with patients?

How do you deal with guilt/self-blame some patients feel?

patient with heart disease or cancer

patient who has trouble changing diet or eliminating smoking (experience guilt about lifestyle).

patient with migraine saw her inability to control pain as a moral failure

One tenet of HH: "We choose our level of health and illness."—how do you see that?

When traditional physicians can't find a somatic cause for a patient's symptoms, they often say, "It's all in your mind." How do you react to that?

How do you see a child and responsibility for health/disease?

Do you exercise regularly, smoke, meditate, eat the diet you prescribe?

How do you feel about your lapses?

Do you feel the insurance structure should be changed to offer incentives for maintaining health?

Does that penalize those who don't alter their lifestyles?

Paradox: acupuncture, body-work leave the patient dependent on the practitioner (as opposed to health teaching, life style modification).

Do you see acupuncture as treating symptoms or cause?

Meaning of "response-ability?"

Some traditional physicians worry that HH physicians will not be as accountable for the quality of care. How do you feel about that?

Do you have any other ideas or thoughts on the consequences of a shift towards the individual assuming more responsibility for his/her own health?

The Holistic Health Movement

How do psychology and nursing relate to holistic health?

Why do you think HH is more interdisciplinary?

Any problems with that in the clinic?

How do you handle the status/power differential between physician and a nurse or a body-worker?

Do you see many sixties values, consciousness pervading the
   movement?
   Were you personally involved in any of the sixties movements?
      Elaborate
   Do you see any areas of potential conflict between the
      humanistic and economic supporters of HH?
   Argument that can't make money on prevention/health teaching (more
      for technical procedures).
How do you see medicine reacting to HH?
   Family medicine, pediatrics, and HH share many of the same goals.
      Why so much mutual antagonism?
   What professional assoc. do you belong to? (for physicians: AMA,
      AHMA, AHH)
   Composition, activities?
Do you see any need for licensing or credentialing within holistic
   health?
What do you see as the future of the HH movement?
   Is it a passing phase, fad?
   Will it result in a shift in the medical model?
   Will there eventually be 2 parallel systems of health and illness care?
      If so, how will they be likely to be structured?

Spiritual
What is your religious affiliation?
How would you describe your spiritual commitment?
   Commitment to helping others?
   Does this ever conflict with making money or other pragamatic con-
      siderations like efficiency?
   Do you see most HH practitioners as having similar spiritual
      commitments?
   What about the patients who come here?

Strains/Problems in the Model
Egalitarianism is highly valued (both relationship with patients
and with colleagues)
   doctor gets more pay than nurse
   doctor has more knowledge than patient (need expert)
Sense ambivalence re professionalism.
   Conflict between valuing intuition and science.
   Professional social relationships not as separate.

Possible dangers with preoccupation with health.

Lifestyles, attitudes resistant to change.

Dangers of moral crusade—lifestyle.

Insurance structure and increased costs.

Moral commitment of many early HH practices—as model is more widely adopted, others may abuse.

Can a practitioner make an adequate income from preventive medicine? (highest fees from technological procedures)

The high costs of the HH modalities are a problem for some patients

Appendix B

Respondent Profiles

Presenting the information on each provider and patient formally interviewed would make some of the more visible leaders and providers easily identifiable. Therefore, this section will provide composite information about these respondents. It must be remembered that countless numbers of patients and a variety of providers were interviewed on a less formal basis.

Breakdown of Respondents
10 physicians
5 psychologists
4 nurses
2 others (1 dentist; 1 office manager)
4 patients

Physicians
Average age 40.2 years (36.8 years not including the two physicians active in the holistic movement, but not currently doing clinical practice).
Sex: 9 males; 1 female.
7 in Family Practice (5 board certified)
1 in Internal Medicine (board certified)
2 in Obstetrics/Gynecology (both board certified)

Nurses
Average age 44.5 years (36.3 years, not including one nurse active in the holistic movement, but not currently doing clinical practice).
Sex: 4 female.
1 holds generic R.N. degree
2 hold B.S. as well (1 also has P.H.N. certificate)
1 holds non-nursing Ph.D.

Psychologists
Average age 41.4 years.
Sex: 4 male; 1 female.

Dentist
Age 37 years.
Sex: male.

Notes

Chapter I

1. One example is the formation of the University of California, Los Angeles Center for Health Enhancement Education and Research, directed by Charles Kleeman, M.D., professor at the School of Medicine. The Center is staffed by physicians, nutritionists, exercise physiologists and psychologists. A twenty-four day program teaches clients how to prevent and reverse disease through proper diet, exercise, and stress reduction. Health newsletters, such as those distributed by the Harvard Medical School and the Public Health School at University of California, Berkeley also illustrate this widespread interest.

2. Talcott Parsons' conceptualization of the sick role, along with its extensions and critiques, will be discussed in Chapter IV. Basically, it consists of a set of two rights (exemption from normal role responsibilities and nonresponsibility for the illness itself) and two responsibilities (seeking professionally competent help and the desire to get well) incumbent on those admitted to the sick role by physicians, who are seen as societal gatekeepers.

3. This is not an extreme form of relativism that denies, for example, any "real" disease. While I believe there is objectively real disease, I also believe that the boundaries of disease are extremely ambiguous. Additionally, I separate "disease" from the "experience of illness," which is far more relative, culturally derived, and experiential than the former.

   My stance is that our reality, what we come to think, feel, and believe, is *socially constructed* in the sense of the sociologies of everyday life, symbolic interaction, and interpretive social science (Berger and Luckmann, 1967; Rabinow and Sullivan, 1979; Conrad and Schneider, 1980), which assumes a shared social and cultural element, as opposed to an individual constructionist approach. This social aspect of the construction of reality implies the patterns and shared meanings necessary to the social science enterprise (while this allows a wide lattitude of variability, it avoids the extreme form of a more individualistic relativism).

   Furthermore, since our reality is socially constructed within a highly pluralistic society, I see that reality as constantly negotiated in micro-political terms. Thus, for example, patients in the primary holistic clinic I studied had more faith in their physicians because those practitioners gave up many symbols of what both parties defined as the distance and authoritarianism of the traditional professional role. Other patients and physicians, who adhere more closely to the traditional allopathic medical model, would define that same shift as an indication of a lack of professionalism, which in turn would denote a lack of competence of the holistic physicians. So the identical symbols signal contradictory meanings to two different groups in American society who may share many similar demographic characteristics (for example, both groups might be upper middle class professionals).

4. Max Weber first explicitly formulated the methodological approach of using "ideal types" to simplify and exaggerate evidence in creating a model to facilitate analysis. While recognizing that such conceptualization is artificial, I agree with his contention that cultural and behavioral analysis cannot avoid the use of typological concepts.

5. Once I established reliable contacts in the movement, primarily three nurses and one physician who had been active in the Association for Holistic Health leadership, I asked who they felt were the most qualified practitioners.

6. The major methodological problem I encountered in this area was that most of the providers who advertised or announced themselves as "holistic" were not those regarded as the most highly competent. The latter group had a much lower profile, both due to awareness of the connotations of the word "holistic" and their aversion to public visibility. They relied more on network referrals for potential clients to learn about their work. Often they practiced in family practice, internal medicine, or "preventive medicine" practices, one even within a very traditional medical school, attempting to combine holistic, preventive principles and modalities in their practice. It took a much longer period in the field, while developing extensive contacts in the movement, to locate those physicians, usually with medical specialty board certification, who practiced the highest quality integration of approaches.

7. One of the few unbiased and also empirically documented overviews of the holistic health movement is Phyllis H. Mattson's book, *Holistic Health in Perspective* (Mattson, 1982). Although she is a medical anthropologist and conducted her field research in a different geographical location, her data closely parallel mine in most areas (Lowenberg, 1980, 1985). Such closely parallel results provide an interesting rebuttal to the supposedly "subjective" nature of the process of field research. On a more limited scale, the work of Gordon (1980, 1981, 1982), Goldstein et al. (1985, 1987), and Glasser (1983) also supplies a form of replication for portions of my findings, extending the degree of their representativeness.

8. I returned to this setting later, both to obtain taped transcriptions of dentist-patient interaction and for more focused interviewing.

9. Refer to appendix for description of respondents and for additional details of interview content.

10. Because of the duration of the study and the richness of the data gathered during its various stages, the vast bulk of the data had to be omitted or presented in abbreviated form. It was a continual temptation to include additional examples; however, I was aware of the limits to readers' patience. Additionally, in an interpretive methodological approach, the data is used illustratively, rather than to document assertions quantitatively.

Chapter II

1. Berliner and Salmon refer to this as scientific medicine (Berliner and Salmon, 1979; Salmon, 1984); however, I will avoid that term because of its impli-

cation that all aspects of allopathic medicine are scientifically based, while all aspects of holistic medicine have no empirical backing.

2. These parameters were first presented at a Pacific Sociological Association conference (Lowenberg, 1980). For the most comprehensive summaries of holistic health characteristics, see especially Gordon (1980) and Mattson (1982). Also refer to Ardell (1976); Otto and Knight (1979); Berliner and Salmon (1980); Kopelman and Moskoff (1981); Gordon et al. (1984); and Salmon (1984).

3. This poses another interesting paradox. While holistic practitioners may at times treat symptoms outside a causal framework, the popularized ideology stresses that holistic health treats the cause, rather than "merely treating symptoms like allopathic medicine." For example, traditional acupuncture restores balance, which in turn decreases symptoms. Thus a different causal framework is used, rather than one totally abandoning causation.

4. The social causation postulated by this model was already noted very early in the phenomenon of voodoo death in other cultures. Observations on voodoo death and the "will to live" initially interested some researchers in these directions.

5. Evarts G. Loomis, M.D. founded Meadowlark, another early and influential holistic health center. Ardell claims it is the oldest (it was established in 1958 as a center promoting self-healing and self-exploration). Ardell describes Loomis' visits to several of Europe's health spas as influencing the directions he concentrates on. Besides the healing environment they create at Meadowlark, many workshops are offered on topics such as nutrition, meditation, body work, music and art, dream work, and journal writing (Ardell, 1977: 20–21; Loomis, 1979).

6. Cassell discusses the dispute throughout the history of medicine between those who view disease as a generalized phenomenon versus diseases as localized entities (Cassell, 1986a). What I am calling allopathic medicine represents the ontological conception of disease, which views diseases as invading entities which are then localized in parts of the body. Holistic medicine is of the school of the physiological conception of disease, which sees disease causation in terms of an imbalance between the person and his environment. While the ontological view has most recently been dominant in Western scientific medicine, he asserts that the last fifty years has again seen a shift towards the physiological or ecological perspective (Cassell, 1986a:19–20).

7. This notion of self responsibility is the major departure between the holistic view and that of the Marxist, political economist view of illness. The Marxist view paints a picture of the patient as victim as much as does the traditional medical model. In the former case, the patient is the victim of the capitalist, profit oriented system, rather than a random victim of externally invading illness (Waitzkin and Waterman, 1974; Navarro, 1976). The holistic model rejects both these views, substituting an image of a patient with much more individual control over his reality, including his state of health or illness.

8. Two of the most comprehensive compendia of holistic modalities are *The Holistic Health Handbook*, compiled by the Berkeley Holistic Health Center, and Leslie J. Kaslof's *Wholistic Dimensions in Healing* (Bauman et al., 1978; Kaslof, 1978).

Chapter III

1. Alfonse T. Masi also indicates growing physician support for holistic and public health approaches in a 1978 editorial in the *Journal of Chronic Disease*, titled "An Holistic Concept of Health and Illness: A Tricentennial Goal for Medicine and Public Health" (Masi, 1978).
2. Ironically, this shift in the radical perspective may have, combined with the pervasive emphasis on cost containment measures, worked to withdraw access from already underserved groups. A Robert Wood Johnson Foundation report, "Access to Health Care in the United States: Results of a 1986 Survey," concludes that there has been significant deterioration in access to medical care for the nation's poor and minority groups. Some of the improved access indications of the foundation's 1982 survey had been reversed by 1986 (Johnson Foundation: 1986).
3. It is ironic that Dubos' work, cited so frequently by holistic health proponents, also develops the argument that the idea of attaining perfect health will always remain a mirage (Dubos, 1959). According to his ecological perspective, whenever one set of medical conditions is conquered, another set of problems replaces it. Yet many holistic pronouncements set up expectations that a person can reach a level of super health that may be impossible to attain, at least for the population as a whole.
4. McKeown used historical evidence to demonstrate that the recent decline of mortality, the main evidence of improvement in health, was due to the reduction of deaths from infectious disease (McKeown, 1976:8–9). However, his analysis of the data indicated that only ten percent of that improvement in mortality could be attributed to medical intervention. McKeown concludes that the improvement of health during the past three centuries was primarily due to the provision of food, protection from hazards, and population limitations (ibid:197). The primary reason behind the improvement was the improvement in nutritional status resulting from the increased availability of adequate food supplies.
5. Lewis Thomas represents those arguing that there is no evidence that health has deteriorated in the United States, and that Americans are probably somewhat healthier since 1950, despite public perceptions to the contrary (Thomas, 1979: 95–96).
6. Linda Aiken adds a further dimension to the argument of diminished effectiveness of medical care by documenting the inadequacies of medical treatment for chronic illness. She demonstrates the divergence in needs of patients with chronic illness from the acute treatment model. Physicians trained in acute care modalities organize ambulatory care around an emphasis on episodic treatment and specialty care (Aiken, 1976:239).
7. During the past twenty years, awareness of the problematic nature of specialization has grown, and various attempts to encourage primary care have been launched. Jeter writes that general practitioners declined in number due to the AMA reaction to the Flexner Report. Then in the 1950s, the AMA, aware of public concern about fragmented medicine and overspecialization, tried to encourage an increase in medical school graduates entering general family practice (Jeter, 1981:73). Knowles also sees a renewed interest in general or family practice (Knowles, 1977b:3). Despite the numerous writ-

ings attempting to encourage family practice and primary care, however, those groups have still not been accorded the status of specializations such as surgery or neurology.

8. Freidson argues that the consequences of this shift in public opinion have been grossly exaggerated. Citing public opinion poll data, he asserts that while there has been a definite decline in the public's trust, that decline is part of a shift of decreased confidence in all American institutions. In describing this as a shift rather than a major reversal, Freidson writes, "Neither medicine itself nor the health care institutions in which its members work are the objects of widespread and deep hostility or doubt, but they have become the objects of more questioning and challenge" (Freidson, 1986:65). Despite the increase in consumer dissatisfaction, he argues that the medical profession continues to retain both its monopoly within the health care system and its basic "cultural authority" (ibid:71).

9. While acknowledging the increase in consumerism, Freidson warns us not to exaggerate the potential of the consumer movement to drastically alter the medical profession's power and autonomy within the health care system (Freidson, 1985:18).

10. At the same conference, Robert Mendelsohn, M.D., who wrote *Confessions of a Medical Heretic*, gave an even more dramatic and sarcastic presentation, and he was continually interrupted by applause. Not only were his anti-physician comments greeted enthusiastically, but a tremendous burst of applause broke out when he said, "If your parent is dying, bring them home." A similar reaction greeted his statement that he now works with medical students who do deliveries at home. This illustrates the overlap between the constitutive meanings and affinities of those involved in the holistic, hospice, and home birthing movements.

11. Ozonoff and Ozonoff write that medical manuals for the lay public were popular in the United States from its inception. They argue that the majority of the contemporary self-help books accept the content and emphasis of Western scientific medicine, stressing the cure of illness and relief of symptoms. These are augmented, however, by some newer books which follow the holistic paradigm and the new genre of consumer guidebooks (Ozonoff and Ozonoff, 1977:7–8). The vast majority of the holistic literature analyzed here *does* depart dramatically from the content and underlying philosophical assumptions of allopathic medicine; in fact, that literature can be seen as directly attacking almost all those assumptions.

12. Social movements are basically conceptualized more loosely and reflexively than the classical view of a social movement as an association of people working to bring about changes in society. Emphasis is instead placed on transformations in ideas, beliefs, meanings, and consciousness, as well as concrete behavior, as they indicate changes in the society's normative values. The bias of this book is thus in a direction moving away from classical definitions toward those stressing cultural change at the level of symbolic meanings and consciousness. This presupposes a reflexivity of movement participants on the shared nature of transformation (Gusfield, 1978:15).

This more global, less rigid perspective on social movements originally derives from Blumer's conceptualization of expressive, general, and specific social movements (Blumer, 1939:255–278). In Blumer's analysis, cultural

drifts provide the background out of which emerge general social movements. Similarly, specific social movements derive from the setting of general social movements (Blumer, 1939:258).

Gusfield also describes the undirected phase of a social movement as characterized by the reshaping of perspectives and values which occurs outside
of specific associational contexts. As he writes, "The followers are partisans
but need not be members of any association which advocates the change
being studied" (Gusfield, 1968:445). Clients and holistic health movement
followers in this context can thus include the countless people of all ages who
have made drastic alterations in their lifestyles in relation to exercise, nutrition, stress reduction and meditation.

13. For a more detailed discussion of the free clinics, see Rosemary Taylor's
essay on "Free Medicine" (Taylor, 1979). Case and Taylor's collection, *Co-
ops, Communes and Collectives*, presents a thorough analysis of these new
left attempts at cultural and organizational change (Case and Taylor, 1979).

14. Fred Davis describes the different subjective experience of time in the sixties
hippie subculture. His portrayal of the radical shift in time-perspective towards a present orientation emphasizing immediacy provides yet another example of a more specific link to the core meanings constituting the Holistic
Health model (Davis, 1967:14–16).

15. Please see the two articles by Goldstein et al. for data on how self-defined
holistic physicians become interested in holistic health and how incorporating
this approach affects their clinical practice (Goldstein et al., 1985; Goldstein
et al., 1987).

16. The fact that the *New England Journal of Medicine* published the first chapter
of Norman Cousin's book, along with his documentation of the approximately three thousand letters Cousins subsequently received from physicians
applauding and supporting his approach, also demonstrates the attitudinal
support many physicians feel for holistic approaches (Cousins, 1979:
125–126).

17. As the holistic model diffuses into mainstream medicine, it also raises issues
of cooptation. Do holistic physicians want control (thus they would define
cooptation as failure), or is their goal to transform medicine by introducing
a more humanitarian, health-oriented set of principles? In the latter case,
Medicine's cooptation of Holistic Health might be defined as success in transforming major institutional structures.

18. While, in this book, I also utilize the concepts of "ideology" and "rhetoric,"
I do not attach any pejorative connotation to them. All subcultural systems
have an ideology and accompanying rhetoric (this includes sociology, as well
as both allopathic medicine and holistic health). The ideology includes the
constitutive ideas, meanings, values, and world view of participants. On the
other hand, to Stalker and Glymour, the concepts rhetoric and ideology appear to be a tool one uses to discredit ideas they devalue. Thus, to them,
ideology refers to false ideas which must be "exposed." This latter view was
commonly used in the classical, Marxist-based Sociology of Knowledge.
More recently, the field of Sociology of Knowledge has incorporated a more
relativistic and phenomenological stance.

19. Jacqueline Fawcett, a leading nurse theorist, asserts that within nursing there
is now a consensus that the central concepts of the discipline are person,

environment, health, and nursing (Fawcett, 1984:5). As she writes, "The connections among the four metaparadigm concepts are clearly made in the following statement presented by Donaldson and Crowley (1978, p. 119): 'Nursing studies the wholeness or health of humans, recognizing that humans are in continuous interaction with their environment.' This statement may be considered the major proposition of nursing's metaparadigm" (ibid.:6). This proposition reflects the strong overlap between conceptual nursing models and the holistic health model.

20. This figure-ground notion was developed through gestalt theory, primarily by Kohler and Lewin (Asch, 1968). The specific application of figure-ground contrast to this area came from discussions with Fred Davis during 1984 (also refer to Davis, 1979:57).

Chapter IV

1. The major critique levied on ethnographic research is its supposed subjectivity. When Mattson's book was published, I had been working on this research for three years. It is interesting to note that two researchers, unknown to each other and in different disciplines (Medical Anthropology does draw from much of the same literature and methodology as Medical Sociology), would undertake field studies of holistic health practice in different California cities and derive such similar data.

2. Names and details of the description will be fictionalized to protect the participants' anonymity. The substitutions will attempt to maintain the integrity of the data without compromising confidentiality. The identities of all participants interviewed are handled in the same anonymous manner as those in the settings; however, names are used when speakers have made presentations in public forums.

3. The dentist in the secondary setting, and almost every physician I interviewed, had similar reactions to the term "holistic health."

4. I was especially struck by the choice of that picture because in an earlier set of field notes I had commented that when Dr. A checks the pulses during an acupuncture treatment, he holds the patient's hand in a way that seems to symbolize caring and nurturing through touch.

5. It must be remembered that, to another group of patients, those symbols which represent humane caring in this clinic would symbolize professional incompetence. To that more traditional group, symbols such as a white uniform and highly visible technical equipment represent the ideal of technically professional competence in medical care and therefore inspire confidence.

6. The discrepancy between terms of reference for the physicians versus the nurses, psychologists, and ancillary staff replicates the natural office usage. The nurses and psychologists are exclusively referred to by first name, both by patients and other staff. On the other hand, while the physicians are always referred to by first name by other staff members, some patients refer to them by first name, while others use "Dr. A." It is recognized that this discrepancy may not only indicate gender-based status differentials, but the greater degree of status many patients continue to ascribe to the physician role. In the case of the psychologists, one is male and the other is female;

yet, neither is referred to as "Dr. C." This again demonstrates the deep connection between language and social stratification.

7. The majority of the physicians in the interview sample, including one in the primary setting, were born Jewish, although only two described themselves as practicing Jews (one of these had converted to Judaism in adulthood). Seven of the most visible physicians/movement leaders in the local area studied are Jewish (six by birth), while five are not. Despite the small sample, this is interesting in terms of Goldstein et al.'s findings that half of their exploratory sample of holistic physicians were of Jewish origin (they speculate that this finding may be atypical because their sample was from the Los Angeles area) (Goldstein, 1985:320). The majority of both the nurses and the psychologists are not Jewish, however. When asked about "spiritual" rather than "religious" commitments, respondents indicated more active involvement. At the time of interview, most of the physicians were, or had been in the past, involved with Eastern spiritual systems such as Buddhism, Yoga, Arica, and Eckankar.

8. Mattson summarized demographic data on 166 patients in a Northern California holistic health center. In that sample, she found the following characteristics:

   AGE: 21% under 29; 39% 30–39; 14% 40–49; 11% 50–59; 13% 60 plus. SEX: 30% male; 68% female. MARITAL: 34% married; 40% single; 13% divorced; 5% widowed. EDUCATION: 4% high school or less; 26% some college; 39% BA; 19% MA; 7% PhD, MD. OCCUPATION: 35% professional; 17% helping; 15% clerical; 7% housewife; 8% student; 10% other. See Mattson for a more comprehensive overview (Mattson, 1982:116–122).

9. At one of the other local holistic clinics where I conducted interviews, they estimate that 40% of their patients come with a specific condition, usually chronic. That group is not very interested in health promotion, at least not in the initial period. The director estimated that 30% of their patients require both health education and promotion, and intervention for specific problems. He described another 30% as coming to "fine tune" their emotions or their bodies. Many of their patients, especially those in the third group, are highly educated and motivated, and he feels this contributes to their high success rate.

10. Rosemary Taylor argues that the most consistent theme in the consumer dissatisfaction with medicine that stimulates searches to alternative healing systems is dissatisfaction with the practitioner-patient relationship (Taylor, 1984:204–205). The responses of this group of patients definitely supports her claims.

11. The integration of approaches observed in this setting is supported by Goldstein et al.'s findings that most of the holistic physicians they studied had reached a sophisticated integration of holistic approaches into mainstream clinical practice. Additionally, those "holistic techniques" most frequently used by their sample of physicians were all heavily emphasized in this practice: patient education, psychological counseling, nutritional counseling, and meditation (Goldstein et al., 1985:340).

12. Preventive care, patient education, and self-responsibility generate less income than more traditional and technologically-based medical approaches. Insurance companies do not value, and often will not reimburse, preventive approaches, so that too much emphasis in this direction is ultimately less

lucrative for practitioners. On the other hand, it is possible that the structure of payment will change to reward preventive approaches in the next decade.

13. Dr. A had tried establishing a "wellness program" earlier. Although they do a great deal of wellness education in the clinic, they received literally no response when he advertised a stand-alone wellness program. Dr. A explained that as soon as people heard the program would cost 300–400 dollars, they lost interest. He spoke of people's willingness to spend money once they're sick, but not to prevent becoming sick. It was hard for him to comprehend, given the cost of a single day's stay in a hospital.

14. In a similar holistic clinic, they also talk of their emphasis on self-care. Besides the lifestyle change aimed at improving the individual's level of physical health, one of the psychologists speaks of their "emotional fitness program." He sees this presentation as less threatening to people than discussing mental health in terms of mental illness. By talking of interventions aimed at "emotional self-care" or "emotional fitness," he finds their clients experience less stigma and are more open to seeking help. Although this clinic offers many types of psychologically-based approaches (examples are rolfing and meditation techniques), they present them "educationally."

15. The cost for the initial hour assessment was $85 in 1983. Many patients saw this amount, along with the costs of the initial laboratory work as high; however, it was comparable to rates for family practice in the surrounding community. Again, when healthy or experiencing a minor problem, people resist spending such amounts, as opposed to equivalant costs when facing major, acute illness.

16. During one occasion, where I assisted when Nurse B was ill, I became aware that one part of my role-performance departed from Gail's behavior in the same situations. I realized that when I interacted with patients, I was somewhat "too professional." Both Gail and Rose are definitely professional; however, there was a much larger component of more social, joking, intimate talk than my style. At a point where I worked in a pediatric office (twenty years ago), my interactional style was considered extremely warm and informal in terms of the norm; yet, there was a definite difference in the "required" or appropriate levels of both warmth and formality of the role here. This was an example of using participation as further data to document my observations.

On four occasions during the field work, I assisted when one of the nurses was sick. On those days, my research role moved to participant-as-observer (Gold, 1969:35). Besides giving me access to that type of performative data, it expanded my access to both backstage behavior within the setting and to observing physician-patient interactions more extensively.

17. After about a month and a half in the setting, I hugged both Gail and Suzie before leaving for the day. I had become aware of feeling subtle pressure because I distance myself more than is normative for this setting, and I made a conscious effort to "reach out" more.

18. At one of the other holistic clinics where I interviewed two physicians and a psychologist, staff members described their relationships as "more like a family." They uniformly spoke about how they "all take care of each other," and mentioned that the "healing energy" they strive to maintain in the clinic affects practitioners as well as clients.

19. These social occasions, like the staff meetings, provided more direct access

to the backstage behavior, as well as meanings and world views of the staff members. For instance, Dr. A drove a Volvo stationwagon, and Rose (Nurse A) drove a Volkswagon bug. Another example is the nutritious food served at most of these gatherings, such as the beach picnic. On the other hand, when the receptionist invited everyone to her apartment for dinner, the lasagna was prepared with meat, and wine was available for those who wanted it (both of those breaches were discussed by some participants, so it definitely departed from their usual patterns).

20. The interested reader is referred to the following citations for a more comprehensive analysis of the sick role: Parsons, 1951:428–479; Parsons and Fox, 1958; Twaddle, 1972; Siegler and Osmond, 1973; Seagal, 1976.

21. Haug and Levin write that, although the sick-role concept has been widely criticized, even the critiques have accepted the power differential as given. It is only in the last decade that researchers began to postulate a competing model of the doctor-patient relationship involving more equal power and negotiation (Haug and Levin, 1981:213).

22. Although this setting was a private practice clinic, it epitomized many of the same kinds of caring on the part of providers described in the holistic health centers located in churches, which Tubesing, Sullivan, and Glasser see as symbolizing centers of both community and spirituality (Tubesing, 1978; Sullivan, 1983; Glasser, 1983).

Chapter V

1. Rosemary Taylor argues that these types of expressive qualities within the physician-patient relationship assume the most importance when the efficacy of medicine is questioned (Taylor 1984:208).

2. Shiloh's study of "Equalitarian and Hierarchical Patients" raises a further issue (1972). If two groups of patients exist with divergent perceptions of their relation to the hospital and medical staff, the variety of practitioner-patient relationships specified by Szasz and Hollender may be important for individual, as well as structural, differences. This would also be supported by Balint's observations on the different interaction styles of physicians (1960). Thus, clinical coldness and detachment may inspire confidence in one group of patients, while warm, expressive communication may induce confidence in the group of patients seeking holistic care. It would be interesting to compare this group of patients with those utilizing more conventional medical settings in terms of their scores on the Krantz Health Opinion Survey (Krantz, Baum, and Wideman, 1980).

3. The physician is the focus of the analysis here, despite the broader participation of other team members, because of the large comparative pool of data on physician-patient interactions in traditional medical settings.

4. Eric Cassell also describes the new consumerist client as frequently skeptical and mistrusting of physicians' motives and judgment (Cassell, 1986:185). Eliot Freidson, on the other hand, argues that there has only been a partial and relative decline in the respect and trust of the medical profession. In fact, he contends that medicine remains the American institution with the most public confidence (Freidson, 1985:111–113).

5. The actual term "placebo salience" for this well-documented phenomenon was suggested by Fred Davis during discussions in November 1984.
6. I had not been aware of how wedded to "physician" and "patient" roles I was until this became apparent while analyzing the transcripts.
7. Because of the exploratory nature of this study, detailed sociolinguistic analyses of physician-patient interactions in these settings and more traditional medical settings were not conducted. That would be the next step in specifying more precisely the magnitude of differences between the interactional outcomes of the two models. The representativeness of both sets of physicians used would be crucial methodologically to the success of such a study.
8. This clinical situation also involved some backstage talk of the dental technicians. The client's talk was seen as "pretty weird," and their joking comments were the only instance of moral condemnation I observed in that setting. None of this was visible or audible to the patient.

Chapter VI

1. Philip Brickman has conceptualized a framework of four models of helping. In the moral model, people are seen as having the responsibility for both creating and solving their problems. In the compensatory model, people are not blamed for creating their problems; however, they are held responsible for solving them. In the medical model, individuals are not held responsible for either causing or solving their problems. The enlightenment model blames people for causing their problems, but does not hold them responsible for solving them (Cronenwett and Brickman, 1983:84–88). While the addition of the compensatory and enlightenment models allows for a higher degree of analytical complexity, Brickman's medical and moral models correspond to those discussed in this analysis.
2. This is a major area of divergence from the views of the community clinic movement. David Hayes-Bautista, who equates the Community clinic with the holistic health model, sees the pathogenic location outside the individual. Similar to McKinley's left reformist perspective, Hayes-Bautista views individual illness as a reflection of societal illness. This attribution of blame to unemployment, racism, malnutrition, and pollution exempts the individual from any attribution of blame (Hayes-Bautista, 1977:83).
3. In 1983 a *Los Angeles Times* column estimated approximately forty life insurance companies offered discounts for healthy habits. Six companies were cited as offering disability insurance discounts for non-smokers and joggers. Some of the companies were reported to require aerobic exercise for a minimum of twenty minutes daily, four days a week for discounts (Weaver, 1983:13).
4. Kopelman and Moskop argue persuasively about the moral components of a holistic health perspective, while denying that traditional medicine imputes moral judgments. It must be noted that they hold positions within a medical school department.
5. Salmon has referred to what I call the "ideology of choice" as a "lifestyles ideology" (Salmon, 1984:258). While the two phenomena overlap, they are

not identical. Both specify causal links between lifestyle behavior and illness; however, the "ideology of choice" implies a more explicit individual choice in "creating" a far wider range of diseases.

6. This response was by far the most extreme of any practitioners or patient/ clients interviewed. It was made in an interview outside the setting by one of the two staff members in Mar Vista Clinic with the most extreme views. The comment was made in response to a question on how she saw a child and responsibility. No other practitioner interviewed or observed indicated such extreme beliefs; however, I suspect such views might be expressed more frequently among practitioners at the more radical end of the holistic health continuum.

7. This finding directly contradicts Kopelman and Moskop's contention that moral evaluations take place within holistic medicine, while traditional physicians do not make those moral judgments (Kopelman and Moskop, 1981).

8. Again, these views reflect the *participants'* perceptions and beliefs.

9. It could be argued that the levels of compassionate acceptance observed may derive from the Western monistic tradition. These practitioners, however, almost exclusively attributed it to Eastern spiritual disciplines and an overarching Eastern world view, and they framed it within those concepts.

10. Another interesting cultural example is the increasing incidence of bulimia among adolescents and young adults. Being overweight is a highly stigmatized, visible sign of lack of moral grace. The health effects of bulimic behavior are far more dangerous than excessive weight; yet, the priority is placed on the visible aspects of maintaining the appearance of health, rather than health itself.

11. Joseph Kotarba documents similar experiences in his work on chronic pain (Kotarba, 1983).

12. My own reactions during the field research made me painfully aware of this kind of self condemnation. While observing in the clinic, I frequently found myself thinking that I "really should" eliminate sugar and chocolate from my diet. I was also almost continually aware of the excessive stress in my life. During one instance, where the staff surprised one of the psychologists with a Baskin-Robbins mud pie (rich ice cream cake) for his birthday, I noticed how relieved I felt.

13. This could have been rhetoric, however, as this particular physician came through as one of the most caring, sensitive, and spiritually committed physicians I interviewed. His reputation in the traditional medical and nursing communities also reflects that assessment.

14. Whenever I discussed even peripheral aspects of this problem with a colleague facing cancer, he became extremely angry about the blame and guilt that followed from this ideology, and repeatedly emphasized how it "must be exposed."

Chapter VII

1. The professions, including medicine, have traditionally upheld an ethic of obligation. Basically, the professional was obligated to provide services for clients, whether or not he or she felt like caring for them. Thus a lawyer was

obligated to defend even reprehensible criminals, and ministers were professionally obligated to try to save sinners. Similarly, physicians held the obligation and responsibility to heal even those patients who had played a part in causing their own illness (the patients, in turn, were obligated to cooperate and to want to get well). This professional commitment, with its related sense of obligation, may be breaking down with the new more individualistic lifestyle focus and the "ideology of choice." The providers in this study whose compassion buffered the levying of blame continued to hold that strong ethic of obligation, which was integrally embedded in a monistic world view, almost always framed in Eastern terms.

2. Several authors have alluded to this aspect of increasing medicalization with movement towards lifestyle intervention. Guttmacher specifically notes the potential of holistic health to medicalize much of everyday life (Guttmacher, 1979). Crawford also writes that the new health movements and their accompanying world view may ultimately expand medical power in his article "Healthism and the Medicalization of Everyday Life" (Crawford, 1980). Arney and Bergen develop a parallel argument in *Medicine and the Management of Daily Living* (Arney and Bergen, 1984). And Conrad specifically warns of this phenomenon in relation to the current preventive focus in health care (Conrad, 1984).

3. While this conceptualization accepts a gradual historical process of medicalization of deviance, and now postulates a swing of the pendulum away from medicalization towards demedicalization, there is an alternate possibility. The evidence can be interpreted to indicate that the concept of exemption from responsibility in mental illness was never actually dominant except with a small but powerful elite.

4. This process parallels the policy strategy of deinstitutionalization in mental illness in California. Movement towards a community based treatment system was justified with humanitarian considerations of the negative effects of institutionalization; yet, Scull argues persuasively that the actual rationale for the program direction was economic considerations (Scull, 1977).

5. Salmon also argues, in describing the new health policy based on lifestyle modification, that those who become sick are being scapegoated for causing their problems; he concludes that this strategy is due to the prevailing economic restraints (Salmon, 1984).

6. Undertaking a major analysis of these themes would require a separate work. See Tipton's *Getting Saved From the Sixties* (1982), Bellah's "The New Consciousness and the Berkeley New Left" (1976), and particularly Marsella et al.'s compilation, *Culture and Self· Asian and Western Perspectives* (Marsella, DeVos, and Hsu, 1985).

7. The initial section of Tipton's book summarizes those historical strands, as does Bellah's work, to an extent impossible here (Tipton, 1982; also Bellah, 1976). See also *Habits of the Heart: Individualism and Commitment in American Life* for the fullest discussion (Bellah, Madsen, Sullivan, Swidler, and Tipton, 1985).

8. One can argue that there are new Western views incorporating interconnectedness, such as those embodied in the new physics and recent variants of systems theory. I see these developments as influenced by that same diffusion of Eastern world views.

9. Lock presents an example from her fieldwork in Japan. Japanese socialization is oriented towards harmony and the attainment of a "flexible, compliant personality which is able to subordinate ego needs to those of the group" (Lock, 1978:162). Similarly, family and group affiliation take precedence over individual needs. The system of Japanese medicine she studied was holistic; however, it was embedded in a network of responsibilities to others. For example, the Japanese family actively participates in the illness and recovery process. Similarly, the period of illness is taken "as a chance for reflection and for consolidation and promotion of group bonds—one of the most basic values in Japanese society" (ibid.:167).

10. However, Bellah notes that, although such monistic beliefs are diametrically apposed to utilitarian individualism, there are elements of Christian theology which stress the unity of being with a consequent compassion and love for all beings (Bellah, 1976:347).

11. A detailed discussion of the subtle meanings of karma in Eastern thought cannot be undertaken here, and any such detail would go beyond the meanings attributed to the concept by participants in the holistic movement. Without being embedded in the larger constellation of values and symbolic ideas, however, "karma" can become translated into blaming the victim, as in the example of the nurse who assigned the child a causal role in child abuse because it "chose to be incarnated into that family."

12. As Wei-ming argues in his discussion of the differences in conceptions of selfhood between Confucian thought and American self-growth systems, the part of Confucian learning omitted here is the disciplined ritual practice and structure of obligations to others (Wei-ming, 1985:232–3). Similarly Chu distinguishes between the American self, which is characterized by the strong sense of individualism, and the traditional Chinese self, which is more oriented to significant others, as well as anchored in family and community relationships (Chu, 1985:257–258). DeVos describes the parallel submersion of individuality in favor of cooperation and peaceful relationships within Japanese culture (DeVos, 1985:164).

13. Muriel Gillick analyzes the popularity of jogging in terms of similar ideas (Gillick, 1984). In an article titled "Health Promotion, Jogging, and the Pursuit of the Moral Life," she develops the theme that upright living has symbolically become a means to personal and social redemption.

14. Similarly, some early examinations of the current medical system in China indicate parallel tensions and contradictions as a Western way is superimposed on the Eastern system. Renee Fox and Judith Swazey's pilot study demonstrated the constant tensions and dualities between approaches based on Eastern and Western traditions. Using a critical care unit at Tianjin's First Central Hospital as a case study, they observed the attempt to integrate sophisticated Western medicine into the existing system of traditional medicine (Fox and Swazey, 1982).

15. It can be argued that an Eastern world view tolerates a greater amount of ambiguity than the Western mode. Eastern conceptions have always emphasized balance between opposing forces, rather than separation and polarized opposites.

References

Achterberg, J., and F. Lawlis. 1982. Imagery and health intervention. *Topics in Clinical Nursing*, 3,4:55–60.

Aiken, L. 1976. Chronic illness and responsive ambulatory care. In D. Mechanic (ed.), *Growth of Bureaucratic Medicine*, New York: John Wiley and Sons.

Aiken, L. H., and D. Mechanic (eds.). 1986. *Applications of Social Science to Clinical Medicine and Health Policy*. New Brunswick, NJ: Rutgers University Press.

Alonzo, A. 1985. Health as situational adaptation: A social psychological perspective. *Social Science and Medicine*, 21, 12:1341–1344.

Altman, D. E. 1986. Two views of a changing health care system. In L. H. Aiken and D. Mechanic (eds.), *Applications of Social Science to Clinical Medicine and Health Policy*, 100–112. New Brunswick, NJ: Rutgers University Press.

Andrews, L. B., and L. S. Levin. 1979. Self-care and the law. *Social Policy*, 9:44–49.

Angell, M. 1985. Disease as a reflection of the psyche. *New England Journal of Medicine*, 312, 24:1570-1572.

Antonovsky, A. 1980. *Health, Stress and Coping*. San Francisco: Jossey-Bass.

Antonovsky, A. 1987. *Unraveling the Mystery of Health*. San Francisco: Jossey-Bass.

Ardell, D. B. 1977. *High Level Wellness: An Alternative to Doctors, Drugs, and Disease*. Emmaus, PA: Rodale Press.

Ardell, D. B. 1976. From omnibus tinkering to high level wellness: the movement toward holistic health. *American Journal of Health Planning*, 1,2: 15–34.

Arney, W. R., and B. J. Bergen. 1984. *Medicine and the Management of Living*. Chicago: University of Chicago Press.

Asch, S. E. 1968. Gestalt theory. In D. L. Sills (ed.), *International Encyclopedia of the Social Sciences*, Vol. 6, 158–175. New York: Macmillan.

Association of Holistic Health. 1983. *Membership Brochure* San Diego, California.

Association of Holistic Health. 1979. *Statement of Purpose*. San Diego, California.

Aubert, V., and S. L. Messinger. 1972. The criminal and the sick. In E. Freidson and J. Lorber (eds.), *Medical Men and Their Work*, 288–308. Chicago: Aldine Publishing Co.

Dahr, R. T. 1982. Holistic or wholistic health: A philosophy of practice in gerontological nursing. *Journal of Gerontological Nursing*, 8, 5:262.

Balint, M. 1960. *The Doctor, His Patient and the Illness*. New York: International University Press.

Ballantine, R. 1982. The nutritional dimension. In T. Deliman and J. S. Smolowe
(eds.), *Holistic Medicine: Harmony of Body Mind Spirit*, 41–67. Reston,
VA: Reston Publishing Company.

Banks, J. A. 1972. *The Sociology of Social Movements*. London: Macmillan.

Bauman, E. 1978. Introduction to holistic health. In Berkeley Holistic Health
Center (ed.), *The Holistic Health Handbook*, 17–19. Berkeley, CA: And/
Or Press.

Bellah, R. N. 1976a. The new consciousness and the Berkeley new left. In C. Y.
Glock and R. N. Bellah (eds.), *The New Religious Consciousness*, 77–92.
Berkeley: University of California Press.

Bellah, R. N. 1976b. New religious consciousness and the crisis in modernity. In
C. Y. Glock and R. N. Bellah (eds.), *The New Religious Consciousness*,
333–352. Berkeley: University of California Press.

Bellah, R. N., R. Madsen, W. M. Sullivan, A. Swidler, and S. M. Tipton. 1985.
Habits of the Heart: Individualism and Commitment in American Life.
Berkeley: University of California Press.

Bendix, R. 1968. Max Weber. In D. L. Sills (ed.), *International Encyclopedia
of the Social Sciences*, Vol. 16, 493–502. New York: Macmillan.

Benson, H. 1975. *The Relaxation Response*. New York: William Morrow
and Co.

Benson, H. 1979. *The Mind/Body Effect*. New York: Berkley Books.

Benson, H., and M. D. Epstein. 1980. The placebo effect: a neglected asset in
the care of patients. In A. C. Hastings et al. (eds.), *Health for the Whole
Person*, 179–185. Boulder, CO: Westview Press.

Benson, H., J. B. Kotch, K. D. Crassweller, and M. M. Greenwood. 1981.
Historical and clinical considerations of the relaxation response. *Journal of
Holistic Health*, 6:3–10.

Berger, B. M. 1967. Hippie morality—more old than new. *Trans-Action*, 19–27.

Berger, B. M. 1981. *The Survival of a Counterculture: Ideological Work and
Everyday Life Among Rural Communards*. Berkeley: University of California Press.

Berger, P. L., and T. Luckmann. 1967. *The Social Construction of Reality: A
Treatise in the Sociology of Knowledge*. Garden City, NY: Doubleday and
Company.

Berkeley Holistic Health Center. 1978. *The Holistic Health Handbook: A Tool
for Attaining Wholeness of Body, Mind, and Spirit*. Berkeley, CA: And/Or
Press.

Berliner, H. S. 1984. Scientific medicine since Flexner. In J. W. Salmon (ed.),
Alternative Medicines: Popular and Policy Perspectives, 191–228. New
York: Tavistock Publications.

Berliner, H. S., and J. W. Salmon. 1980. The holistic alternative to scientific medicine: History and analysis. *International Journal of Health Services*, 10,1:133–147.

Berliner, H. S., and J. W. Salmon. 1979. The holistic health movement and scientific medicine: The naked and the dead. *Socialist Review*, 9,1:31–52.

Betz, M., and L. O'Connell. 1983. Changing doctor-patient relationships and the rise in concern for accountability. *Social Problems*, 31, 1:84–95.

Blattner, B. 1981. *Holistic Nursing*. Englewood Cliffs, NJ: Prentice-Hall.

Bloom, S. W., and R. W. Wilson. 1979. Patient-practitioner relationships. In H. B. Freeman, S. Levine, and L. G. Reeder (eds.), *Handbook of Medical Sociology*, 275–297. Englewood Cliffs, NJ: Prentice-Hall.

Bloomfield, H. H., and R. B. Kory. 1978. *The Holistic Way to Health and Happiness*. New York: Simon and Schuster.

Blotcky A. D., and B. I. Tittler. 1982. Psychosocial predictors of physical illness: Toward a holistic model of health. *Preventive Medicine*, 11, 5:602–611.

Blue Shield of California 1982. *The Blue Shield of California Guide to Staying Well*. Chicago: Contemporary Books, Inc.

Blumer, H. 1939. Collective behavior. In R. Park (ed.), *An Outline of the Principles of Sociology*, 220–280. New York: Barnes and Noble.

Bogdan, R., and S. J. Taylor. 1975. *Introduction to Qualitative Research Methods: A Phenomenological Approach to the Social Sciences*. New York: John Wiley and Sons.

Bosk, C. L. 1979. *Forgive and Remember: Managing Medical Failure*. Chicago: University of Chicago Press.

Boulding, K. 1966. The concept of need for health services. *Milbank Memorial Fund Quarterly*, 44, 3:202–223.

Brenner, P. 1978. *Health is a Question of Balance*. New York: Vantage Press.

Brenner, P. 1981a. Healing Through Communication. Workshop presented at Mandala/Association of Holistic Health Conference, August 29, San Diego, California.

Brenner, P. 1981b. Life is a Shared Creation. Presentation at Mandala/Association of Holistic Health Conference, August 30, San Diego, California.

Brenner, P. 1984. A personal trajectory. In J. S. Gordon, D. T. Jaffe and D. E. Bresler (eds.), *Mind, Body and Health: Toward an Integral Medicine*, 178–187. New York: Human Sciences Press.

Bresler, D. E. 1980. Chinese medicine and holistic health. In A. C. Hastings et al. (eds.), *Health for the Whole Person*, 407–419. Boulder, CO: Westview Press.

Brint, A. I., and P. A. Wright. 1978. The Berkeley Holistic Health Center. In Berkeley Holistic Health Center (ed.), *The Holistic Health Handbook*, 226–236. Berkeley, CA: And/Or Press.

Brown, B. B. 1984. *Between Health and Illness: New Notions of Stress and the Nature of Well Being*. Boston: Houghton Mifflin Company.

Brown, H. N., and N. E. Zinberg. 1982. Difficulties in the integration of psychological and medical practices. *American Journal of Psychiatry*, 139, 12: 1576–1580.

Bulen, E. 1979. *Holistic Health Focus*, 2, 1:2.

Callan, J. P. 1979. Holistic health or holistic hoax? *JAMA*, 241, 11:1156.

Capra, F. 1975. *The Tao of Physics*. Berkeley, CA: Shambhala.

Capra, F. 1981. Physics and holistic health: a new understanding of reality. *Journal of Holistic Health*, 6:30–36.

Capra, F. 1982. Introduction. In L. Dossey, *Space, Time and Medicine*. Boulder, CO: Shambhala.

Carlson, R. J. 1975. *The End of Medicine*. New York: John Wiley and Sons.

Carlson, R. 1978. Public policy and legal implications of holistic health on the state and national level. *Journal of Holistic Health*, 3:83–89.

Carlson, R. 1980. The future of health care in the United States. In A. C. Hastings et al. (eds.), *Health for the Whole Person*, 483–495. Boulder, CO: Westview Press.

Carlson, R. J. 1984. The whole society: Medicine in an unhealthy world. In J. S. Gordon, D. T. Jaffe, and D. E. Bresler (eds.), *Mind, Body and Health: Toward an Integral Medicine*, 249–256. New York: Human Sciences Press.

Carlson, R. J., and R. Cunningham (eds.). 1978. *Future Directions in Health Care: A New Public Policy*. Cambridge, MA: Ballinger Publishing Co.

Case, J., and R. C. R. Taylor. 1979. Introduction. In J. Case and R. C. R. Taylor (eds.), *Co-ops, Communes and Collectives: Experiments in Social Change in the 1960s and 1970s*. New York: Pantheon Books.

Cassell, E. J. 1986a. Ideas in conflict: The rise and fall (and rise and fall) of new views of disease. *Daedalus*, 115, 2:19–42.

Cassell, E. J. 1986b. The changing concept of the ideal physician. *Daedalus*, 115,2:185–208.

Chow, E. P. Y. 1979. Chinese medicine: contributions to wholistic healing. In H. A. Otto and J. W. Knight (eds.), *Dimensions in Wholistic Healing*, 391–401. Chicago: Nelson-Hall.

Chrisman, N. J. 1977. The health seeking process: An approach to the natural history of illness. *Culture, Medicine and Psychiatry*, 1:351–378.

Chu, G. C. 1985. The changing concept of self in contemporary China. In A. J. Marsella, G. DeVos, and F. L. K. Hsu (eds.), *Culture and Self: Asian and Western Perspectives*, 252–277. New York: Tavistock Publications.

Chung, A. W. 1980. China's contribution to holistic health. *Journal of Holistic Health*, 5:105–111.

Clark, C. C. 1983. Women and arthritis: Holistic/wellness perspectives. *Topics in Clinical Nursing*, 4, 4:45–55.

Clark, F. V. 1978. Transpersonal psychology. In L. J. Kaslof (ed.), *Wholistic Dimensions in Healing*, 276–279. New York: Doubleday.

Cmich, D. E. 1984. Theoretical perspectives on holistic health. *Journal of School Health*, 54, 1:30–32.

Cockerham, W. C. 1986. *Medical Sociology*. Englewood Cliffs, NJ: Prentice-Hall.

Cogswell, B. E., and M. B. Sussman (eds.) 1981. *Family Medicine: A New Approach to Health Care*. New York: Haworth Press.

Connelly, D. M. 1979. *Traditional Acupuncture: The Law of the Five Elements*. Columbia, MD: The Centre for Traditional Acupuncture.

Conrad, P. 1984. Pitfalls of prevention. *The Disability and Chronic Disease Quarterly*, 4, 2:1–2.

Conrad, P., and J. W. Schneider. 1980. *Deviance and Medicalization: From Badness to Sickness*. St. Louis: C. V. Mosby Company.

Cousins, N. 1979. *Anatomy of an Illness as Perceived by the Patient*. New York: W. W. Norton and Company.

Cousins, N. 1983. *The Healing Heart*. New York: W. W. Norton and Company.

Crawford, R. 1977. You are dangerous to your health: The ideology and politics of victim blaming. *International Journal of Health*, 7, 4:663–680.

Crawford, R. 1980. Healthism and the medicalization of everyday life. *International Journal of Health Services*, 10, 3:365–388.

Crawford, R. 1981. Individual responsibility and health politics. In P. Conrad and R. Kern (eds.), *The Sociology of Health and Illness: Critical Perspectives*, 468–481. New York: St. Martin's Press.

Cronenwett, L., and P. Brickman. 1983. Models of helping and coping in childbirth. *Nursing Research*, 32, 2:84–88.

Davidson, K. 1981. Positive thought becomes cancer weapon: many discount effectiveness of patients' images of battling cells. *Los Angeles Times*, April 4, Part II:1.

Davidson, P. O., and S. M. Davidson (eds.). 1980. *Behavioral Medicine: Changing Health Lifestyles*. New York: Brunner/Mazel.

Davis, F. 1963. *Passage Through Crisis*. New York: Bobbs-Merrill Co.

Davis, F. (ed.) 1966. *The Nursing Profession*. New York: John Wiley and Sons.

Davis, F. 1967. Why all of us may be hippies someday. *Trans-Action*, 10–18.

Davis, F. 1972a. Uncertainty in medical prognosis, clinical or functional. In F. Davis, *Illness, Interaction and the Self*, 92–102. Belmont, CA: Wadsworth Publishing Co.

Davis, F. 1972b. Deviance disavowal: the management of strained interaction by the visibly handicapped. In F. Davis, *Illness, Interaction and the Self*, 130–150. Belmont, CA: Wadsworth Publishing Co.

Davis, F. 1979. *Yearning for Yesterday: A Sociology of Nostalgia*. New York: Free Press.

Deliman, T., and J. S. Smolowe (eds.). 1982. *Holistic Medicine: Harmony of Body Mind Spirit*. Reston, VA: Reston Publishing Company.

DeVos, G. 1985a. Dimensions of the self in Japanese culture. In A. J. Marsella, G. DeVos, and F. L. K. Hsu (eds.), *Culture and Self: Asian and Western Perspectives*, 141–184. New York: Tavistock Publications.

DeVos, G., A. J. Marsella, and F. L. K. Hsu. 1985b. Introduction: Approaches to culture and self. In A. J. Marsella, G. DeVos, and F. L. K. Hsu (eds.), *Culture and Self: Asian and Western Perspectives*, 2–23. New York: Tavistock Publications.

Dossey, L. 1982a. *Space, Time and Medicine*. Boulder, CO: Shambhala.

Dossey, L. 1982b. Consciousness and health: What's it all about? *Topics in Clinical Nursing*, 3, 4:1–6.

Dossey, L. 1982c. Consciousness and caring: Retrospective 2000. *Topics in Clinical Nursing*, 3, 4:53–83.

Doty, J. 1981. Setting Up a Holistic Health Center. Workshop at Mandala/Association of Holistic Health Conference, August, San Diego, California.

Douglas, J. D. 1976. *Investigative Social Research*. Beverly Hills, CA: Sage Publications.

Driessen, J. 1978. Health sharing: comments on the characteristics of holistic health. *Holistic Health Focus*, 1, 4:2.

Dubos, R. 1959. *Mirage of Health*. New York: Anchor Books.

Dubos, R. 1979. Introduction. In N. Cousins, *Anatomy of an Illness*, 11–23. New York: W. W. Norton and Company.

Duhl, L. J. 1980. The Social Context of Health. In A. C. Hastings et al. (eds.), *Health for the Whole Person*, 39–48. Boulder, CO: Westview Press.

Duval, M. K. 1977. The provider, the government, and the consumer. In J. M. Knowles (ed.), *Doing Better and Feeling Worse: Health in the United States*, 185–192. New York: W. W. Norton and Company.

Ehrenreich, B., and D. English. 1973. *Complaints and Disorders: The Sexual Politics of Sickness*. New York: The Feminist Press.

Ehrenreich, J. (ed.) 1978. *The Cultural Crisis of Modern Medicine*. New York: Monthly Review Press.

Ehrenreich, J., and B. Ehrenreich. 1978. Medicine and social control. In J. Ehrenreich (ed.), *The Cultural Crisis of Modern Medicine*, 39–80. New York: Monthly Review Press.

Emerson, R. W. 1949. The transcendentalist. In G. F. Whicher (ed.), *The Transcendentalist Revolt Against Materialism*, Boston: D. C. Heath and Co. (Reprint of his original lecture delivered in 1842).

Engel, G. L. 1977. The need for a new medical model: a challenge for biomedicine. *Science*, 196, 4286:129–135.

Engel, G. L., and Schmale, A. H. 1967. Psychoanalytic theory of somatic disorder: conversion, specificity, and the disease onset situation. *Journal of the American Psychoanalytic Association*, 18:355.

Epstein, S. S. 1978. *The Politics of Cancer*. San Francisco: Sierra Club Books.

Epstein, S. S. 1982. Ecology: A Medical Political Perspective. Presentation at Mandala/Association of Holistic Health Conference, August 28, San Diego, California.

Evans, R. W. 1983a. Health care technology and the inevitability of resource allocation and rationing decisions, Part 1. *JAMA*, 249, 16:2047-2053.

Evans, R. W. 1983b. Health care technology and the inevitability of resource allocation and rationing decisions, Part 2. *JAMA*, 249, 17:2208-2219.

Fawcett, J. 1984. *Analysis and Evaluation of Conceptual Models*. Philadelphia: F. A. Davis Co.

Ferguson, T. 1980. Medical self-care: Self-responsibility for health. In A. C. Hastings et al. (eds.), *Health for the Whole Person*, 87–99. Boulder, CO: Westview Press.

Fink, D. L. 1976. Holistic health: Implications for health planning. *American Journal of Health Planning*, 1:23–31.

Fisher, S., and A. D. Todd (eds.). 1983. *The Social Organization of Doctor-Patient Communication*. Washington, DC: Center for Applied Linguistics.

Flaster, D. J. 1983. *Malpractice*. New York: Charles Scribner's Sons.

Flynn, P. 1980. *Holistic Health : The Art and Science of Care*. Bowie, MD: Robert J. Brady Co.

Fox, R. C. 1977. The medicalization and demedicalization of American society. In J. H. Knowles, M.D. (ed.), *Doing Better and Feeling Worse*, 9–22. New York: W. W. Norton and Company.

Fox, R. C. 1984. "Reflections and Opportunities in the Sociology of Medicine." Presentation at the Awards Ceremony, Section on Medical Sociology, 1984 American Sociological Association Meetings, August 29, San Antonio, Texas.

Fox, R. C., and J. P. Swazey. 1982. Critical care at Tianjin's First Central Hospital and the fourth modernization. *Science*, 217, 20:700–705.

Frank, J. D. 1974. *Persuasion and Healing*. New York: Schocken Books.

Frank, J. D. 1981. *Holistic Medicine: A View From the Fence*. Los Angeles: The Holmes Center.

Freidson, E. 1960. Client control and medical practice. *American Journal of Sociology*, 65, 4:374–382.

Freidson, E. 1965. Disability as social deviance. In S. Sussman (ed.), *Sociology and Rehabilitation*, Washington, DC: American Sociological Association.

Freidson, E. 1970a. *Professional Dominance*. New York: Atherton.

Freidson, E. 1970b. *Profession of Medicine*. New York: Dodd-Mead.

Freidson, E. 1973. Prepaid group practice and the new 'demanding patient'. *Milbank Memorial Fund Quarterly*, 473–488.

Freidson, E. 1985. The reorganization of the medical profession. *Medical Care Review*, 42, 1:11–35.

Freidson, E. 1986. The medical profession in transition. In L. H. Aiken and D. Mechanic (eds.), *Applications of Social Science to Clinical Medicine and Health Policy*, 63–79. New Brunswick, NJ: Rutgers University Press.

Freund, P. E. S. 1982. *The Civilized Body: Social Domination, Control and Health*. Philadelphia: Temple University Press.

Gartner, A., and F. Riessman. 1979. *Self-Help in the Human Services*. San Francisco: Jossey-Bass.

Gerard, R. 1978. Integral psychology and esoteric healing. *Journal of Holistic Health*, 3:33–36.

Gerth, H. H., and M. C. Wright. 1946. *From Max Weber: Essays in Sociology*. New York: Oxford University Press.

Geyman, J. P. 1984. Holistic health care: Neither new nor coherent. *The Journal of Family Practice*, 19, 6:727–728.

Giller, R. M. 1978. Introduction to wholistic healing groups and centers. In L. J. Kaslof (ed.), *Wholistic Dimensions in Healing: A Resource Guide*, Garden City, NY: Doubleday and Company, Inc.

Gillick, M. R. 1984. Health promotion, jogging and the pursuit of the moral life. *Journal of Health Politics, Policy and Law*, 9, 3:369–387.

Glasser, M. L. 1983. *Understanding the Patient Experience With Alternative Health Care: The Example of the Wholistic Health Center*. Ph.D. dissertation, University of Illinois at Urbana-Champaign.

Glasser, W. 1982. Reality Therapy: Taking Control of our Lives Through Stations of the Mind. Presentation at Mandala/Association of Holistic Health Conference, August 29, San Diego, California.

Glock, C. Y., and R. N. Bellah (eds.). 1976. *The New Religious Consciousness*. Berkeley: University of California Press.

Gluck, L. 1978. *Holistic Health Focus*, 1, 2:2.

Glymour, C., and D. Stalker. 1983. Engineers, cranks, physicians, magicians. *New England Journal of Medicine*, 308, 16:960–964.

Gold, R. L. 1969. Roles in sociological field observations. In G. J. McCall and J. L. Simmons (eds.), *Issues in Participant Observation*, 30–39. Reading, MA: Addison-Wesley Publishing.

Goldstein, M. S., D. T. Jaffe, D. Garell., and R. E. Berke. 1985. Holistic doctors: Becoming a nontraditional medical practitioner. *Urban Life*, 14, 3: 317–344.

Goldstein, M. S., D. T. Jaffe, C. Sutherland, and J. Wilson. 1987. Holistic physicians: Implications for the study of the medical profession. *Journal of Health and Social Behavior*, 28, 2:103–119.

Gordon, J. S. 1980a. The paradigm of holistic medicine. In A. C. Hastings et al. (eds.), *Health for the Whole Person*, 3–27. Boulder, CO: Westview Press.

Gordon, J. S. 1980b. Holistic health centers. In A. C. Hastings et al. (eds.), *Health for the Whole Person*, 467–478. Boulder, CO: Westview Press.

Gordon, J. S. 1981. Holistic medicine: toward a new medical model. *Journal of Clinical Psychiatry*, 42, 3:114–120.

Gordon, J. S. 1982. Holistic medicine: Advances and shortcomings. *Western Journal of Medicine*, 136, 6:546–551.

Gordon, J. S. 1984. Alternatives in mental health. In J. S. Gordon, D. T. Jaffe, and D. E. Bresler (eds.), *Mind, Body and Health: Toward an Integral Medicine*, 235–248. New York: Human Sciences Press.

Gordon, J. S., D. T. Jaffe, and D. E. Bresler (eds.). 1984. *Mind, Body and Health: Toward an Integral Medicine*. New York: Human Sciences Press.

Gordon, R. 1978. Separateness: a key to pathology. *Journal of Holistic Health*, 3:133–140.

Green, E., and A. Green. 1982. Science and the Human Potential. Presentation given at Mandala/Association for Holistic Health Conference, August 29, San Diego, California.

Grisell, R. D. 1979. Kundalini yoga as healing agent. In H. A. Otto and J. W. Knight (eds.), *Dimensions in Wholistic Healing*, 441–462. Chicago: Nelson-Hall.

Grossinger, R. 1982. *Planet Medicine: From Stone Age Shamanism to Post-Industrial Healing*. Boulder, CO: Shambhala.

Gusfield, J. R. 1963. *Symbolic Crusade: Status Politics and the American Temperance Movement*. Chicago: University of Illinois Press.

Gusfield, J. R. 1968. The study of social movements. In D. L. Sills (ed.), *International Encyclopedia of the Social Sciences, Vol. 14*, 445–452. New York: Macmillan Co.

Gusfield, J. R. 1975. *Community: A Critical Response*. New York: Harper and Row.

Gusfield, J. R. 1978a. The Modernity of Social Movements: Public Roles and Private Parts. Draft prepared for Thematic Session presented at the American Sociological Association meetings, September 4, San Francisco, California.

Gusfield, J. R. 1978b. Historical problematics and sociological fields: American liberalism and the study of social movements. *Research in Sociology of Knowledge, Sciences and Art*, 1:121–149.

Gusfield, J. R. 1980. Foreword. In P. Conrad and J. W. Schneider (eds.), *Deviance and Medicalization*, v–x. St. Louis: C. V. Mosby.

Gusfield, J. R. 1981. *The Culture of Public Problems: Drinking-Driving and the Symbolic Order*. Chicago: University of Chicago Press.

Gusfield, J. R. 1983. Stigma and Redemption: Themes in the Medicalization of Drinking-Driving Offenders. Paper presented at the Alcohol Epidemiology Section, International Council on Alcohol and Addictions, June 21, Padova, Italy.

Guttmacher, S. 1979. Whole in body, mind and spirit: holistic health and the limits of medicine. *Hastings Center Report*, 9:15–21.

Hackler, T. 1981. Holistic medicine: the maintenance of 'wellness'; an assault on 'dis-ease'. *United Mainliner*, 25, 2:92–96.

Hames, C. C., and D. H. Joseph. 1986. *Basic Concepts of Helping: A Holistic Approach* (2nd ed.). Norwalk, CT: Appleton-Century-Crofts.

Hastings, A. C., J. Fadiman, and J. S. Gordon (eds.). 1980. *Health for the Whole Person: The Complete Guide to Holistic Medicine*. Boulder, CO: Westview Press.

Haug, M. R., and B. Lavin. 1981. Practitioner or patient—who's in charge? *Journal of Health and Social Behavior*, 22, 3:212–228.

Haug, M. R., and B. Lavin. 1983. *Consumerism in Medicine: Challenging Physician Authority*. Beverly Hills, CA: Sage Publications.

Hayes-Bautista, D. E. 1977. Marginal patients, marginal delivery systems and health systems plans. *American Journal of Health Planning*, 1, 3:36–44.

Hayes-Bautista, D. E., and D. S. Harveston. 1977. Holistic health care. *Social Policy*, 7:7–13.

Hine V. H. 1982. Holistic dying: The role of the nurse clinician. *Topics in Clinical Nursing*, 3, 4:45–54.

Hirschhorn, L. 1979. Alternative services and the crisis of the professions. In J. Case and R. C. R. Taylor (eds.), *Co-ops, Communes and Collectives: Experiments in Social Change in the 1960s and 1970s*, 153–193. New York: Pantheon Books.

Holden, C. 1978. Holistic health concept gaining momentum. *Science*, 200: 1029.

Holden, C. 1980. Behavioral medicine: an emergent field. *Science*, 209, 4455: 479–481.

Holmes, T. H. 1980. Stress: the new etiology. In A. C. Hastings, et al. (eds.), *Health for the Whole Person*, 345–356. Boulder, CO: Westview Press.

Holmes, T. H., and R. H. Rahe. 1967. The social readjustment rating scale. *Journal of Psychosomatic Research*, 11:213–218.

Howard, J. 1975. Humanization and dehumanization of health care: a conceptual view. In J. Howard and A. Strauss (eds.), *Humanizing Health Care*, 57–102. New York: John Wiley.

Howard, J., and A. Strauss (eds.). 1975. *Humanizing Health Care*. New York: John Wiley.

Hsu, F. L. K. 1985. The self in cross-cultural perspective. In A. J. Marsella, G. DeVos, and F. L. K. Hsu (eds.), *Culture and Self: Asian and Western Perspectives*, 24–55. New York: Tavistock Publications.

Hughes, E. C. 1958. *Men and Their Work*. New York: Free Press.

Illich, I. C. 1976. *Medical Nemesis*. Toronto: Bantam Books.

Jaffe, D. T. 1980a. The holistic perspective. *Holistic Health Focus*, 3.

Jaffe, D. T. 1980b. *Healing From Within*. New York: Bantam Books.

Jaffe, D. T. 1984a. Self-management and behavioral medicine: Seizing control of self-defeating behavior. In J. S. Gordon, D. T. Jaffe, and D. E. Bresler (eds.), *Mind, Body and Health: Toward an Integral Medicine*, 167–177. New York: Human Sciences Press.

Jaffe, D. T. 1984b. The role of family therapy in treating physical illness. In J. S. Gordon, D. T. Jaffe, and D. E. Bresler (eds.), *Mind, Body and Health: Toward an Integral Medicine*, 211–224. New York: Human Sciences Press.

Jampolsky, G. G. 1979. *Love is Letting Go of Fear*. Millbrae, CA: Celestial Arts.

Jampolsky, G. G. 1980. A Course in Miracles. Workshop given jointly with Hugh Prather at Mandala/Association of Holistic Health Conference, San Diego, California.

Jampolsky, G. G. 1981. A Course in Miracles. Workshop given with Hugh Prather at Mandala/Association of Holistic Health Conference, San Diego, California.

Jeter, K. 1982. Family medicine and holistic health: an analytic essay. In B. E. Cogswell and M. B. Sussman (eds.), *Family Medicine: A New Approach to Health Care*, 73–80. New York: Haworth Press.

Johnson, F. 1985. The western concept of self. In A. J. Marsella, G. DeVos, and

F. L. K. Hsu (eds.), *Culture and Self: Asian and Western Perspectives*, 92–138. New York: Tavistock Publications.

Johnson, M. M., and H. W. Martin. 1965. A sociological analysis of the nurse role. In J. K. Skipper and R. C. Leonard (eds.), *Social Interaction and Patient Care*, 29–29. Philadelphia: J. B. Lippincott Company.

Kahn, H., and A. J. Wiener. 1967. *The Year 2000*. New York: Macmillan.

Kane, J. 1979. Insurance and the abandonment of responsibility. *The Coevolution Quarterly*, 146–150.

Kane, J. 1980a. Symptom as metaphor. *New Age*, 24–26.

Kane, J. 1980b. Yoga and medicine: a healing partnership. *Yoga Journal*, 26–58.

Kane, J. 1983. Unwhole healers: A doctor's diagnosis of the medical profession. *Whole Life Times*, 1–4.

Kane, R. J. 1980. Iatrogenesis: Just what the doctor ordered. *Journal of Community Health*, 5, 3:149–158.

Kasl, S. V. 1986. The detection and modification of psychosocial and behavioral risk factors. In L. H. Aiken and D. Mechanic (eds.), *Applications of Social Science to Clinical Medicine and Health Policy*, 359–391. New Brunswick, NJ: Rutgers University Press.

Kaslof, L. J. (ed.) 1978. *Wholistic Dimensions in Healing*. New York: Doubleday.

Keppel, B. 1982. 'Wellness': a new focus in hospitals. *Los Angeles Times*, I:1.

Kirsch, J. 1977. Can your mind cure cancer? *New West*, 40–45.

Kleinman, A., and J. L. Gale. 1982. Patients treated by physicians and folk healers: A comparative outcome study in Taiwan. *Culture, Medicine and Psychiatry*, 6:405–423.

Kleinman, S. 1982. Actors' conflicting theories of negotiation: The case of a holistic health center. *Urban Life*, 11, 3:312–327.

Knowles, J. H. 1977a. Responsibility for health. *Science*, 198, 4322:1103.

Knowles, J. H. (ed.). 1977b. *Doing Better and Feeling Worse: Health in the United States*. New York: W. W. Norton and Company.

Kobasa, S. C., S. R. Maddi, and S. Kahn. 1982. Hardiness and health: a prospective study. *Journal of Personality and Social Psychology*, 42, 1:168–177.

Kopelman, L., and J. Moskop. 1981. The holistic health movement: a survey and critique. *The Journal of Medicine and Philosophy*, 6, 2:209–235.

Kosa, J., and I. K. Zola. 1975. *Poverty and Health*. Cambridge, MA: Harvard University Press.

Kotarba, J. A. 1975. American acupuncturists: the new entrepreneurs of hope. *Urban Life*, 4, 2:149–177.

Kotarba, J. A. 1983a. Social control function of holistic health care in bureaucratic settings: The case of space medicine. *Journal of Health and Social Behavior*, 24, 3:275–287.

Kotarba, J. A. 1983b. *Chronic Pain: Its Social Dimensions*. Beverly Hills, CA: Sage Publications.

Krantz, D. S., A. Baum, and M. V. Wideman. 1980. Assessment of preferences for self-treatment and information in health care. *Journal of Personality and Social Psychology*, 39, 5:977–990.

Krieger, D. 1975. Therapeutic touch: the imprimatur of nursing. *American Journal of Nursing*, 75, 5:784–787.

Krieger, D. 1979. Therapeutic touch and contemporary applications. In H. A. Otto and J. W. Knight (eds.), *Dimensions in Wholistic Healing*, 297–306. Chicago: Nelson-Hall.

Krieger, D. 1984. Therapeutic touch and the metaphysics of nursing. In J. S. Gordon, D. T. Jaffe, and D. E. Bresler (eds.), *Mind, Body and Health: Toward an Integral Medicine*, 107–116. New York: Human Sciences Press.

Kronenfeld, J. J., and C. Wasner. 1982. The use of unorthodox therapies and marginal practitioners. *Social Science and Medicine*, 16:1119-1125.

Kuhn, T. S. 1970. *The Structure of Scientific Revolutions* (2nd ed.). Chicago: The University of Chicago Press.

Lackner, J. 1979. Integrating holistic health in society. *Journal of Holistic Health*, 4:29–34.

Laing, R. D. 1967. *The Politics of Experience*. New York: Ballantine Books.

Lalonde, M. 1974. *A New Perspective on the Health of Canadians*. Ottawa: Government of Canada.

Lee, J. A. 1976. Social change and marginal therapeutic systems. In R. Wallis and P. Morley (eds.), *Marginal Medicine*, New York: Free Press.

Lee, P. R. 1976. The frontiers of health planning. *American Journal of Health Planning*, 1, 2:1–6.

Lee, T. N. 1978. Chinese medicine: a paragon of holistic medicine. *Journal of Holistic Health*, 3:61–65.

Lemert, E. M. 1951. *Sociopathic Behavior*. New York: McGraw-Hill.

Lemert, E. M. 1967. *Human Deviance, Social Problems and Social Control*. Englewood Cliffs, NJ: Prentice-Hall.

LeShan, L. 1959. Personality states as factors in the development of malignant disease: a critical review. *Journal of the National Cancer Institute*, 22:1–18.

LeShan, L. 1974. *The Medium, the Mystic and the Physicist*. New York: Ballantine Books.

LeShan, L. 1977. *You Can Fight For Your Life*. New York: Jove Publications.

LeShan, L., and R. E. Worthington. 1956. Personality as a factor in the pathogenesis of cancer: a review of the literature. *British Journal of Medical Psychology*, 29:49–56.

Light, D. W. 1986. Surplus versus cost containment: The changing context for health providers. In L. H. Aiken and D. Mechanic (eds.), *Applications of Social Science to Clinical Medicine and Health Policy*, 519–542. New Brunswick, NJ: Rutgers University Press.

Lippin, R. 1978. Holistic health trends. Letter to the Editor, *Journal of Occupational Medicine*, 20, 2:75.

Livingston, R. B. 1980. Specialization in medicine need not exclude holistic health. *Journal of Holistic Health*, 5:10–19.

Lock, M. M. 1978. Scars of experience: The art of moxibustion in Japanese medicine and society. *Culture, Medicine and Psychiatry*, 2, 2:151–175.

Lockheed, T. 1984. Holistic health—a uniting force for nurses. *Canadian Nurse*, 80, 11:24–25.

Lofland, J. 1971. *Analyzing Social Settings*. Belmont, CA: Wadsworth Publishing Company, Inc.

Lofland, J. 1976. *Doing Social Life: The Qualitative Study of Human Interaction in Natural Settings*. New York: John Wiley and Sons.

Lofland, J., and R. Stark. 1965. Becoming a world-saver: A theory of conversion to a deviant perspective. *American Sociological Review*, 30, 6:862–875.

Lofland, L. M. 1978. *The Craft of Dying*. Beverly Hills, CA: Sage Publications.

Loomis, E. G. 1979. The wholistic health and growth center concept: the background and history of the Meadowlark experience. In H. A. Otto and J. W. Knight (eds.), *Dimensions in Wholistic Healing*, 91–102. Chicago: Nelson-Hall.

Lopata, H. Z. 1979. Expertization of everyone and the revolt of the client. In J. R. Folta and E. Deck (eds.), *A Sociological Framework for Patient Care*, 127–141. New York: John Wiley and Sons.

Lowenberg, J. S. 1979. Holistic Health: Medical Model or Marginal Offshoot of the Future? Unpublished manuscript.

Lowenberg, J. S. 1980a. Holistic Health: An Analysis of the Movement. Paper presented at annual meeting of Pacific Sociological Association, April 12, San Francisco.

Lowenberg, J. S. 1980b. Holistic Health and the Movements of the Sixties: Strands of Continuity. Unpublished manuscript.

Luker, K. 1975. *Taking Chances: Abortion and the Decision Not to Contracept*. Berkeley: University of California Press.

Luker, K. 1984. *Abortion and the Politics of Motherhood*. Berkeley: University of California Press.

Madsen, R. P. 1984. *Morality and Power in a Chinese Village*. Berkeley: University of California Press.

Manbridge, J. J. 1979. The agony of inequality. In J. Case and R. C. R. Taylor (eds.), *Co-ops, Communes and Collectives. Experiments in Social Change in the 1960s and 1970s*, 194–214. New York: Pantheon Books.

Manderscheid, R. W. 1980. Implications of Biopsychosocial Relationships. Paper presented at AAAS Annual Meeting, Symposium title: Behavioral Medicine: The Biopsychosocial Interface, January 7, San Francisco, California.

Marsella, A. J., G. DeVos, and F. L. K. Hsu. 1985 (eds.). *Culture and Self: Asian and Western Perspectives*. New York: Tavistock Publications.

Martin, E. J. 1986. Holistic nursing practice: An idea whose time has come. *Journal of Professional Nursing*, 2, 2:78.

Masi, A. T. 1978. An holistic concept of health and illness: a tricentennial goal for medicine and public health. *Journal of Chronic Disease*, 31:563–572.

Mattson, P. H. 1982. *Holistic Health in Perspective*. Palo Alto, CA: Mayfield Publishing Co.

McCall, G. J., and J. L. Simmons (eds.). 1969. *Issues in Participant Observation*. Reading, MA: Addison-Wesley Publishing Co.

McCarthy, J. D., and M. N. Zald. 1973. *The Trend of Social Movements in America: Professionalization and Resource Mobilization*. Morristown, NJ: General Learning Press.

McGuire, M. B. 1983. Words of power: Personal empowerment and healing. *Culture, Medicine and Psychiatry*, 7, 3:221–240.

McKeown, T. 1978. Behavioral and environmental determinants of health and their implication for public policy. In R. J. Carlson and R. Cunningham (eds.), *Future Directions in Health Care: A New Public Policy*, 21–38. Cambridge, MA: Ballinger Publishing Co.

McKeown, T. 1979. *The Role of Medicine: Dream, Mirage or Nemesis?* Princeton, NJ: Princeton University Press.

McKinley, J. B. 1979. A case for refocusing upstream: the political economy of illness. In E. G. Jaco (ed.), *Patients, Physicians, and Illness* (3rd ed.), 9–26. New York: Free Press.

Mead, M. 1956. Nursing: primitive and civilized. *American Journal of Nursing*, 56, 8:1001.

Mechanic, D. 1962. The concept of illness behavior. *Journal of Chronic Diseases*, 15:189–194.

Mechanic, D. 1968. *Medical Sociology*. New York: Free Press.

Mechanic, D. 1975. Preface. In R. J. Carlson, *The End of Medicine*.

Mechanic, D. 1976. *The Growth of Bureaucratic Medicine: An Inquiry into the Dynamics of Patient Behavior and the Organization of Medical Care*. New York: John Wiley.

Mechanic, D. 1985. The public perception of medicine. *New England Journal of Medicine*, 312, 3:181–183.

Mehan, H., and H. Wood. 1975. *The Reality of Ethnomethodology*. New York: John Wiley.

Mendelsohn, R. S. 1979. *Confessions of a Medical Heretic*. New York: Warner Books.

Merton, T. 1965. *The Way of Chuang Tzu*. New York: New Directions.

Miles, R. B. 1978. Humanistic medicine and holistic health care. In Berkeley Holistic Health Center (ed.), *The Holistic Health Handbook*, 20–24. Berkeley, CA: And/Or Press.

Miles, R. B. 1984. The rituals of childbirth. In J. S. Gordon, D. T. Jaffe, and D. E. Bresler (eds.), *Mind, Body and Health: Toward an Integral Medicine*, New York: Human Sciences Press.

Miller, E. E. 1978. *Feeling Good: How to Stay Healthy*. Englewood Cliffs, NJ: Prentice-Hall.

Miller, E. E. 1982. Looking Inward: The Forever Journey. Workshop presented at Mandala/Association of Holistic Health Conference, September 1, San Diego, California.

Miyamoto, S. F. 1979. Social movements in the field of medicine. In J. R. Folta and E. Deck (eds.), *A Sociological Framework for Patient Care*, 79–88. New York: John Wiley and Sons.

Moberg, D. 1979. Experimenting with the future: Alternative institutions and American socialism. In J. Case and R. C. R. Taylor (eds.), *Co-ops, Communes and Collectives: Experiments in Social Change in the 1960s and 1970s*, 274–312. New York: Pantheon Books.

Moerman, D. 1980. Physiology and Symbol: Anthropology of Symbolic Healing. Paper presented at meetings of the American Association for Advancement of Science, January 5, San Francisco.

Moll, J. A. 1982. High-level wellness and the nurse. *Topics in Clinical Nursing*, 3, 4:61–67.

Morse, S. J. 1982. In defense of the insanity defense. *Los Angeles Times*, Part II:7.

Nader, R. 1981. Creating the holistic environment. *Journal of Holistic Health*, 6:11–16.

Navarro, V. 1976. *Medicine Under Capitalism*. New York: Prodist.

Ng, L., D. Davis, and R. Manderscheid. 1978. The health promotion organization: a practical intervention designed to promote healthy living. *Public Health Reports*, 93, 5:446–455.

Ng, L., D. L. Davis, R. W. Manderscheid, and J. Elkes. 1981. Toward a conceptual formulation of health and well-being. In L. Ng and D. L. Davis (eds.), *Strategies for Public Health: Promoting Health and Preventing Disease*, 44–58. New York: Van Nostrand Reinhold Company.

Oppenheim, M. 1978. The cure for America's health-care crisis is plain common sense. *Los Angeles Times*, January 8. Part II:6.

Oppenheim, M. 1980. Sounding board: Healers. *New England Journal of Medicine*, 303:1117-1120.

Ornstein, R. 1972. *The Psychology of Consciousness*. New York: Penguin.

Ornstein, R., and D. Sobel. 1987. The healing brain. *Psychology Today*, 21, 3:38–52.

Otto, H. A., and J. W. Knight (eds.). 1979a. *Dimensions in Wholistic Healing: New Frontiers in the Treatment of the Whole Person*. Chicago: Nelson-Hall.

Otto, H. A., and J. W. Knight. 1979b. Wholistic healing: Basic principles and concepts. In H. A. Otto and J. W. Knight (eds.), *Dimensions in Wholistic Healing*, 3–28. Chicago: Nelson-Hall.

Oyle, I. 1979. *The New American Medicine Show*. Santa Cruz, CA: Unity Press.

Ozonoff, V. V., and D. Ozonoff. 1977. On helping those who help themselves. *Hastings Center Report*, 7–10.

Parkes, C. M. 1972. *Bereavement: Studies of Grief in Adult Life*. New York: International Universities Press.

Parsons, T. 1951. *The Social System*. New York: The Free Press.

Parsons, T. 1968. Christianity. In D. L. Sills (ed.), *Encyclopedia of the Social Sciences*, Vol.2, 425–446. New York: Macmillan.

Parsons, T., and R. Fox. 1958. Illness, therapy and the modern urban family. In G. Jaco (ed.), *Patients, Physicians, and Illness* (1st ed.), New York: The Free Press. [Originally in *The Journal of Social Issues*, 8, 4 (1952):2–3, 31–44.]

Pearlin, L. I., M. A. Lieberman, E. G. Menaghan, and J. T. Mullan. 1981. The stress process. *Journal of Health and Social Behavior*, 22, 4:337–356.

Pelletier, K. R. 1977. *Mind as Healer, Mind as Slayer: A Holistic Approach to Preventing Stress Disorders*. New York: Dell Publishing Co.

Pelletier, K. R. 1979. *Holistic Medicine: From Stress to Optimum Health*. New York: Delacorte Press.

Polidora, J. 1977. Holistic Physiology of Mind/Body. Presentation at Mandala/ Association of Holistic Health Conference, September 3, San Diego, California.

Polidora, J. 1978. Holistic physiology of mind/body. *Journal of Holistic Health*, 3:75–83.

Rabinow, P., and W. M. Sullivan. 1979. *Interpretive Social Science*. Berkeley: University of California Press.

Rachman, S. J., and C. Philips. 1980. *Psychology and Behavioral Medicine*. New York: Cambridge University Press.

Read, D. A. 1983. Holistic health from the inside. *Journal of School Health*, 53, 6:382–385.

Reed, W. L. 1979. Holistic health: A focus for socio-medical research. *Journal of Holistic Health*, 4:115–119.

Reeder, L. G. 1978. The patient-client as consumer. In H. D. Schwartz and C. S. Kart (eds.), *Dominant Issues in Medical Sociology*, 111–117. Reading, MA: Addison-Wesley Publishing Co.

Reilly, D. T. 1983. Young doctors' views on alternative medicine. *British Medical Journal*, 287:337–339.

Relman, A. 1979. Holistic medicine. *New England Journal of Medicine*, 300, 6:312.

Robert Wood Johnson Foundation. 1987. *Access to Health Care in the United States: Results of a 1986 Survey*, Special Report Number 2, Princeton, NJ.

Romanucci-Ross, L., D. E. Moerman, and L. R. Tancredi. 1983. *The Anthropology of Medicine: From Culture to Method*. South Hadley, MA: Bergin and Garvey Publishers.

Rosch, P. J., and H. M. Kearney. 1985. Holistic medicine and technology: A modern dialectic. *Social Science and Medicine*, 21, 12:1405-1409.

Roszak, T. 1969. *The Making of a Counter Culture*. New York: Doubleday and Co.

Roth, J. A. 1972. Some contingencies of the moral evaluation and control of clientele: The case of the hospital emergency service. *American Journal of Sociology*, 77:839–856.

Roth, J. A. 1977. *Health Purifiers and Their Enemies*. New York: Prodist.

Ruzek, S. K. 1981. The women's self-help health movement. In P. Conrad and R. Kern (eds.), *The Sociology of Health and Illness: Critical Perspectives*. New York: St. Martin's Press.

Salk, J. 1978. Health and disease: A biological and metabiological model. *Journal of Holistic Health*, 3:120–128.

Salmon, J. W. (ed.). 1984a. *Alternative Medicines: Popular and Policy Perspectives*. New York: Tavistock Publications.

Salmon, J. W. 1984b. Defining health and reorganizing medicine. In J. W. Salmon (ed.), *Alternative Medicines: Popular and Policy Perspectives*, 252–288. New York: Tavistock Publications.

Salmon, J. W., and H. S. Berliner. 1980. Health policy implications of the holistic health movement. *Journal of Health Politics, Policy and Law*, 5, 3:535–553.

Samuels, M., and H. Bennett. 1973. *The Well Body Book*. New York: Random House.

Samuels, M., and H. Bennett. 1974. *Be Well*. New York: Random House Inc./ The Bookworks.

Samuels, M., and H. Bennett. 1983. *Well Body, Well Earth: The Sierra Club Environmental Health Sourcebook*. San Francisco: Sierra Club Books.

Samuels, M., and N. Samuels. 1982. *The Well Child Book*. New York: Summit Books.

Savage, D. G. 1988. Alcoholics may be denied some VA aid, court rules, *Los Angeles Times*, April 22, Part I: 1–15.

Scarf, M. 1980. Images that heal: A doubtful idea whose time has come. *Psychology Today*, 32:32–46.

Schaffner, K. F. 1981. Introduction, reductionism and holism in medicine. *The Journal of Medicine and Philosophy*, 6, 2:93–100.

Schatzman, L., and A. L. Strauss. 1973. *Field Research: Strategies for a Natural Sociology*. Englewood Cliffs, NJ: Prentice-Hall.

Schiff, M. 1973. Neo-transcendentalism in the new left counter-culture: A vision of the future looking back. *Comparative Studies of Society and History*, 15, 2:130–142.

Schulman, S. 1958. Basic functional roles in nursing: Mother surrogate and healer. In E. G. Jaco (ed.), *Patients, Physicians, and Illness*, 528 537. New York: The Free Press.

Schwartz, H., and J. Jacobs. 1979. *Qualitative Sociology*. New York: The Free Press.

Schwartz, H. D., and C. S. Kart (eds.). 1978. *Dominant Issues in Medical Sociology*. Reading, MA: Addison-Wesley.

Scull, A. T. 1977. *Decarceration: Community Treatment and the Deviant—A Radical View*. Englewood Cliffs, NJ: Prentice-Hall.

Segall, A. 1976. The sick role concept. *Journal of Health and Social Behavior*, 17, 2:163–169.

Selye, H. 1956. *The Stress of Life*. New York: McGraw-Hill.

Selye, H. 1979. Holistic health research—A top priority. *Journal of Holistic Health*, 4:11–18.

Shapiro, J., and D. H. Shapiro. 1979. The psychology of responsibility: some second thoughts on holistic medicine. *New England Journal of Medicine*, 301, 4:211–212.

Shealy, C. N. 1979. Foreword. In I. Oyle, *The New American Medicine Show*, xi–xiii. Santa Cruz, CA: Unity Press.

Shiloh, A. 1972. Equalitarian and hierarchical patients. In E. Freidson and J. Lorber (eds.), *Medical Men and Their Work*, 249–266. Chicago: Aldine.

Shukla, H. C., G. F. Solomon, and R. E. Doshi. 1979. The relevance of some Ayurvedic (traditional Indian medical) concepts to modern holistic health. *Journal of Holistic Health*, 4:125–131.

Siegler, M., and H. Osmond. 1973. The sick role revisited. *Hastings Center Studies*, 1:41–58.

Siegler, M., and H. Osmond. 1974. *Models of Madness, Models of Medicine*. New York: Macmillan.

Simonton, O. C., S. Mathews-Simonton, and J. L. Creighton. 1978. *Getting Well Again*. Toronto: Bantam Books.

Skipper, J. 1965. The role of the hospital nurse: Is it instrumental or expressive?. In J. K. Skipper and R. C. Leonard (eds.), *Social Interaction and Patient Care*, 40–50. Philadelphia: J. B. Lippincott.

Smith, T. 1983. Alternative medicine. *British Medical Journal*, 287, 6388:307.

Smuts, J. C. 1926. *Holism and Evolution*. New York: Macmillan.

Spear, J. 1977. A Functional Attitudinal Clearing Program Actualizing Holistic Health. Presentation at Mandala/Association of Holistic Health Conference, September 4, San Diego, California.

Stalker, D. and C. Glymour (eds.). 1985. *Examining Holistic Medicine*. Buffalo, NY: Prometheus Books.

Starr, P. 1978. Medicine and the waning of professional sovereignty. *Daedalus*, 107, 1:175–193.

Starr, P. 1979. The phantom community. In J. Case and R. C. R. Taylor (eds.), *Co-ops, Communes and Collectives: Experiments in Social Change in the 1960s and 1970s*, 245–273. New York: Pantheon Books.

Starr, P. 1981. The politics of therapeutic nihilism. In P. Conrad and R. Kern (eds.), *The Sociology of Health and Illness*, 434–448. New York: St. Martin's Press.

Stone, H. 1979. Wholistic healing: Historic base and short history. In H. A. Otto and J. W. Knight (eds.), *Dimensions in Wholistic Healing*, 29–38. Chicago: Nelson-Hall.

Strode, W. S. 1979. An emerging medicine: Creating the new paradigm. In H. A. Otto and J. W. Knight (eds.), *Dimensions in Wholistic Healing*, 65–77. Chicago: Nelson-Hall.

Sudnow, D. 1967. *Passing On*. Englewood Cliffs, NJ: Prentice-Hall.

Sullivan, W. M. 1983. A new ecology of healing: medicine and religion in "wholistic" care. Unpublished manuscript.

Sun Bear. 1980. Making Medicine: a Native American Perspective. Workshop at Mandala/Association of Holistic Health Conference, August, San Diego, California.

Svarstad, B. L. 1986. Patient-practitioner relationships and compliance with prescribed medical regimens. In L. H. Aiken and D. Mechanic (eds.), *Applications of Social Science to Clinical Medicine and Health Policy*, 438–459. New Brunswick, NJ: Rutgers University Press.

Svihus, R. 1978. Healing is the patient's responsibility too. *Holistic Health Focus*, 1, 6, (November):1.

Swearingen, R. L. 1984. The physician as the basic instrument. In J. S. Gordon, D. T. Jaffe, and D. E. Bresler (eds.), *Mind, Body and Health: Toward an Integral Medicine*, 101–106. New York: Human Sciences Press, Inc.

Szasz, T. S. (1970) *The Manufacture of Madness*. New York: Harper.

Szasz, T. and M. Hollender. 1978. The basic models of the doctor-patient relationship, in H. D. Schwartz and C. S. Kart (eds.), *Dominant Issues in Medical Sociology*, 100–107. Reading, MA: Addison-Wesley Publishing.

Taub, E. A., and B. Taub. 1979. Integrative medicine. *Holistic Health Focus*, 2, 2:4–6.

Taub, E. A., and B. Taub. 1982. Becoming a Health Facilitator. Workshop at Mandala/Association of Holistic Health Conference, September 1, San Diego, California.

Taylor, R. 1979. Free medicine. In J. Case and R. C. R. Taylor (eds.), *Co-ops, Communes and Collectives: Experiments in Social Change in the 1960s and 1970s*, 17–48. New York: Pantheon Books.

Taylor, R. 1982. The politics of prevention. *Social Policy*, 13, 1:32–41.

Taylor, R. 1984. Alternative medicine and the medical encounter in Britain and the United States. In J. W. Salmon (ed.), *Alternative Medicines: Popular and Policy Perspectives*, 191–228. New York: Tavistock Publications.

Taylor, S. E., R. R. Lichtman, and J. V. Wood. 1982. Breast cancer patients respond to family support. *U.C.L.A. This Week*, 3, 7:1–4.

Tesh, S. N. 1988. *Hidden Arguments: Political Ideology and Disease Prevention Policy*. New Brunswick, NJ: Rutgers University Press.

Thomas, L. 1979. On the science and technology of medicine. In G. L. Albrecht and P. C. Higgins (eds.), *Health, Illness, and Medicine*, 94–107. Chicago: Rand McNally.

Tipton, S. M. 1982. *Getting Saved From the Sixties*. Berkeley: University of California Press.

Todd, M. C. 1977. The need for a holistic approach in medicine. *The Journal of Holistic Health*, 2:7–10.

Travis, J. W. 1977. *Wellness Workbook*. Mill Valley, CA: Wellness Resource Center.

Travis, J. W. 1978. Wellness education and holistic health— how they're related. *Journal of Holistic Health*, 3:25–32.

Travis, J. W. 1981. *Wellness Workbook For Helping Professional*. Mill Valley, CA: Wellness Associates.

Travis, J. W. 1984. The role of wellness education and holistic health. In J. S. Gordon, D. T. Jaffe, and D. Bresler (eds.), *Mind, Body and Health: Toward an Integral Medicine*,188–198. New York: Human Sciences Press, Inc.

Tubesing, D. A. 1978. A practical approach to creating wholistic health centers. *Journal of Holistic Health*, 3:66–74.

Turner, R. H. 1969. The theme of contemporary social movements. *British Journal of Sociology*, 20:390–405.

Turner, R. J. 1981. Social support as a contingency in psychological well-being. *Journal of Health and Social Behavior*, 22, 4:357–367.

Twaddle, A. C. 1972. The concepts of the sick role and illness behavior. *Advances in Psychosomatic Medicine*, 8:162–179.

Twaddle, A. C. 1973. Illness and deviance. *Social Science and Medicine*, 7, 10:751–762.

Twaddle, A. C. 1974. The concept of health status. *Social Science and Medicine*, 8, 1:29–38.

Twaddle, A. C., and R. M. Hessler. 1986. Power and change: The case of the Swedish Commission of Inquiry on health and sickness care. *Journal of Health Politics, Policy and Law*, 11,1:19–40.

Vaillant, G. E. 1979. Natural history of male psychological health: Effects of mental health on physical health. *New England Journal of Medicine*, 301, 23:1249-1253.

Vanderpool, H. Y. 1984. The holistic hodgepodge: A critical analysis of holistic medicine and health in America today. *Journal of Family Practice*, 19, 6:773–781.

Vayda, E. 1978. Health policy in Canada: The Lalonde report and emerging patterns. In R. J. Carlson and R. Cunningham (eds.), *Future Directions in Health Care: A New Public Policy*, 189–200. Cambridge, MA: Ballinger Publishing Co.

Waitzkin, H. B., and B. Waterman. 1974. *The Exploitation of Illness in Capitalist Society*. Indianapolis, IN: Bobbs-Merrill Educational Publishing.

Wallis, R., and P. Morley (eds.). 1976. *Marginal Medicine*. New York: Free Press.

Walton, S. 1979. Holistic medicine. *Science News*, 116, 24:410–412.

Ward, C. 1979. The child is father to the man. *Holistic Health Focus*, 2, 1.

Weaver, P. 1983. Putting a premium on healthy habits, *Los Angeles Times*, November 18, 1983, Part V:13.

Weber, M. 1958. *The Protestant Ethic and the Spirit of Capitalism*. New York: Charles Scribner's Sons.

Wechsler, R. 1987. A new prescription: Mind over malady. *Discover*, 8, 2:50–61.

Weed, L. 1982. The Present Status of the Computer for Optimizing Health and the Way of the Future for Medical Problem Solving. Presentation at Mandala/Association for Holistic Health Conference, August, San Diego, California.

Wei-ming, T. 1985. Selfhood and otherness in Confucian thought. In A. J. Marsella, G. DeVos, and F. L. K. Hsu (eds.), *Culture and Self: Asian and Western Perspectives*, 231–252. New York: Tavistock Publications.

Weil, A. 1983. *Health and Healing: Understanding Conventional and Alternative Medicine*. Boston: Houghton Mifflin Co.

Whorton, J. C. 1985. The first holistic revolution: Alternative Medicine in the Nineteenth Century. In D. Stalker and C. Glymour (eds.) *Examining Holistic Medicine*, 29–48. Buffalo, NY: Prometheus Books

Wildavsky, A. 1977. Doing better and feeling worse: The political pathology of health policy. In J. H. Knowles (ed.), *Doing Better and Feeling Worse: Health in the United States*, 105–124. New York: W. W. Norton and Company.

Wilf, R. T. 1978. Childbirth: An overview. In L. J. Kaslof (ed.), *Wholistic Dimensions in Healing*, 8–10. New York: Doubleday.

Will, G. F. 1982. Obliterating the idea of responsibility. *Los Angeles Times*, June 23, Part II:7.

Williams, J. 1976. The wholistic approach. *San Francisco, Sunday Examiner and Chronicle: California Living Magazine*, 30:30–34.

Williams, S. M. 1985. Holistic nursing. In D. Stalker and C. Glymour (eds.), *Examining Holistic Medicine*, 49–63. Buffalo, NY: Prometheus Books.

Wolinsky, F. D., and S. R. Wolinsky. 1981. Expecting sick-role legitimation and getting it. *Journal of Health and Social Behavior*, 22:229–242.

Wollman, L., E. DiCyan, G. Goldberg, and A. Hastings. 1980. Holistic approachs to oral health and dentistry. In A. C. Hastings, et al. (eds.), *Health for the Whole Person*, 333–340. Boulder, CO: Westview Press.

World Health Organization 1958. *The First Ten Years of the World Health Organization*. Geneva: Palais des Nations.

Yahn, G. 1979. The impact of holistic medicine, medical groups, and health concepts. *Journal of the American Medical Association*, 242, 20:2202-2205.

Zborowski, M. 1952. Cultural components in response to pain. *Journal of Social Issues*, 8:16–30.

Zola, I. 1966. Culture and symptoms: An analysis of patients' presenting complaints. *American Sociological Review*, 31: 615–630.

Zola, I. 1978. Medicine as an institution of social control. In J. Ehrenreich (ed.), *The Cultural Crisis of Modern Medicine*, 80–101. New York: Monthly Review Press.

Zola, I. K. 1983. *Socio-Medical Inquiries*. Philadelphia: Temple University Press.

Zukov, G. 1979. *The Dancing Wu Li Masters*. New York: William Morrow.

Index

Acknowledgment is made for permission to quote from the following works.

Donald B. Ardell, *High Level Wellness: An Alternative to Doctors, Drugs, and Disease.* Quoted with permission of Donald B. Ardell, Ph.D., who holds the copyright. Originally published by Rodale Press, it is currently published by Ten Speed Press.

Rudolph Ballantine, "The Nutritional Dimension," in *Holistic Medicine: Harmony of Body Mind Spirit,* ed. Tracy Deliman and John S. Smolowe. Copyright © 1982. Quoted by permission of Appleton & Lange.

Barbara Blattner, *Holistic Nursing.* Copyright © 1981. Quoted by permission of Appleton & Lange. (Quotation from page 40 also used by permission of W. W. Norton & Company, Inc., who hold the rights to Rollo May's *Man's Search for Himself,* 1953, whose ideas informed that section.)

Samuel W. Bloom and R. W. Wilson, "Patient-practitioner Relationships," in *Handbook of Medical Sociology,* ed. B. Freeman, S. Levine, and L. G. Reeder. Copyright © 1979 by Prentice-Hall, Inc. Quoted by permission of Prentice-Hall, Inc.

Harold H. Bloomfield, M.D. and Robert B. Kory, *The Holistic Way to Health and Happiness,* copyright © 1978 by Harold H. Bloomfield, M.D. and Robert B. Kory. Quoted by permission of Simon and Schuster, A Fireside Book.

Paul Brenner, M.D., *Health is a Question of Balance.* Copyright © 1978. Quoted by permission of the author, who holds all rights to the material.

Paul Brenner, "A Personal Trajectory," in *Mind, Body and Health: Toward an Integral Medicine,* ed. James S. Gordon, Dennis T. Jaffe, and David E. Bresler. Copyright © 1984. Quoted by permission of Human Sciences Press.

David E. Bresler, "Chinese Medicine and Holistic Health," in *Health for the Whole Person,* ed. Arthur C. Hastings, James Fadiman, and James S. Gordon. Copyright © 1980 by Westview Press. Reprinted by permission of Westview Press.

Fritjof Capra, "Introduction," in *Space, Time, and Medicine,* by Larry Dossey, M.D. Boulder, Colorado: Shambhala Publications, 1982.

Rick J. Carlson, *The End of Medicine.* Copyright © 1975 by John Wiley & Sons, Inc. Reprinted by permission of John Wiley & Sons, Inc.

Effie Poy Yew Chow, "Chinese Medicine: Contributions to Wholistic Healing," in *Dimensions in Wholistic Healing,* ed. Herbert A. Otto and James W. Knight. Copyright © 1978. Quoted by permission.

Frances V. Clark, "Transpersonal Psychology," in *Wholistic Dimensions in Healing,* ed. Leslie J. Kaslof. New York: Doubleday/Dolphin, 1978. Copyright © Leslie J. Kaslof. Reprinted by permission of Leslie J. Kaslof.

William C. Cockerham, *Medical Sociology,* 3rd edition. Copyright © 1986 by Prentice-Hall, Inc. Quoted by permission of Prentice-Hall, Inc.

Peter Conrad and Joseph W. Schneider. *Deviance and Medicalization: From Badness to Sickness.* Copyright © 1980. Permission granted to quote excerpts by Charles E. Merrill Publishing Co.

Tracy Deliman and John S. Smolowe, "Ideas in Holism," in *Holistic Medicine: Harmony of Body Mind Spirit,* ed. Tracy Deliman and John S. Smolowe, M.D. Copyright © 1982. Excerpt quoted with permission from Appleton & Lange.

Larry Dossey, M.D., *Space, Time and Medicine.* Boulder, CO: Shambhala Publications, 1982.

Rene Dubos, "Introduction," in Norman Cousins, *Anatomy of an Illness*. Copyright ©
1979. Quoted by permission of W. W. Norton & Company, Inc.

John Ehrenreich, "Introduction," in *The Cultural Crisis of Modern Medicine*. Copyright © 1978 by John Ehrenreich. Reprinted by permission of Monthly Review
Foundation.

Jacqueline Fawcett, *Analysis and Evaluation of Conceptual Models*. Copyright © 1984.
Quotation reprinted by permission of F. A. Davis Co.

Renée C. Fox, "The Medicalization and Demedicalization of American Society," in *Doing Better and Feeling Worse*, ed. John H. Knowles, M.D. Copyright © 1977 by
the American Academy of Arts and Sciences.

Eliot Freidson. *Profession of Medicine*. Copyright © 1970. Quotation reprinted by permission of Harper & Row Publishers, Inc.

James S. Gordon, "The Paradigm of Holistic Medicine," and "Holistic Health Centers,"
in *Health for the Whole Person*, ed. Arthur C. Hastings, James Fadiman and James
S. Gordon. Copyright © 1980 by Westview Press. Reprinted by permission of
Westview Press.

Ronald D. Grissel, "Kundalini Yoga as Healing Agent," in *Dimensions in Wholistic
Healing*, ed. Herbert A. Otto and James W. Knight. Copyright © 1979. Quoted by
permission.

Joseph R. Gusfield. "The Study of Social Movements," in *International Encyclopedia of
the Social Sciences*, ed. David L. Sills. Copyright © 1968 by Crowell Collier and
Macmillan, Inc. Reprinted by permission of the Macmillan Publishing Company.

Joseph R. Gusfield, *Community: A Critical Response*. Copyright © 1975. Quoted by permission of Harper & Row Publishers, Inc.

Joseph R. Gusfield, "Foreword," in Peter Conrad and Joseph W. Schneider, *Deviance
and Medicalization: From Badness to Sickness*. Copyright © 1980. Permission
granted to quote excerpts by Charles E. Merrill Publishing Co.

Joseph R. Gusfield, "Stigma and Redemption: Themes in the Medicalization of Drinking-
Driving Offenders." Paper presented at the Alcohol Epidemiology Section, International Council on Alcohol and Addictions, June 21, 1983, Padova, Italy. Permission
to quote granted by Joseph R. Gusfield.

Ivan C. Illich, *Medical Nemesis*. Copyright © 1976. Permission granted for quotation by
Pantheon Books, a division of Random House, Inc.

Dennis T. Jaffe, *Healing From Within*. Copyright © 1980. Permission granted for quotation by Alfred A. Knopf, Inc.

Dennis T. Jaffe, "Self-Management and Behavioral Medicine: Seizing Control of Self-
Defeating Behavior," in *Mind, Body and Health: Toward an Integral Medicine*, ed.
James S. Gordon, Dennis T. Jaffe, and David E. Bresler. Copyright © 1984.

Gerald G. Jampolsky, *Love is Letting Go of Fear*. Copyright © 1979 by Gerald G. Jampolsky and Jack O. Keeler.

Kris Jeter, "Family Medicine and Holistic Health: An Analytic Essay," in *Family
Medicine: A New Approach to Health Care*, ed. Betty E. Cogswell and Marvin B.
Sussman. Copyright © 1982. Permission for quotation granted by the Haworth
Press, Inc.

Frank Johnson, "The Western Concept of Self," in *Culture and Self: Asian and Western
Perspectives*, ed. Anthony J. Marsella, George DeVos, and Francis L. K. Hsu.
Copyright © 1985. Permission for quotation granted by Tavistock Publications.

Jeff Kane, M.D., "Unwhole Healers: A Doctor's Diagnosis of the Medical Profession," in

Whole Life Times, January/February 1983, pp. 1–4. Quoted by permission of Jeffrey H. Kane, M.D.

Jonathan Kirsch. "Can Your Mind Cure Cancer?" in *New West,* January 3, 1977.

Dolores Krieger. "Therapeutic Touch and the Metaphysics of Nursing," in *Dimensions in Wholistic Healing,* ed. Herbert A. Otto and James W. Knight. Copyright © 1979. Quoted by permission.

Edwin M. Lemert, *Sociopathic Behavior.* Copyright © 1951. Quotation excerpted by permission of McGraw-Hill Publishers.

Ronald W. Manderscheid, "Implications of Biopsychosocial Relationships." Paper presented at AAAS Annual Meeting in San Francisco, January 7, 1980. Quoted by permission of the author.

Phyllis H. Mattson, *Holistic Health in Perspective.* Copyright © 1982. Quoted by permission of Mayfield Publishing Co.

John D. McCarthy and Mayer N. Zald, *The Trend of Social Movements in America: Professionalization and Resource Mobilization.* Copyright © 1973.

David Mechanic, *Medical Sociology.* Copyright © 1968 by David Mechanic. Reprinted by permission of The Free Press, a division of Macmillan, Inc.

Thomas Merton, *The Way of Chuang Tzu.* Copyright © 1965 by The Abbey of Gethsemani. Reprinted by permission of New Directions Publishing Corporation.

Lorenz K. Y. Ng, Devra L. Davis, Ronald W. Manderscheif, and Joel Elkes, "Toward a Conceptual Formulation of Health and Well-Being," in *Strategies for Public Health: Promoting Health and Preventing Disease,* ed. Lorenz K. Y. Ng and Devra L. Davis. Copyright © 1982. Quoted by permission of Van Nostrand Reinhold Company and Wadsworth, Inc.

Mike Oppenheim, M.D., "The Cure for America's Health-Care Crisis is Plain Common Sense," *Los Angeles Times* (San Diego Edition), January 8, 1978: Part II (Editorial Section), p. 6.

Herbert A. Otto and James W. Knight, "Wholistic Healing: Basic Principles and Concepts," in *Dimensions in Wholistic Healing,* ed. Herbert A. Otto and James W. Knight. Copyright © 1979. Quoted by permission.

Irving Oyle, *The New American Medicine Show.* Santa Cruz, CA: Unity Press, 1979.

Talcott Parsons. "Christianity," in *International Encyclopedia of the Social Sciences,* ed. David L. Sills. Copyright © 1968 by Crowell Collier and Macmillan, Inc. Reprinted by permission of Macmillan Publishing Company.

Kenneth Pelletier, *Mind as Healer, Mind as Slayer.* Copyright © 1977 by Kenneth Pelletier. Reprinted by arrangement with Delacorte Press/Seymour Lawrence. All rights reserved.

Kenneth Pelletier, *Holistic Medicine.* Copyright © 1979 by Kenneth Pelletier. Reprinted by arrangement with Delacorte Press/Seymour Lawrence. All rights reserved.

Rancho Loma Linda. "Don't Commit Lifestyle Suicide!" Advertisement in *Los Angeles Times,* October 19, 1981: Part V, p. 8. Reprinted by permission of Loma Linda University, School of Public Health.

Leo G. Reeder. "The Patient-Client as Consumer," in *Dominant Issues in Medical Sociology,* ed. Howard D. Schwartz and Cary S. Kart. Copyright © 1978 by Addison-Wesley Publishing Company, Inc. Quoted by permission of Random House, Inc., who currently controls all rights.

Theodore Roszak, *The Making of a Counter Culture.* Copyright © 1969. Permission for citation by DOUBLEDAY, a division of Bantam, Doubleday, Dell Publishing Group, Inc.

Maggie Scarf, "Images That Heal: A Doubtful Idea Whose Time Has Come," in *Psychology Today Magazine* 32:32–46. Copyright © 1980 by PT Partners, L. P. Reprinted by permission.

Howard D. Schwartz and Cary S. Kart, "The Changing Role of the Patient: The Patient as Consumer," in *Dominant Issues in Medical Sociology,* ed. Howard D. Schwartz and Cary S. Kart. Copyright © 1978 by Addison-Wesley Publishing Company, Inc. Quoted by permission of Random House, Inc., who currently controls all rights.

O. Carl Simonton, Stephanie Mathews-Simonton, and James L. Creighton, *Getting Well Again.* Copyright © 1980. Quoted by permission of Bantam Books, Inc./Bantam Doubleday Dell.

Douglas Stalker and Clark Glymour. "Introduction: Why Examine Holistic Medicine?" in *Examining Holistic Medicine,* ed. Douglas Stalker and Clark Glymour. Copyright © 1980. Quoted by permission of Prometheus Books.

Harold Stone. "Wholistic Healing: Historic Base and Short History," in *Dimensions in Wholistic Healing,* ed. Herbert A. Otto and James W. Knight. Copyright © 1979. Quoted by permission.

Roy Wallis and Peter Morley. "Introduction," in *Marginal Medicine.* Introduction, copyright © 1976 by Roy Wallis and Peter Morley. Reprinted by permission of The Free Press, a division of Macmillan, Inc.

Aaron Wildavsky. "Doing Better and Feeling Worse: The Political Pathology of Health Policy," in *Doing Better and Feeling Worse: Health in the United States,* ed. John H. Knowles. Copyright © 1977 by the American Academy of Arts and Sciences. Quoted by permission of W. W. Norton and Company, Inc., publisher.

George F. Will, "Obliterating the Idea of Responsibility," *Los Angeles Times* (San Diego Edition), June 23, 1982: Part II (Editorial Section), p. 7.

Irving Zola. "Medicine as an Institution of Social Control," in *The Cultural Crisis of Modern Medicine,* ed. John Ehrenreich. Copyright © 1978 by John Ehrenreich. Reprinted by permission of Monthly Review Foundation.